Drug and Alcohol Abuse Prevention

Drug and Alcohol Abuse Reviews

Edited by
Ronald R. Watson

Drug and Alcohol Abuse Prevention

Drug and Alcohol Abuse Prevention

Edited by

Ronald R. Watson

University of Arizona, Tucson, Arizona

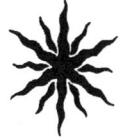

Humana Press • Clifton, New Jersey

Copyright © 1990 by The Humana Press Inc.
Crescent Manor
PO Box 2148
Clifton, NJ 07015 USA

All rights in any form whatsoever reserved.

No part of this book may be reproduced, stored in a retrieval system, or transmitted in any form or by any means (electronic, mechanical, photocopying, microfilming, recording, or otherwise) without written permission from the publisher.

Printed in the United States of America.

The Library of Congress has cataloged this serial title as follows:

Drug and alcohol abuse prevention / edited by Ronald R. Watson
     p. cm. — (Drug and alcohol abuse reviews)
   Includes index.
   ISBN 0-89603-179-9
   1. Drug abuse—United States—Prevention. 2. Alcoholism—United States—Prevention. I. Watson, Ronald R. (Ronald Ross) II. Series.
HV5825.D77627 1991
362.29'17'0973—dc20   90-28904
                                                                   CIP

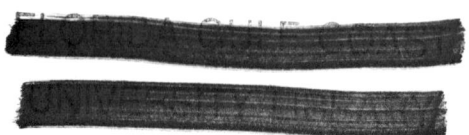

Contents

vii   Preface
ix   Contributors

1   Alcohol Prevention Research:
Confronting the Challenge
Jan Howard, Mary L. Ganikos, and Jane A. Taylor

19   The Role of the Primary Care Practitioner in the Diagnosis and Management of Substance Abuse
George D. Comerci

45   Using the DIS to Diagnose Drug and Alcohol Abuse:
The Effects of Language and Ethnic Status
Robert E. Roberts and Howard M. Rhoades

73   Sensation Seeking, Marijuana Use, and Responses to Prevention Messages:
Implications for Public Health Campaigns
Lewis Donohew, David M. Helm, Patricia Lawrence, and Milton J. Shatzer

95   Evaluation of Girls Clubs of America's Friendly PEERsuasion Program™:
Monitoring Program Implementation
Marcia R. Chaiken

133   Alcohol Use Among LDS and Other Groups Teaching Abstinence
Rick D. Hawks

151 Hispanic Drug Abuse:
Culturally Appropriate Prevention and Treatment
Barbara V. Marin

167 Prevention of Substance Abuse Problems in Women
Barbara W. Lex

223 Effect of Regulation on Alcoholic Beverage
Consumption: *Regression Diagnostics
and Influential Data*
Jon P. Nelson

245 Family Treatment of Alcoholism
Dawn M. Gondoli and Theodore Jacob

263 Changing Drug Use Patterns and Treatment
Behavior: *A Longitudinal Study of Urban Black Youth*
Ann F. Brunswick, Peter A. Messeri, and Angela A. Aidala

313 Using Incentives, Lotteries, and Competitions
in Work-Site Smoking Cessation Interventions
Steven W. Malone and Leonard A. Jason

339 The Etiology and Consequences
of Adolescent Drug Use
David W. Brook and Judith S. Brook

363 Training Teachers for Substance Abuse Prevention
Susan J. Fordney and Randall M. Jones

373 Adolescent Alcohol and Drug Treatment Outcome
Sandra A. Brown, Mariam A. Mott, and Mark G. Myers

405 Index

Preface

A major national goal is to improve our health and advance our opportunities to pursue happiness. Simultaneously, there are increasing health care costs and increasing demands to accomplish more with less financial support. Treatment costs can be reduced and health improved by preventing the toxic effects of drugs.

This first volume of our new series, Drug and Alcohol Abuse Reviews, focuses on stategies to reduce the use and abuse of common compounds known to cause major damage to health: alcohol, tobacco, and illicit drugs such as cocaine and heroin. With the number of deaths attributable to the consumption of alcohol in the US at about 100,000 per year, the annual cost of addictions will be $150 billion by 1995.

A variety of approaches to preventing drug abuse are being applied by governmental agencies and health care providers to reduce costs. These include school-based interventions, driver education programs, media interventions, health warning labels, physician guidance, economic disincentives, restricted availability, punishments and penalties, environmental protections, and social-support approaches.

With such a range of options, it becomes critical to evaluate and choose the most effective systems for a given population. We feel that the present collection of critical survey articles constitutes a thorough examination of the issues and strategies associated with prevention, and trust that readers will find the book exceedingly helpful in understanding and planning what needs to be done.

Ronald R. Watson

Contributors

Angela A. Aidala • *Public Health, Sociomedical Sciences, Columbia University, New York, New York*
David W. Brook • *Department of Psychiatry, Mount Sinai Medical Center, New York, New York*
Judith S. Brook • *Department of Psychiatry, Mount Sinai Medical Center, New York, New York*
Sandra A. Brown • *University of California, San Diego, La Jolla, California*
Ann F. Brunswick • *Public Health, Sociomedical Sciences, Columbia University, New York, New York*
Marcia R. Chaiken • *Health Sciences Center, University of Arizona, Tucson, Arizona*
George D. Comerci • *Department of Pediatrics, University of Arizona, Tucson, Arizona*
Lewis Donohew • *Center for Prevention Research, University of Kentucky, Lexington, Kentucky*
Susan J. Fordney • *The University of Arizona College of Education, Smith Project for Substance Abuse Education, Tucson, Arizona*
Mary L. Ganikos • *National Institute on Alcohol Abuse and Alcoholism, Rockville, Maryland*
Dawn M. Gondoli • *Health Sciences Center, University of Arizona, Tucson, Arizona*
Rick D. Hawks • *Clearfield, Utah*
David M. Helm • *Center for Prevention Research, University of Kentucky, Lexington, Kentucky*
Jan Howard • *National Institute on Alcohol Abuse and Alcoholism, Rockville, Maryland*

Theodore Jacob • *Health Sciences Center, University of Arizona, Tucson, Arizona*

Leonard A. Jason • *Department of Psychology, DePaul University, Chicago, Illinois*

Randall M. Jones • *The University of Arizona College of Education, Smith Project for Substance Abuse Education, Tucson, Arizona*

Patricia Lawrence • *Center for Prevention Research, University of Kentucky, Lexington, Kentucky*

Barbara W. Lex • *Department of Psychiatry, Harvard Medical School, Belmont, Massachusetts*

Steven W. Malone • *Behavioral Medicine Clinic, VA Medical Center–Portland, Portland, Oregon*

Barbara V. Marin • *San Francisco Center for AIDS Prevention Studies, University of California, San Francisco, California*

Peter A. Messeri • *Public Health, Sociomedical Sciences, Columbia University, New York, New York*

Mariam A. Mott • *University of California, San Diego, La Jolla, California*

Mark G. Myers • *University of California, San Diego, La Jolla, California*

Jon P. Nelson • *Department of Economics, The Pennsylvania State University, University Park, Pennsylvania*

Howard M. Rhoades • *The University of Texas Health Science Center at Houston, Houston, Texas*

Robert E. Roberts • *The University of Texas Health Science Center at Houston, Houston, Texas*

Milton J. Shatzer • *Center for Prevention Research, University of Kentucky, Lexington, Kentucky*

Jane A. Taylor • *National Institute on Alcohol Abuse and Alcoholism, Rockville, Maryland*

Alcohol Prevention Research

Confronting the Challenge

Jan Howard, Mary L. Ganikos, and Jane A. Taylor

An estimated 18 million American adults and several million adolescents are experiencing physical, psychological, and social problems from the consumption of alcoholic beverages.[1,2] These problems include traumatic injury, cirrhosis of the liver, certain types of cancer, emotional disorders, interpersonal conflicts, alcohol-related violence, absenteeism, and loss of productivity. Deaths attributable to the consumption of alcohol in the US approx 100,000/yr, and it is predicted that by 1995 the annual cost of alcohol abuse and alcoholism in the US will approach 150 billion dollars.[1,3,*]

Within the federal government, the primary agency dedicated to *research* on alcohol problems is the National Institute on Alcohol Abuse and Alcoholism (NIAAA). The intramural research program of NIAAA, which represents 12% of the budget, involves on-site clinical and laboratory studies of physiology and pharmacology, metabolism and molecular biology, and treatment effectiveness. The extramural program, which utilizes 88% of the budget, supports research initiated by investigators outside NIAAA, who are mainly associated with academic institutions. The extramural effort is di-

---

*This estimate is based on the value of the dollar in 1983.

Drug and Alcohol Abuse Prevention Ed: R. R. Watson ©1990 The Humana Press Inc.

vided into biomedical and neurobehavioral research, epidemiologic and biometric research, and clinical and prevention research, as well as demonstration programs for the homeless.

Implicitly, if not explicitly, all the research activities of NIAAA are directed toward the prevention and curtailment of alcohol abuse and alcoholism. However, the Prevention Research Branch (PRB), within the Division of Clinical and Prevention Research, has the *specific* task of stimulating and monitoring research that focuses on the primary and secondary prevention of alcohol-related problems.[4] Primary prevention attempts to stop the problem from occurring in the first place, whereas secondary prevention attempts to identify persons in the early stages of their problem or illness and to offer educational counseling and guidance, and/or referral to treatment. In conjunction with the Treatment Research Branch of NIAAA, the PRB is responsible for developing *behavioral change research*—studies that test interventions aimed at reducing alcohol abuse and related problems.

Because alcohol abuse is of considerable concern to policymakers within U.S. jurisdictions, a wide variety of preventive interventions are continuously being introduced at national and local levels. Recent universal interventions include raising the minimum drinking age to 21 yrs across the 50 states, and requiring the introduction of health warning labels on containers of all alcoholic beverages produced or distributed for sale in the US.[5] A number of other global prevention strategies were recommended by the Surgeon General's Workshop on Drunk Driving in December 1988, including increased taxes on alcoholic beverages, restraints on advertising, and equal time for counteradvertising.[2] In the private sector, national mobilizations against alcohol abuse are illustrated by the "Just Say 'No'" campaigns and the universal themes of organizations like Mothers Against Drunk Driving.

At the state and local level, preventive interventions are too numerous to count. They encompass laws that define drunk driving and specify appropriate punishments, regulations of Alcohol Beverage Control agencies, tax policies of government jurisdictions, alcohol education programs in public and private schools, server training programs in the hospitality industry, regulations affecting the availability of alcohol, warning signs at points of purchase, guidance practices of primary-care physicians, and employee assistance programs that constructively confront worksite alcohol problems.

Ideally, the introduction of particular prevention strategies should be based on proof of efficacy in comparable contexts and populations. However, proof is frequently elusive, and the pressure to confront and curtail alcohol problems prompts decision-makers to act in the absence of certainty.[6] In the case of the minimum drinking age increase and the introduction of warning labels, a review of relevant theory, data, and experience suggested the utility of these approaches.[7,8] Yet, in many (probably most) situations, the selection of prevention strategies is based on prudent judgments and simple hunches, rather than proof in any meaningful sense of the term. Furthermore, even when the choice of an intervention is based on solid evidence of prior effectiveness, there is no guarantee that it will prove beneficial in the context of its new application.

Natural Experiments

The pressure to act in a climate of uncertainty and the need to learn from experience provide the impetus for so-called "natural experiments" in alcohol prevention research. In essence, a natural experiment is the testing of an intervention that is designed, implemented, and controlled by persons independent of the research enterprise. The investigators are forced to work within and around an experimental environment that is not of their making.

Natural experiments in the alcohol prevention arena have examined the impact of increases[9-11] and decreases[12-14] in the minimum drinking age, varying definitions of drunk or impaired driving,[15,16] varying punishments for drunk driving,[16-18] changes in the price[19,20] and availability[21,22] of alcoholic beverages, organized lobbying by prevention pressure groups,[23] and the introduction of warning labels on containers of alcohol.[24] In the tobacco arena, researchers have studied the effects of advertising constraints and counteradvertising policies on smoking behavior.[25] If the recommendations of the Surgeon General's Workshop on Drunk Driving are implemented, similar studies might be undertaken with respect to alcohol advertising.[2]

Natural experiments have the advantage of testing real interventions in real situations, devoid of the artificiality of laboratory settings, the perceived tentativeness of pilot prevention programs, and the biases introduced by flawed simulations and failed deceptions. In addition, ready-made interventions limit the cost of research to the evaluation of their effectiveness. More important, perhaps, is the fact that evaluations of natural interventions can be used to inform institutionalized correcting processes. Thus, the legislation requiring warning labels also requires that, a year after the law's implementation, the Secretary of the Treasury shall report to Congress any recommended changes in the labels as justified by appropriate investigation.[2] This, in turn, necessitates an immediate comprehensive research effort.

Unfortunately, the advantages of natural experiments are countered by endemic threats to their scientific integrity. Because the interventions involved in such experiments are beyond the immediate control of the investigator, the entire process can be considered program- rather than research-driven. From a scientific standpoint, it may be impossible to define and select an appropriate concurrent control group, particularly if the intervention is universally applied to a specific population. Analogously, it is impossible to allocate communities, groups, or individuals randomly to the intervention and control phenomena. Historical controls may provide the only basis for relevant comparisons, but they cannot control for possible contaminating effects of other life events that occur during the experimental period. Also, in a worst-case scenario, the timing of the natural intervention may not permit the collection of baseline data at all.

Investigators involved in natural experiments might enhance the scientific integrity of their research by building experiments of their own choosing onto the natural study. For example, they might test the interactive effects of systematically introducing other relevant interventions into the experimental context, in ways that permit randomized controlled trials of the "secondary" strategies. The literature suggests that the effectiveness of preventive interventions is increased by the simultaneous introduction of more than one strategy.[26-31] Thus, media approaches by themselves appear to be less effective than a combination of media and interpersonal contacts.[32,33] In this vein, researchers might examine the effect of deliberately combining warning labels with more personal communication about the hazards of alcohol, comparing the impact of the labels alone with the dual approach.[34]

Studies of Investigator-Controlled Interventions

When researchers themselves control the intervention process, they have greater opportunities to protect their research from the intrusion of bias. They have discretion to select appropriate control groups, randomization procedures, target groups, and sequencing patterns for the interventions.

Studies of investigator-initiated strategies to prevent alcohol-related problems are a relatively new domain of inquiry. Yet, a broad range of research technologies and techniques has been employed.

These approaches include laboratory studies of changes in expectancies, intentions, attitudes, and behaviors;[35-38] focus-group tests of marketing interventions;[39] structured observational assessments of interactional strategies;[40] quasi-experimental community studies of server training (Putnam SL, Knoxville, TN, personal communication, 1989), law enforcement (Putnam SL, Knoxville, TN, personal communication, 1989), and media interventions;[32] experimental trials of educational and cognitive-behavioral strategies;[41-45]* and computer simulations of price[19] and availability effects.[46]

On the horizon are community-based experimental designs that involve a sufficient number of population units to provide statistically meaningful conclusions. In the absence of available funding, alternative approaches such as population-based case-control studies[47, 48] and quasi-experimental designs may have to suffice. Thus, NIAAA staff are evaluating the range of methodologies employed in prevention studies of heart disease, cancer, and trauma.

It should, of course, be recognized that successful intervention research does not begin at the point of intervention. It necessarily rests on a foundation of basic research concerning ingredients of behavioral change (and booster effects), risk-taking, individual and political decision-making, and dissemination processes. Important, too, is the development of appropriate methods, data collection systems, and response capabilities[49] for studying natural and investigator-initiated interventions. Meaningful research necessitates the utilization of qualitative as well as quantitative methodologies, including ethnographic observations of drinking and preventive behavior in real-world settings.[27, 40, 50, 51]

A Typology of Prevention Strategies

From a social-psychological perspective, behavioral change can be viewed as a function of socialization, social control, and social support. At the group or institutional level, it may also be the result of selection processes,

---

*I.e., strategies that teach youth to recognize and resist environmental and social influences to drink, and to perceive and reinforce the pervasiveness of peer group norms against drinking.[43,44]

whereby persons with acceptable behavioral patterns are selected into the organizational system (or retained by it) and those with unacceptable behaviors are excluded. Thus, the wide array of prevention or change strategies being developed, implemented, and tested in the alcohol area can be classified into the following categories.*

Socialization Approaches

The concept of socialization refers to the transfer of knowledge, values, and norms from one group or person to another. If the socialization process is successful, the recipient group or individual internalizes what has been formally or informally taught and acts accordingly, through mechanisms of *self*-control.

School-Based Interventions

Prevention programs in grammar and high schools include instruction and training in the hazards of alcohol consumption, values clarification, decision-making, refusal skills, and social-competency skills.[1,51,52] In general, school-based programs, especially the more traditional curricula, have had very limited success.[1,26,51] However, those based on social-learning theory that involve teaching by student peers, sensitizing to normative expectations and social influences, enhancing coping skills, and field experiences that change perceptions of risk (e.g., visits to emergency rooms) offer promise of effectiveness.[1,44,51,53-55] The systematic use of "booster" training also appears beneficial.[26,43,51] At the college level, laboratory and field studies of expectancy and social norm training indicate that students can be effectively taught to anticipate realistically the physiological effects of alcohol consumption, to monitor the progression of these effects, and to regulate or moderate their drinking behavior.[36-38,56]

Driver Education Programs

Two types of educational interventions focus on the prevention of drinking and driving—school-based instruction (primary prevention) and programs for drunk-driving offenders (secondary prevention).[1,57-59] Evaluations of the youth-oriented efforts show mixed success (e.g., increased knowledge about the hazards of drinking and driving, but more permissive

---

*Strategies are placed in the category that seems most appropriate, although certain aspects of a strategy may relate to other categories as well.

attitudes toward such behavior).[1, 58, 60] Yet, research suggests that training in methods of peer intervention may significantly increase student constraints on the drinking and driving of their associates.[58, 61] Although the educational programs for DWI (driving while intoxicated) offenders also show limited success in changing behavior, they may be useful supplements (rather than alternatives) to such deterrents as license revocation.[62]*

Media Interventions

Mass communication is a common approach to the prevention of alcohol problems, alone and in combination with other behavior-change strategies. As indicated earlier, community studies suggest that the effectiveness of media interventions is enhanced by more personal approaches to the socialization process.[32, 33] The choice of media options (e.g., television, radio, or print) should be governed by marketing information regarding the potential exposure and receptivity of the target group.[63-65]

Historical data concerning smoking practices in the US indicate that counter advertising on television was an effective strategy, at least in the short term.[25] The withdrawal of counter ads from television, which coincided with the voluntary termination of cigaret advertising itself, significantly weakened the anti-smoking campaign on electronic media.[25] In the alcohol area, the effects of prevention-oriented messages are not well documented.[63, 66] For example, it has been observed that "very little has been learned about the role of mass communications in drinking-driving despite the expenditure of many millions of dollars for campaigns and substantial amounts for research."[66]

Advertising that promotes the consumption of alcoholic beverages costs well over a billion dollars a year,[63, 67, 68] with unresolved implications for the creation and perpetuation of alcohol-related problems.[63] Mass communication encouraging the use of alcohol extends beyond the advertisements themselves, and includes the projection of positive images of alcohol consumption in the program content of prime-time television.[69] Positive images of alcohol may also stem from producer sponsorship of sporting events, pub nights, drinking contests, and gifts of clothing bearing brand names and logos.[68]

Researchers differ in their opinions about the effects of advertising on alcohol use and abuse.[70] In a recent review article, it was concluded that alcohol advertising shows little impact on alcohol sales or consumption.[71]

---

*DWI offenders who are found to have a chronic alcohol problem may be referred to rehabilitation programs in addition to or in lieu of education.[59]

Yet, others submit that advertising does influence consumption, and perhaps alcohol-related problems as well.[63,68] It is generally agreed that more sophisticated studies need to be conducted "under impartial and independent auspices" to identify clearly the effects of alcohol advertising.[63,68,71] A major difficulty in this type of research is disentangling the impact of advertising from the larger cultural context in which it is embedded.[66,72]

Health Warning Labels

The new warning labels on alcoholic beverages are not simply a form of mass communication about the risks of alcohol consumption. They have the potential of establishing new norms of drinking behavior because they officially project the concerns of the US Government regarding particular hazards of drinking.[5] By making an authoritative statement about these definitive risks (birth defects, impaired driving, impaired operation of machinery, and health problems), warning labels can be considered instruments of socialization and should be studied as such. Apparently, there are no published evaluations of warnings on alcoholic beverages, but studies of labels on such products as saccharin suggest the utility of this approach.[8] The extent of its value may depend on the use of concurrent prevention strategies[34] and the specifics of message content and imagery.[8,34]

Physician Guidance

Studies of preventive interventions by primary-care physicians regarding smoking, nutrition, injuries, weight reduction, and self-examination[73,74] suggest that providers of care could play an important preventive role in the alcohol area as well. These efforts might include anticipatory guidance for youth (and parents) and the establishment, through doctor–patient consensus, of normative constraints on risk-taking behavior.[52,58,75,76] For patients with emergent problems, interventions could also include early detection, counseling, and referral to treatment.[75,77-80]

Social-Control Approaches

Social-control strategies are entwined with the described instruments of socialization that are essentially targeted toward *self*-control. However, social-control interventions go beyond self-control by setting socially defined limits on human discretion. They support the process of self-control, but provide insurance against its failure.

Economic Disincentives

A number of studies indicate that increases in the price of alcoholic beverages are correlated with decreases in such problems as alcohol-related traffic fatalities and cirrhosis.[81,82] Even the consumption of beer by American youth is sensitive to price.[81,83] Taxes on alcoholic beverages have been used primarily as a source of revenue rather than a prevention strategy.[81] However, the Surgeon General's Workshop on Drunk Driving recommended increased taxation as an appropriate means of reducing the drunk-driving problem.[2] Although taxes are not a form of punishment, they do impose limits on the discretion of drinkers to obtain and consume alcoholic beverages.

Other economic disincentives include liability suits against producers[84] and servers[85] of alcohol. Liability suits are partially responsible for the interest of the hospitality industry in server training programs,[85] which may reduce their insurance rates.[85] It is also possible that liability considerations softened the opposition of alcohol producers to warning labels on beverage containers. When product labels forewarn consumers of specified dangers (e.g., birth defects), producers may be absolved of liability for ensuing harm.[86]

Restricted Availability

A growing body of literature indicates that restrictions on the availability of alcoholic beverages reduce alcohol problems[22,70] and that the release of constraints increases problems.[1,70,87] Evaluations of changes in the legal minimum drinking age provide examples of this pattern, especially for the age groups affected by the law.[7,26,88] Ongoing research suggests that raising the drinking age to 21 yrs* does more than delay the onset of alcohol problems,** because it appears to reduce alcohol use among young people up to 25 yrs of age (O'Malley PM, Ann Arbor, MI, personal communication, 1989).

Analogously, other controls on alcohol availability (when implemented together) show promise as prevention strategies—including restrictions on the number and type of places where alcoholic beverages are sold or consumed,[70,91] and a variety of server interventions.[91-94] Server training is a

---

*It is interesting to note that the federal government used economic incentives (or disincentives) to achieve universal state acceptance of the age 21 standard. Funds for highway improvements were made conditional on state compliance with the new age limit.[7]

**For a discussion of the delay concept, *see* references [89] and.[90]

management strategy to moderate customer drinking practices by teaching servers to recognize cues suggestive of inebriation and to curtail or refuse service of alcoholic beverages.[26,27,30] Server constraints may also be directed toward persons at risk of losing self-control, not simply toward persons who are already intoxicated.

Punishments and Penalties

Violations of laws controlling alcohol availability, drunk driving, and other harmful behaviors are punishable by incarceration, fines, and license revocation.[95,96] Punishments that are certain, swift, and severe[1,95,97,98] are likely to be more effective than those that are encumbered by the uncertainties,[95] delays,[95] and mitigations[95] of criminal and civil justice systems. Public perceptions of the probability of punishment may have greater implications for deterrence than the punishment itself.[98] Perceptions are, in turn, influenced by the visibility of the law enforcement process (e.g., by media coverage and sobriety checkpoints on roads and highways[17,98]).

Per se laws, that curtail the discretion of accusers and accused to determine the legality of behavior, may facilitate the implementation of law enforcement efforts.[99] Moreover, license revocation (especially administrative revocation) may have greater deterrence value than jail sentences, [1,95,100] because it is perceived to be a certain and severe sanction.[95] So-called "mandatory" jail sentences can result in so many delays, postponements, dismissals, and burdens on judicial and enforcement systems that their threat value is neutralized.[95,98] By contrast, administrative license revocation[99] is triggered solely by a report of the arrest to the division of motor vehicles. This is done independently of the courts, thereby maximizing the swiftness and certainty of punishment. License revocation is also a more cost-effective countermeasure, placing the bulk of the financial responsibility on the offender rather than society.[99]

Environmental Protections

Another societal approach to the reduction of alcohol-related problems has been labeled "environmental safety measures," frequently mentioned in connection with drunk driving.[26,57] Basically, these interventions recognize the problematic nature of behavioral change and try to protect drinkers and other potential victims from injury.[26,57] These strategies include ignition interlock devices in cars that prevent driving by intoxicated persons, air bags and other cushioning devices, safer highway designs, and safety features on machinery and tools.[26,57] Such interventions have obvious implications for injury control in general, not simply the curtailment of alcohol-induced injuries.[26,57]

Social-Support Approaches

In important respects, social support is a manifestation and extension of social control. Treatment strategies for alcoholism rely heavily on social-support structures, typified by Alcoholics Anonymous and similar systems of therapy.[1] Moreover, in the prevention area, a number of established and emergent strategies are based on principles of social support.

Employee Assistance Programs rely on social networks and job performance to identify workers with incipient problems and to support behavioral change.[101-103] Peer-oriented interventions in school settings legitimize norms against drinking, and support resistance behavior.[41-44] Designated-driver programs entrust the welfare of drinkers and society to prearranged support systems,[57,58] including friends who "don't let friends drive drunk." The availability of free taxis and parent drivers are other cases in point.[57,58]

It can be additionally argued that American society is witnessing and encouraging a shift in the "cultural position of alcohol,"[104] defining it as a potentially dangerous drug that justifies heightened concern and control. If this is true, there may be increasing social support for individuals, groups, and collectivities that work toward the goal of behavioral change. Concurrently, there should be increasing social support for preventive interventions that show a track record of effectiveness. And that record can only be established through scientifically grounded research.

Selection Approaches

Selection strategies appear to be an emergent domain of intervention focused primarily on screening at the point of employment or admission, and certain types of testing. The category might additionally include informal group processes aimed at identifying and isolating persons who violate group norms against drinking or problem drinking. Selection approaches could be considered a form of social control, especially when they serve as vehicles of punishment. However, they also protect the viability of socialization and social-support systems as mechanisms for preventing alcohol problems. Thus, the subtleties of selection processes deserve indepth study, as indicators and catalysts of social change.

References

[1]National Institute on Alcohol Abuse and Alcoholism. Sixth special report to the US Congress on alcohol and health, January 1987. National Institute on Alcohol Abuse and Alcoholism, Rockville, MD (DHHS publication no. [ADM] 87– 1519), 1987.

[2]Office of the Surgeon General. Surgeon General's workshop on drunk driving: proceedings, Washington, DC, December 14–16, 1988. Office of the Surgeon General, Rockville, MD (USGP0:1989-234-994), 1989, 8–11.

[3]National Institute on Alcohol Abuse and Alcoholism. Toward a national plan to combat alcohol abuse and alcoholism: A report to the United States Congress, September 1986. National Institute on Alcohol Abuse and Alcoholism, Rockville, MD, 1986, 26.

[4]US Department of Health and Human Services. National Institute on Alcohol Abuse and Alcoholism (NIAAA), in *Prevention*, 88–89. US Government Printing Office, Washington, DC (in press).

[5]Title VIII of Public Law 100–690.

[6]J. Howard. Prevention research at NIAAA: Confronting the challenge of uncertainty, in Prevention research findings: 1988: Proceedings of the first national conference on prevention research findings: Implications for alcohol and other drug abuse program planning, Kansas City, MO, March 26–30, 1988 (K. H. Rey, C. L. Faegre, and P. Lowery, eds.), Office for Substance Abuse Prevention, Rockville, MD (DHHS publication no. [ADM] 89-1615 [OSAP prevention monograph no. 3]), 1990, 243–252.

[7]US General Accounting Office. Drinking-age laws: An evaluation synthesis of their impact on highway safety. US General Accounting Office, Washington, DC (PEMD-87-10), 1987.

[8]US Department of Health and Human Services. National Institute on Alcohol Abuse and Alcoholism (NIAAA). Review of the research literature on the effects of health warning labels: A report to the US Congress. Department of Health and Human Services, Rockville, MD (contract no. ADM 281-86-0003), 1987.

[9]R. W. Hingson, N. Scotch, T. Mangione, A. Meyers, L. Glantz, T. Heeren, N. Lin, M. Mucatel, and G. Pierce (1983) Impact of legislation raising the legal drinking age in Massachusetts from 18 to 20. *Am. J. Public Health* **73,** 163–170.

[10]A. C. Wagenaar (1983) Preventing highway crashes by raising the legal minimum age for drinking: The Michigan experience 6 years later. *J. Safety Research* **17,** 101–109.

[11]A. C. Wagenaar (1982) Aggregate beer and wine consumption: Effects of changes in the minimum legal drinking age and a mandatory beverage container deposit law in Michigan. *J. Stud. Alcohol* **43,** 469–488.

[12]P. J. Cook and G. Tauchen (1984) The effect of minimum drinking age legislation on youthful auto fatalities, 1970–1977. *J. Leg. Stud.* **13,** 169–190.

[13]R. G. Smart (1977) Changes in alcoholic beverage sales after reductions in the legal-drinking age. *Am. J. Drug Alcohol Abuse* **4**, 101–108.

[14]R. G. Smart and M. Goodstadt (1977) Effects of reducing the legal alcohol-purchasing age on drinking and driving problems: A review of empirical studies. *J. Stud. Alcohol* **38**, 1313–1323.

[15]R. Hingson, T. Heeren, and S. Morelock (1989) Effects of Maine's 1982 .02 law to reduce teenage driving after drinking. *Alcohol, Drugs and Driving* **5**, 25–36.

[16]P. L. Zador, A. K. Lund, M. Fields, and K. Weinberg. Fatal crash involvement and laws against alcohol-impaired driving. Insurance Institute for Highway Safety, Washington, DC, 1988.

[17]R. Hingson, T. Heeren, D. Kovenock, T. Mangione, A. Meyers, S. Morelock, R. Lederman, and N. A. Scotch (1987) Effects of Maine's 1981 and Massachusetts' 1982 driving-under-the-influence legislation. *Am. J. Public Health* **77**, 593–597.

[18]H. L. Ross and R. B. Voas. The New Philadelphia story: The effects of severe penalties for drunk driving. AAA Foundation for Traffic Safety, Washington, DC, 1989.

[19]C. E. Phelps (1988) Death and taxes: An opportunity for substitution. *J. Health Economics* **7**, 1–24.

[20]P. J. Cook and G. Tauchen (1982) The effect of liquor taxes on heavy drinking. *Bell J. Economics* **13**, 379–390.

[21]J. F. Hoadley, B. C. Fuchs, and H. D. Holder (1984) The effect of alcohol beverage restrictions on consumption: A 25-year longitudinal analysis. *Am. J. Drug Alcohol Abuse* **10**, 375–401.

[22]O. Horverak (1983) The 1978 strike at the Norwegian Wine and Spirits Monopoly. *Br. J. Addict.* **78**, 51–66.

[23]M. Wolfson (1989) The citizens' movement against drunken driving and the prevention of risky driving: A preliminary assessment. *Alcohol, Drugs and Driving* **5**, 73–84.

[24]R. Room. Epidemiology of alcohol problems. National Institute on Alcohol Abuse and Alcoholism, grant no. 5 P50 AA05595-09, 1989.

[25]Office on Smoking and Health. Smoking control policies, in Reducing the Health Consequences of Smoking: 25 years of progress: A report of the Surgeon General, 1989. Centers for Disease Control, Rockville, MD (DHHS publication no. [CDC] 89-8411), 1989, 461–636.

[26]J. M. Moskowitz (1989) The primary prevention of alcohol problems: A critical review of the research literature. *J. Stud. Alcohol* **50**, 54–88.

[27]R. F. Saltz (1988) Research in environmental and community strategies for the prevention of alcohol problems. *Contemporary Drug Problems* **Spring**, 67–81.

[28]H. D. Holder (1988) A public health model for the prevention and reduction of alcohol problems. Testimony given to the Governmental Affairs Committee, US Senate, June 29, 1988.

[29]M. D. Klitzner. Part 2: An assessment of the research on school-based prevention programs, in Report to Congress on the nature and effectiveness of Federal, State, and local drug prevention/education programs, October 1987. US Department of Education in conjunction with US Department of Health and Human Services, Washington, DC (USGP0:1988-201-668:60223),1987, i–47.

[30]H. D. Holder (1987) Environmental restrictions and effective prevention policy, in Control issues in alcohol abuse prevention: strategies for states and communities. *Advances in Substance Abuse* **S1**, 405–432.

[31]H. D. Holder and L. Wallack (1986) Contemporary perspective for the prevention of alcohol problems: an empirically-derived model. *J. Public Health Policy* **7**, 324–339.

[32]J. K. Worden, B. S. Flynn, D. G. Merill, J. A. Waller, and L. D. Haugh (1989) Preventing alcohol-impaired driving through community self-regulation training. *Am. J. Public Health* **79**, 287–290.

[33]N. Maccoby, J. W. Farquhar, P. D. Wood, and J. Alexander (1977) Reducing the risk of cardiovascular disease: Effects of a community-based campaign on knowledge and behavior. *J. Community Health* **3**, 100–114.

[34]Program announcement: Measuring the impact of alcohol warning labels. National Institute on Alcohol Abuse and Alcoholism, Rockville, MD (Request for applications AA-89-06 [Catalog of Domestic Assistance No. 13.273]), 1989.

[35]L. S. Bensley. Identifying precursors to problem drinking. National Institute on Alcohol Abuse and Alcoholism, grant no. 5 RO1 AA06319-05, 1989.

[36]J. S. Baer, D. R. Kivlahan, K. Fromme, and G. A. Marlatt. Secondary prevention of alcohol abuse with college student populations: A skills-training approach, in *Issues in Alcohol Use and Misuse by Young Adults* (G. Howard, ed.), Notre Dame University, Notre Dame (in press).

[37]D. R. Kivlahan, D. B. Coppel, K. Fromme, E. Williams, and G. A. Marlatt (1990) Secondary prevention of alcohol-related problems in young adults at risk, in *Prevention and Early Intervention: Biobehavioral Perspectives* (K. D. Craig and S. M. Weiss, eds.), Springer Press, NY, pp. 287–300.

[38]S. G. Curry and G. A. Marlatt (1987) Building self-confidence, self-efficacy and self-control, in *Treatment and Prevention of Alcohol Problems: A Resource Manual* (W. M. Cox and R. L. Rondebush, eds.), Academic, NY, pp. 117–137.

[39]M. B. Mazis. Evaluating health warning labels for alcoholic beverages. National Institute on Alcohol Abuse and Alcoholism, grant no. 1 RO1 AA08383-01, 1989.

[40]M. Hennessy and R. F. Saltz (1989) Adjusting for multimethod bias through selection modeling. *Evaluation Rev.* **13**, 380–399.

[41]W. B. Hansen. Adolescent alcohol prevention trial. National Institute on Alcohol Abuse and Alcoholism, grant no. 5 RO1 AA06201-05, 1989.

[42]T. E. Dielman. Countering pressures related to adolescent alcohol misuse. National Institute on Alcohol Abuse and Alcoholism, grant no. 5 RO1 AA06324-06, 1989.

[43]P. C. Campanelli, T. E. Dielman, J. T. Shope, A. T. Butchart, and D. S. Renner (1989) Pretest and treatment effects in an elementary school-based alcohol misuse prevention program. *Health Educ. Q.* **16,** 113–130.

[44]W. B. Hansen, J. W. Graham, B. H. Wolkenstein, B. Z. Lundy, J. Pearson, B. R. Flay, and C. A. Johnson (1988) Differential impact of three alcohol prevention curricula on hypothesized mediating variables. *J. Drug Educ.* **18,** 143–153.

[45]R. H. Hopkins, A. L. Mauss, K. A. Kearney, and R. A. Weisheit (1988) Comprehensive evaluation of a model alcohol education curriculum. *J. Stud. Alcohol* **49,** 38–50.

[46]H. D. Holder and J. O. Blose (1987) Reduction of community alcohol problems: Computer simulation experiments in three counties. *J. Stud. Alcohol* **48,** 124–135.

[47]N. S. Weiss (1983) Control definition in case-control studies of the efficacy of screening and diagnostic testing. *Am. J. Epidemiol.* **118,** 457–460.

[48]A. S. Morrison (1982) Case definition in case-control studies of the efficacy of screening. *Am. J. Epidemiol.* **115,** 6–8.

[49]National Institute on Alcohol Abuse and Alcoholism. Report of the Ad Hoc Extramural Science Advisory Board meeting of the workshop on prevention research, November 18, 1987. National Institute on Alcohol Abuse and Alcoholism, Rockville, MD, 1989.

[50]R. E. Sykes. Regulation of alcohol abuse among tavern patrons II. National Institute on Alcohol Abuse and Alcoholism, grant no. 2 RO1 AA06489-03, 1989.

[51]J. Howard, J. A. Taylor, M. L. Ganikos, H. D. Holder, D. F. Godwin, and E. D. Taylor (1988) An overview of prevention research: Issues, answers, and new agendas. *Public Health Rep.* **103,** 674–683.

[52]Program announcement: Research on the prevention of alcohol abuse among children, adolescents, and young adults. National Institute on Alcohol Abuse and Alcoholism, Rockville, MD, 1988.

[53]W. H. Bruvold and T. G. Rundall (1988) A meta-analysis and theoretical review of school based tobacco and alcohol intervention programs. *Psychol. Health* **2,** 53–78.

[54]E. Bernstein and W. G. Woodall (1987) Changing perceptions of riskiness in drinking, drugs, and driving: An emergency department-based alcohol and substance abuse prevention program. *Ann. Emergency Med.* **16,** 1350–1354.

[55]N. S. Tobler (1986) Meta-analysis of 143 adolescent drug prevention programs: Quantitative outcome results of program participants compared to a control or comparison group. *J. Drug Issues* **16,** 537–567.

[56]G. A. Marlatt. Prevention of alcohol problems in college students. National Institute on Alcohol Abuse and Alcoholism, grant no. 5 RO1 AA05591-07, 1989.

[57]B. G. Simons-Morton and D. G. Simons-Morton. Controlling injuries due to drinking and driving: The context and functions of education, in Surgeon General's workshop on drunk driving: Background papers, Washington, DC, December 14–16, 1988. Office of the Surgeon General, Rockville, MD, 1989, 77–92.

[58]M. Klitzner. Youth impaired driving: Causes and countermeasures, in Sur-

geon General's workshop on drunk driving: Background papers, Washington, DC, December 14–16, 1988. Office of the Surgeon General, Rockville, MD, 1989, 192–206.

[59]F. Klajner, L. C. Sobell, and M. C. Sobell (1984) Prevention of drunk-driving, in *Prevention of Alcohol Abuse* (P. M. Miller and T. D. Nirenberg, eds.), Plenum, NY, pp. 441–468.

[60]P. M. Kohn, M. S. Goodstadt, G. M. Cook, M. Sheppard, and C. Godwin (1982) Ineffectiveness of threat appeals about drinking and driving. *Accid. Anal. Prev.* **14**, 457–464.

[61]A. J. McKnight and K. McPherson (1986) Evaluation of peer intervention training for high school alcohol safety education. *Accid. Anal. Prev.* **18**, 339–347.

[62]K. Stewart and V. S. Ellingstad. Rehabilitation countermeasures for drinking drivers, in Surgeon General's workshop on drunk driving: Background papers, Washington, DC, December 14–16, 1988. Office of the Surgeon General, Rockville, MD, 1989, 234–246.

[63]C. K. Atkin. Mass communication effects on drinking and driving, in Surgeon General's workshop on drunk driving: Background papers, Washington, DC, December 14–16, 1988. Office of the Surgeon General, Rockville, MD, 1989, 15–35.

[64]L. E. Hewitt and H. T. Blane (1984) Prevention through mass media communication, in *Prevention of Alcohol Abuse* (P. M. Miller and T. D. Nirenberg, eds.), Plenum, NY, pp. 281–323.

[65]J. L. Hochheimer (1981) Reducing alcohol abuse: A critical review of educational strategies, in *Alcohol and Public Policy: Beyond the Shadow of Prohibition* (M. H. Moore and D. R. Gerstein, eds.), National Academy Press, Washington, DC, pp. 286–335.

[66]J. B. Haskins (1985) The role of mass media in alcohol and highway safety campaigns. *J. Stud. Alcohol* **S10**, 184–191.

[67]US General Accounting Office. Alcohol warning labels: Current rules may allow health warnings to go unnoticed. US General Accounting Office, Washington, DC (GAO/HRD-89-118), 1989.

[68]American Medical Association Board of Trustees (1986) Alcohol advertising, counteradvertising, and depiction in the public media. *JAMA* **256**, 1485–1488.

[69]L. Wallack (1984) Television programming, advertising, and the prevention of alcohol-related problems, in *Toward the Prevention of Alcohol Problems: Government, Business and Community Action* (D. R. Gerstein, ed.), National Academy Press, Washington, DC, pp. 79–109.

[70]M. J. Ashley and J. G. Rankin (1988) A public health approach to the prevention of alcohol-related health problems. *Annu. Rev. Public Health* **9**, 233–271.

[71]R. G. Smart (1988) Does alcohol advertising affect overall consumption? A review of empirical studies. *J. Stud. Alcohol* **49**, 314–323.

[72]S. Olson and D. R. Gerstein (1985) *Alcohol in America: Taking Action to Prevent Abuse.* National Academy Press, Washington, DC.

[73]Guide to clinical preventive services: Report of the US preventive services task force. Washington, DC (Prepublication copy), 1989.

[74]Final report of the Industrywide Network for Social, Urban and Rural Efforts (INSURE) Project. INSURE, Washington, DC, 1988.

[75]Program announcement: Research on economic and socioeconomic issues in the prevention, treatment, and epidemiology of alcohol abuse and alcoholism. National Institute on Alcohol Abuse and Alcoholism, Rockville, MD,1989.

[76]R. L. DuPont (1983) Teenage drug use: Opportunities for the pediatrician. *J. Pediatr.* **102,** 1003–1007.

[77]P. Wallace, S. Cutler, and A. Haines (1988) Randomised controlled trial of general practitioner intervention in patients with excessive alcohol consumption. *Br. Med. J.* **297,** 663–668.

[78]K. L. Kumpfer. Prevention of substance abuse: A critical review of risk factors and prevention strategies. Prepared for the American Academy of Child Psychiatry's project prevention: An intervention initiative, September, 1988.

[79]T. F. Babor, E. B. Ritson, and R. J. Hodgson (1986)Alcohol-related problems in the primary health care setting: A review of early intervention strategies. *Br. J. Addict.* **81,** 23–46.

[80]R. M. Cavanaugh (1986) Personal and confidential history from adolescents: An opportunity for prevention. *J. Adolesc. Health Care* **7,** 118–122.

[81]D. Coate and M. Grossman (1987) Change in alcoholic beverage prices and legal drinking ages: Effects on youth alcohol use and motor vehicle mortality. *Alcohol Health Research World* **12,** 22–25,59.

[82]P. Cook (1981) The effect of liquor taxes on drinking, cirrhosis and auto accidents, in *Alcohol and Public Policy: Beyond the Shadow of Prohibition* (M. H. Moore and D. R. Gerstein, eds.), National Academy Press, Washington, DC, pp. 255–285.

[83]H. Saffer and M. Grossman (1987) Beer taxes, the legal drinking age, and youth motor vehicle fatalities. *J. Legal Studies* **16,** 351–374.

[84]R. B. Schmitt. Suit against distiller tests liability for birth defects. *The Wall Street Journal* May 15, 1989, B1 (col. 3).

[85]A. J. McKnight. Factors influencing the effectiveness of server education in leading to alcohol intervention. *J. Stud. Alcohol* (in press).

[86]H. A. Waxman. Speech on HR 5120: The Anti-drug Abuse Act. Congressional Record; November 10, 1988: E 3729.

[87]J. O. Blose and H. D. Holder (1987) Liquor-by-the-drink and alcohol-related traffic crashes: A natural experiment using time-series analysis. *J. Stud. Alcohol* **48,** 52–60.

[88]R. J. Bonnie (1985) Regulating conditions of alcohol availability: Possible effects on highway safety. *J. Stud. Alcohol* **S10,** 129–143.

[89]P. Asch and D. T. Levy (1987) Does the minimum drinking age affect traffic fatalities? *J. Policy Analysis and Management* **6,** 180–192.

[90]M. A. Males (1986) The minimum purchase age for alcohol and young-driver fatal crashes: A long-term view. *J. Legal Studies* **15,** 181–211.

[91]J. F. Mosher and D. H. Jernigan (1989) New directions in alcohol policy. *Annu. Rev. Public Health* **10,** 245–279.

[92]R. F. Saltz. Server intervention and responsible beverage service programs, in Surgeon General's workshop on drunk driving: Background papers, Washington, DC, December 14–16, 1988. Office of the Surgeon General, Rockville, MD,1989, 169–179.

[93]E. S. Geller, N. W. Russ, and W. A. Delphos (1987) Does server intervention make a difference? *Alcohol Health Research World* **11,** 64–69.

[94]N. W. Russ and E. S. Geller (1987) Training bar personnel to prevent drunken driving: A field evaluation. *Am. J. Public Health* **77,** 952–954.

[95]J. L. Nichols and H. L. Ross. The effectiveness of legal sanctions in dealing with drinking drivers, in Surgeon General's workshop on drunk driving: Background papers, Washington, DC, December 14–16, 1988. Office of the Surgeon General, Rockville, MD, 1989, 93–112.

[96]Distilled Spirits Council of the United States, Inc. Summary of State laws and regulations relating to distilled spirits: Twenty-fifth edition. DISCUS, Inc., Washington, DC, 1985.

[97]S. Farrell (1989) Policy alternatives for alcohol-impaired driving. *Health Educ. Q.* **16,** 414–427.

[98]H. L. Ross (1985) Deterring drunken driving: An analysis of current efforts. *J. Stud. Alcohol* **S10,** 122–128.

[99]P. F. Waller (1985) Licensing and other controls of the drinking driver. *J. Stud. Alcohol* **S10,** 150–160.

[100]H. L. Ross. What is the best way to reduce drunken driving? Loss of license a better choice. *Washington Times* Sept. 19, 1989, 3(col. 3–5).

[101]W. J. Sonnenstuhl and H. M. Trice (1987) The social construction of alcohol problems in a union's peer counseling program. *J. Drug Issues* **17,** 223–254.

[102]N. R. Kurtz. Dynamics of the identification and referral process in work organizations, in Occupational alcoholism: A review of research issues: Proceedings of a workshop, Reston, VA, May 22–24, 1980. National Institute on Alcohol Abuse and Alcoholism, Rockville, MD (DHHS publication no. [ADM] 82-1184 [Research monograph no. 8]), 1982, 273–314.

[103]W. Reichman and D. W. Young. Psychodynamics of the return and followup process in the work organization, in Occupational alcoholism: A review of research issues: Proceedings of a workshop, Reston, VA, May 22–24, 1980. National Institute on Alcohol Abuse and Alcoholism, Rockville, MD (DHHS publication no. [ADM] 82-1184 [Research monograph no. 8]), 1982, 331–349.

[104]R. Room (1987) Relating drinking and drugs to injury control: Perspectives and prospects. *Public Health Rep.* **102,** 617–620.

The Role of the Primary Care Practitioner in the Diagnosis and Management of Substance Abuse

George D. Comerci

The Problem

Substance abuse has become a major threat and cause of disability for persons of all ages, races, and socioeconomic levels. Neither educational achievement, domicile, nor family background and make-up are guarantees against either direct involvement in substance abuse or the consequences of abuse by others. It is evident that the primary care health practitioner, regardless of his/her focus of clinical practice, will encounter persons who are directly or indirectly affected by substance abuse. It is equally clear that the primary care practitioner must be prepared to identify such individuals, and to provide them with effective treatment and, if indicated, appropriate referral.

Age

The harmful effects of substance abuse are experienced by persons of all ages. Substance abuse during pregnancy not only threatens the life of the mother, but has a deleterious effect on the developing fetus and, by increasing obstetrical complications, the outcome of pregnancy.[1,2] Because of the easy access to both licit and illicit drugs of abuse, infants and young children are increasingly exposed to the risk of accidental poisoning, which in some instances is the result of the intentional administration of substances of abuse by parents or other caretakers.[3,4] There has been a downward trend in the number of high school students using drugs, but children are beginning experimentation with drugs, including alcohol and tobacco, at an earlier age.[5] The number of students using drugs by the sixth grade has tripled since 1975. Twenty-two percent of high school seniors in 1988 reported that they had first used alcohol, 11% marijuana, and 0.6% cocaine, while they were in the seventh to eighth grades. Two percent first tried cocaine when they were in the ninth grade. Perhaps most publicized is the dramatic increase over the last three decades in substance abuse by older adolescents and young adults, where it is the greatest cause of disability and perhaps death. The leading causes of death in this age group are accidents, homicide, and suicide.[6] Over half of all accidents in the under 21 age group are the result of motor vehicle fatalities, of which 51% are related to alcohol abuse.[7] In the 15–24 age group, 30% of homicides and 20% suicides are alcohol related[8,9] (see Table 1). Other drugs certainly play a role as well.

Although there is a decrease in substance use and abuse during the third decade of life, a disturbing increase in abuse, especially alcohol, occurs in the "older" population (over age 55) and with retirement.[10] This presents almost insurmountable problems for the families of such individuals as well as physicians who provide medical care for them. This problem is especially difficult in the elderly, to a large extent because of the physiological changes of aging and psychosocioeconomic factors.

Socioeconomic

Regardless of whether an individual resides in a poor urban or rural community, or whether financially secure socially and educationally privileged, and living in an affluent community, the threat of substance abuse is present. Although there exist many predisposers to substance abuse and although the frequency of substance abuse is greater in certain communities, families, and individuals, there is no individual entirely protected from or free of the influence of substance abuse. Theorists emphasize the interaction of individual personality and coping styles, family and peers, and the environment, as etiological factors for substance abuse and dependence. From these theories derives the concept of the high-risk individual. Ideally, families, communities, neighborhoods, and schools provide resources necessary for successful coping and have a positive influence on the individual's health and

Table 1
Adolescent Mortality Ages 15–24 Years, n = 38 Million[6-9]

Cause of death	Rate per 100.000	Absolute number/year	Percent alcohol related
Accidents[a]	51.2	20,480	40
Homicide	14.2	5680	30
Suicide	13.1	5240	20
Malignancy	5.4	2160	0
Automotive[a]	39	15,600	45

[a]Automotive deaths under age 21 yr.[7] = 51%.

welfare. When adequate models for success are present and when success seems attainable because opportunities for education, employment, and rewards exist, the alternatives to drug abuse increase. Conversely, when these resources do not exist, the risk for drug abuse increases. This view is supported by the very high rates of substance abuse among those who live in certain underserved rural areas and inner-city neighborhoods, among those who drop out of school and those that are unemployed.[11]

The Health and Economic Consequences of Substance Abuse

Immediate and Short-Term Consequences

Some of the short-term harmful consequences of alcohol and other drug abuse in the adolescent and young adult have already been addressed. A complete discussion of the entire range of immediate and short-term negative effects of substance abuse are beyond the scope of this discussion. It will suffice to comment merely on some of the major personal and social problems created by the abuse of psychoactive substances.

The use of alcohol and other mind-altering substances, such as marijuana, cocaine, LSD, PCP, opiates, inhalants, and numerous other chemicals, is associated directly with accidental death and injury. The proportion of fatalities involving an alcohol intoxicated driver for all age groups in 1987 was 40%. In that year, 24,000 Americans died and an additional 534,000 were injured in alcohol-related traffic accidents.[7] Moreover, alcohol use is associated with 25–35% of all injuries among automobile drivers, and with a high percentage of injuries and deaths attributed to fire, drowning, and falls. It has been implicated in half of all homicides in the US and in many adult suicides.[12] Death from intentional and unintentional overdosing is significant.

Deaths and injuries result from substance abuse associated with military and industrial accidents, including those involving public transportation, other utilities, and commercial shipping. The human suffering and grief imposed by these tragedies is incalculable, the lost human potential and productivity inestimable, and the harmful effects on the environment irredeemable. The economic burden imposed by drug-related absenteeism and lost productivity, medical expenses, and crime has been estimated at well over $200 billion a year.[10,13] When the costs of drug testing programs, incarceration and rehabilitation, drug interdiction, including police and legal activities, property damage, and public education programs are added, the total cost is astronomical.

It is impossible to measure the effect of substance abuse on individual growth and development precisely. Chronic and heavy marijuana use has been shown to be a cause of severe loss of motivation in young people. Cognitive development is slowed in adolescents using alcohol, marijuana, and other drugs, and the effect of substance abuse and dependence on psychosocial maturation is clear.[14,15] For many who become involved in drug abuse, education is interrupted and rarely do dependent young people return to school.

The spread of infections by sexual transmission and intravenous drug abuse, including Hepatitis B and AIDS, is now a major public health problem. Perinatal and obstetrical infections are widespread with significant morbidity and mortality, as well as psychosocial and economic consequences.

Long-Term Consequences

The long-term consequences of drug abuse include congenital disorders, metabolic and cardiovascular complications, chronic lung disease and malignancies, and the effects of these problems on family and community. Alcohol and tobacco contribute more to morbidity and mortality than do any other legal or illicit psychoactive substances. In the US, tobacco use alone (including smokeless tobacco use) contributes to more than 300,000 premature deaths each year; causes of these deaths include coronary heart disease, chronic bronchitis and emphysema, and cancer of the lung, larynx, pharynx, oral cavity, esophagus, and other organs.[16,17] Despite this evidence, many adults continue to smoke. Alcohol use and alcoholism are also associated with adverse effects on cardiovascular function and with an increased risk of oral and upper gastrointestinal cancers.[18]

Why Primary Care Physician Involvement?

The need for involvement of primary care physicians in the prevention, identification, intervention, and treatment of substance abuse is underscored by the previous discussion and statistics. Primary care physicians, because of their relationship with patients and families, their education and clinical training, and the position they hold in the community can play a key role in combating the problem of substance abuse. No other person has license to delve into the personal lives of others to the extent that a physician has. Anticipating confidentiality, empathic concern, and nonjudgmental acceptance, patients are willing to share their personal problems with a physician. Moreover, information regarding substance abuse has a direct bearing on one's health, and therefore revealing such information is acknowledged by the patient as legitimate and necessary. Consequently, this places the physician in a position ideal for identification of those who are abusing substances or are physically or psychologically dependent. The primary care physician is in the best position to initiate treatment and, depending on the seriousness of the problem, to make appropriate referrals and coordinate medical care. Because of their ongoing relationship with families, primary care practitioners are able to identify possible predisposing familial factors, such as a family history of alcohol or other drug abuse, abnormal child-rearing practices, and high risk family lifestyles. This information can serve as the basis for targeted anticipatory guidance or intervention aimed at changing behavior and prevention. The nature of primary care practice allows the physician, as a part of his/her usual practice, to educate and support the individual patient and family.[19,20]

The Role of the Primary Care Practitioner

It is clear that the role of the primary care physician with regard to substance abuse is multiple and variable. It covers a spectrum from the management of the emergency overdose or untoward drug reaction to that of a responsible citizen. The emphasis of this chapter will not be on the emergency management of the acute drug intoxication or overdose. This chapter will emphasize the role of the primary care physician as diagnostician, counselor, and case manager and how it varies depending on the stage of substance abuse. It will include:

1. Anticipatory guidance for those individuals and families with a high potential for abuse;
2. Recognition of the substance abuser and those at risk;
3. Immediate intervention;
4. Referral and coordination of care; and
5. Family support and education, and resources.

Anticipatory Guidance

Identifying persons most likely to experiment with or to begin abusing drugs requires an awareness of and sensitivity to what may be considered to be predictors or predisposing factors for substance abuse. For the physician who cares for infants and children, an awareness of those child-rearing practices that may result in a high potential for substance abuse might allow for very early intervention. Table 2 lists those parental attitudes and child-rearing practices considered to be abnormal or inappropriate, and the feelings that they engender in offspring.[21,22] Table 3 lists the personality characteristics and other factors that have been shown to be predictive of substance abuse and dependence in adolescents and young adults.[23,24] To gain an appreciation of the possible association between child-rearing and the potential for substance abuse, the physician can relate those feelings engendered by certain childhood experiences (e.g., type of child-rearing) and those individual characteristics and factors that have been found to be predictive of substance abuse.

Drugs may be abused as a means of coping with unpleasant or painful emotions, often the outcome of abnormal or inappropriate child-rearing or childhood experiences. For example, a person might abuse amphetamines in order to relieve dysthymia or depressive feelings, or use marijuana in order to reduce anxiety. Two types of stress-reducing skill can be utilized: one aimed at coping with a variety of daily living stressors, and the other used to defend against the temptation to experience the pleasure of an illicit substance. This suggests that substance abuse is the result of a general deficiency in coping skill and that adolescents with poor generic coping skills, when faced with the pressure or temptation to use a drug, are more likely to succumb than those with good skills. Clinically, it is evident that young persons who have difficulty delaying gratification, who have not had experi-

Table 2
Inappropriate Parental Attitudes and Child-Rearing Practices
and Their Parental Consequences

Parental attitude or behavior

1. Overpermissive/oversubmissive/overindulgent: Unable or unwilling to set limits, rarely punish or deny child privileges or gratification
2. Neglectful/belittling: Parent(s) who shows lack of responsibility or actual emotional or physical abuse of their children
3. Overcoersion/distrust/punitiveness: Rigid, demanding, very high and controlled standards for children; perfectionistic, compulsive, often belittling and/or punitive (child cannot possibly satisfy), conflict and turmoil
4. Rejection/belittlement: Feelings of not wanting or not loving the child openly or subtly conveyed by parent(s). Ambivalent feelings conveyed or actual neglect or belittling behavior; child may be scapegoat or "black sheep" or actually unwanted; distrustful: parent (s) has little faith and tends to assume child has same weakness as parent(s)
5. Symbiotic: Abnormally close tie between one parent, usually the mother and a child; prevents normal contact with peers and outside world; "you and I against the world" attitude
6. Vicarious: The parent(s) lives through the child; pressure on child to achieve in areas important to parent; parent(s) derives pleasure from child's activities, "good" or "bad"
7. Inconsistent: Opposite of rigidity, rules constantly changing; parent(s) unpredictable in their response; often marital disharmony, alcohol and other drug abuse
8. Overprotective: shielding child from ordinary or imaginary hazards of living; parent(s) often has phobias; may be narrow or generalized fear; parent(s) may have guilt and fear of retribution and therefore overprotective

Adolescent reaction or behavior

1. Overpermissive/oversubmissive/overindulgent: Need for immediate gratification; inability to deal with adversity; expects much reward without effort or responsibility. Inability to accept discipline; impulsive behavior; poor self-control; inability to control aggressive or risk-taking behaviors; boredom and blasé with intensified need for stimulation, excitement, thrills and pleasure; disdain and contempt for parents and authority; blameful of parents and others for his/her shortcomings and problems; unwillingness to accept consequences of actions
2. Neglectful/belittlement: Low self-esteem; heightened need for peer and social acceptance; poor bonding with parents, family, and community

(continued)

Table 2 *(continued)*

3. Overcoersion/distrust/punitiveness: Hypercritical of self, drives self ("workaholic"); rebellious and resistant (to protect individuality); poor self-esteem, depression, withdrawal; anger and rebellious towards parents and authority; poor bonding
4. Rejection/belittlement: Feels unwanted/unloved; yearns for friendships and peer/social acceptance and approval; may retaliate and rebel—evoke further rejection.
5. Symbiotic: Damaged self-concept and low self-esteem; feels inadequate; may react in anger when realizes handicap
6. Vicarious: At first compliance, then anxiety, and finally rebellion or withdrawal; self-concept suffers since never quite lives up to parent's expectation; socialization may suffer because of narrowing of activities
7. Inconsistent: Low self-esteem: Poor bonding; not able to trust or rely on others; seeks out others (individuals, groups, "gangs") to substitute for parents; often becomes angry and rebellious. Indefinite values and goals
8. Overprotective: Fearful with lowered self-esteem, or anger at having been so restricted associated with rebellion at parent(s) who have caused the adolescent's fears and bad feelings about himself.

ence dealing with adversity, and who are impulsive seem to be more likely to engage in abuse.

Research data underscore the importance of individual personality and coping styles, family and peers, and their interaction as etiological factors for substance abuse and dependence.[25] From these theories derives the concept of the high-risk individual. Current prevention programs rely heavily on this theoretical framework. Characteristics that constitute a high-risk profile include: low religiosity, low self-esteem, indefinite values, poor interpersonal relations, poor coping skills, and low resistance to pressures to use drugs. Persons who have:

1. Made positive attachments with their families, teachers, and peers;
2. Developed adequate coping skills; and
3. School and community models of competent coping and adequate resources and opportunities

are more likely to deal with stress effectively and less likely to resort to problem behaviors, including drug abuse.[26]

Parental guidance with regard to child-rearing, although probably one of the more difficult interventions to accomplish, is an important first step that primary care physicians can take as a substance abuse prevention strategy.

Table 3
Predictors and Predisposing Factors for Substance Abuse[a]

Low self-esteem
Indefinite values
Poor interpersonal relations
High need for acceptance by others
High need for social approval
Poor bonding to parents, family, and community
Low religiosity
Inadequate coping and communication skills
Inability to accept discipline
Unwillingness to accept consequences of his/her actions
Difficulty delaying gratification/need for immediate gratification
Lacking experience in dealing with adversity
Impulsivity
Poor grade-school performance
Learning disabilities and attention disorders
Childhood behavioral and emotional disorders
Childhood antisocial and aggressive behavior
Early use of alcohol and tobacco
Friends and/or siblings who use alcohol, tobacco, and other drugs
Frequent moves to a new community and school
Parents and/or other family members who abuse substances or are chemically dependent

[a]Compare to Table 2: Adolescent Reaction or Behavior.

Such anticipatory guidance for young parents should include the following suggestions:

1. Refrain from modeling alcohol and other drug using behavior;
2. Decrease media exposure of children to "do drug and alcohol" messages;
3. Decrease the availability of drugs and alcohol in the home; and
4. Increase limit setting on all unacceptable behaviors of infants and children, and plan to establish appropriate restrictions on adolescent drug use and drug-associated activities.

Another difficult but important strategy is prenatal counseling against drinking and drug use and abuse during pregnancy.

Children of substance abusers are at a very high risk. Both genetic and environmental factors play a role. Children of alcoholics are four to five times more likely to become alcohol dependent than are other children. Twin studies have shown that identical twins show a higher concordance for alcohol abuse than nonidentical twins. Adoption studies have found that adopted boys with one alcoholic biological parent are three to four times more likely to abuse alcohol than adoptees with biological parents who did not abuse alcohol.[27,28,29] The physician must educate such parents in which there is a history of alcohol or other drug abuse about the vulnerability of their offspring. They should be told that every effort must be made to remove alcohol and other addicting substances from the home and environment, and that parental modeling of alcohol and other drug use should be minimized if not eliminated.

There is much that can be done in the way of education and guidance by the primary care practitioner. Parents should be told that they serve as models for the way their children will relate to drugs, including alcohol. A child is more likely to use tobacco, alcohol, and other drugs if he or she grows up in a home in which parents and other family members smoke, drink, or abuse both licit and illicit substances. Parental attitudes of acceptance of drug use and abuse, and those of other authority figures, such as teachers, will tend to make the child more accepting as well, resulting in an increased likelihood of abuse by the child.

Education of the parent and child, therefore, begins with the first prenatal visit and should continue through childhood, adolescence, and young adulthood. This critical period when standards of behavior and values are being assimilated and developed is a unique opportunity for primary care practitioners to influence the future behavior of the individual and his/her vulnerability to substance abuse. During childhood and the prepubertal period, physicians can talk directly with children regarding what they have learned about drugs and drug abuse. Questions listed in Table 4 provide the basis for discussion regarding the meaning of drug abuse, the dangers of drugs, and what to do if someone offers them drugs or tries to force them to use drugs, including alcohol and tobacco. Parents should be encouraged to talk with their children and adolescents about alcohol, tobacco, and other drug use and abuse. They should examine their own practices and attitudes to determine the degree to which they are asking their children to "do what I say, not what I do." Children should understand that medications are used for specific reasons and know the difference between taking drugs as medication, as opposed to taking drugs for excitement, pleasure, or to alter performance.

Table 4
Questions Concerning Drugs for the School Aged Child

Have your teachers ever talked about drugs at school?
What have you learned about drugs at school?
Have you and your friends ever talked about drugs?
Do you understand the word "drugs"? What does it mean?
Have you ever wondered why some people use drugs?
Why do you think grown-ups say that drugs are harmful?
Has anyone ever tried to sell you drugs or tried to force you to take drugs?

Recognition of the Substance Abuser and Those at Risk of Abuse

Current patterns of drug abuse make it more likely that the primary care physician will encounter substance abuse in his/her clinic or office rather than in the emergency department. It is true, however, that accidental trauma associated with intoxication or drunkenness often will be the reason a physician encounters a substance abuser and, for the astute clinician, certainly provides the opportunity for diagnosis and intervention. More often, the patient will present the problem to the physician because the abuse of substances causes serious interference with school, work, and/or family relations. Physical illness complicating substance abuse is less likely to be the reason for a visit to a physician by an adolescent or young adult than it is for an older individual. Often substance abuse is suspected at the time of a routine health maintenance visit or visit for an illness unrelated to substance abuse. More often the younger patient is seen because there are problems at school, including academic failure, truancy, or antisocial acting out behaviors. The physician must have a high index of suspicion of drug abuse if the opportunity for diagnosis is not to be missed.

The Kinds and Stages of Substance Abuse

Drug use may be experimental, recreational, circumstantial, intensive, and compulsive.[30] *Experimental* drug abuse is primarily the result of curiosity or a desire to learn the feeling of a "high" (euphoria) or a new experience. The abuse is short-term, unplanned, and may involve one or more drugs. *Recreational* drug use is no less substance abuse, but its purpose is to experience a "high" in a social setting and among friends and acquaintances who wish to share the experience. It is noncompulsive use, voluntary, and planned. The drugs used may be "gateway" drugs, (alcohol, cigarets, and marijuana), or drugs with a higher addictive potential, such as cocaine, heroin, and others. However, most users of "gateway" drugs go on to experiment with other drugs, and some become dependent on them.[31] Cigaret smoking, especially for girls, is an important marker for subsequent abuse of illicit drugs.[25]

Circumstantial drug use is the taking of a drug to achieve a purpose. Examples include the use of a stimulant drug to remain awake, alcohol to relieve anxiety, or propranolol to control a tremor. Drugs used in religious ceremonies might be considered circumstantial use. *Intensive* drug use is the daily use of a substance because of a need to achieve relief or maintain a level of performance. *Compulsive* drug use is characterized by dependency and high-dose, high-frequency use. Examples are alcoholics, heroin addicts, and compulsive users of other psychoactive drugs, such as cocaine.

In children and adolescents, a five stage progression to chronic use or dependence, outlined in Table 5, is known to occur.[31,32] The patient's presentation to the physician will vary depending on the stage of abuse. The therapeutic role of the primary care physician will differ depending on the patient's stage of use or abuse. Behavioral manifestations at each stage of development are quite characteristic, and provide the basis for suspecting and/or making the diagnosis. The *stages of drug abuse* include: the *potential*, the *experimentation* stage, the stage of *regular use, preoccupation with the euphoria (the "high"),* and *"burn-out."* Persons in the stage of *high potential* (Stage 0) for abuse have personality traits and family, genetic, and environmental factors that may indicate a high risk or likelihood of future use and abuse. It is a stage in which the physician can exercise his/her influence and power to prevent drug abuse through education and guidance. The role of the primary care physician during the stage of *high potential* has been described above in the discussion on anticipatory guidance. The stage of *experimentation* (Stage 1) is one in which the young person learns what it is like to experience a "high" or the euphoria associated with addictive drugs. Poor judgment by a young adolescent even in this early stage of abuse may be lethal. It is a stage in which alcohol, tobacco, and marijuana are used. Unfortunately, as "gateway" drugs, their use often leads to stage 2, the stage of *regular use* and continued seeking of the euphoria. There is now regular buying or stealing of drugs and an increase in frequency of abuse, sometimes alone. Stage 3 is an advanced stage in which there is a *preoccupation* with the euphoria produced by drugs, or the "high." The young person experiences marked dysphoria without drugs

Table 5
The Stages and Evolution of Substance Abuse

Stages of abuse and their description

Stage 0: The Potential: A preabuse stage in which the child/adolescent has a high potential for abuse; he/she is curious about drug use, and is vulnerable to experimentation (see Table 1)

Stage 1: Experimentation: Learning the euphoria; what it is like to be "high'; mild euphoria with quick return to baseline mood; good feeling with few if any consequences

Stage 2: Early Regular Use: Seeking the euphoria definite euphoria and excitement followed by anxiety, discomfort, and guilt.

Stage 3: Late Regular Use: Preoccupation with; the "High"; preoccupied with drug use and procurement, with wide mood swings. Now dependent on (addicted to) substances of abuse

Stage 4: End Stage of Drug Addition: Deterioration and "burnout"; use of drugs/alcohol to "maintain" and avoid dysphoria

Kinds of drugs and pattern of abuse

Stage 0: None. Alcohol and/or drugs at home and available; models for alcohol/drug abuse in environment

Stage 1: Tobacco, marijuana, and alcohol obtained from friends; learning to use drugs to alter mood; learning what it is like to be euphoric ("high"); drug use increases to regular weekend use

Stage 2: Seeks effects of using: Acquire their own supply; regularly seeks the euphoria; use of stimulants, sedatives, in addition to marijuana, alcohol and tobacco

Stage 3: Marked dysphoria without drugs and/or withdrawal symptoms; in distress; questioning his/her control over drugs; depression, suicidal thoughts; daily use of harder drugs (cocaine, opiates) and hallucinogens, alone as well as with other persons

Stage 4: Drug/alcohol use to "maintain" and avoid dysphoria (to feel normal); use of drugs all of the time; use of any and all drugs available, or that can be stolen, bartered or bought; overdoses

Manifestations

Stage 0: Need for immediate gratification: Decreased impulse control; need for acceptance by peers; bored and blasé; Angry rebellion directed at parents/authority

Stage 1: Little change in behavior, "avoidance lying"

Stage 2: Definite change in behavior, dress, friends, and school performance; mood swings, "conning", and regular lying. Increase in frequency of use, sometimes alone; regular buying or stealing of drugs

(continued)

Table 5 *(continued)*

Stage 3: Stealing, prostitution, selling to obtain "fix"; family fights, pathologic lying, school failure; "Cool," aloof, no straight friends; questioning his/her control over drugs; depression, suicidal thoughts; increased risk-taking, self-destructive activities; overdosing begins

Stage 4: Physical and mental deterioration with paranoia, angry aggression, dropout, flashbacks, amnesia, and overdoses; guilt, withdrawal, depression, shame, remorse; increased risk-taking behaviors, self-destructive, suicidal

---

and, depending on the drug, withdrawal symptoms. Feeling that control is being lost, depression, shame, and guilt are experienced, and suicidal thoughts are not uncommon. In the final stage of *"burn-out"* (Stage 4), he/she is now drug-dependent and is using "any and all drugs all of the time." Feelings of isolation, withdrawal, and severe depression are common. There is physical and mental deterioration with paranoia and physical signs of malnutrition and debilitation.

A knowledge of the determinants of substance abuse, and the kinds and stages of abuse will enable a physician to recognize the warning signs of abuse whether they be early or late. The use of previsit questionnaires can generate a large amount and variety of clinical information. Table 6 lists examples of routine questions for use as a questionnaire that are specific to substance abuse and suitable for an adolescent or young adult. Similar questionnaires can be used for adults. In addition to the usual historical data obtained during a regular visit, there are open-ended questions intended to provide in-depth information that may indicate advanced substance abuse. The open-ended questions listed in Table 7 are asked during an interview or the physical examination, and are inappropriate for a questionnaire. Questions should be modified for use with an adult patient. Responses can then be used as lead-ins to more productive dialogue with the patient. A questionnaire for the parents or spouse of a patient known to be abusing drugs can be used to delve deeper than one used for the patient during a routine or health maintenance visit (*see* Table 8). The questions can be modified for use by a spouse. Persons in the advanced stages of substance abuse are more likely to be uncooperative and to give incomplete or inaccurate answers, in which case a parent's questionnaire or one suitable for a spouse should be used. It is intended to identify behaviors associated with substance abuse that the patient is unlikely to disclose.

Table 6
Questionnaire Items Relevant to Substance Abuse

	Yes	No
1. Do you smoke cigarets?		
2. Do you smoke marijuana?		
3. Do you often feel "bummed out," down, or depressed?		
4. Do you ever use drugs or alcohol to feel better?		
5. Do you ever use drugs or alcohol when you are alone?		
6. Do your friends get drunk or get high at parties?		
7. Do you get drunk or get high at parties?		
8. Do your friends ever get drunk or get high at rock concerts?		
9. Do you ever get drunk or get high at rock concerts?		
10. Have your school grades gone down recently? Problems at work?		
11. Have you flunked any subjects recently? Have you been fired from a job?		
12. Have you had recent problems with your coaches or advisors at school? Problems with supervisors at work?		
13. Do you feel that your friends, parents, or spouse just do not seem to understand you?		

Table 7
Open-Ended Questions Intended to Provide a Basis
for Further Exploration of Advanced Substance Abuse

1. What do your friends do at parties? Do you go the the parties? Do you drink? Get drunk? Get high?
2. Do you drive drunk? Stoned? Have you ridden with a driver who was drunk or stoned? Could you call home and ask for help? What would your parents say? Do?
3. Do you go to rock concerts? Do you drink there? Do you get high? Who drives after the concert?
4. After drinking, have you ever forgotten where you had been or what you had done?
5. Have you recently dropped some old friends and started going with a new group?
6. Do you feel that lately you are irritable, "bitchy," or moody?
7. Do you find yourself getting into more frequent arguments with your friends? Brothers and sisters? Parents?
8. Do you have a girlfriend/boyfriend? How is that going? Are you having more fights/arguments with him/her lately? Have you recently broken up?
9. Do you find yourself being physically abusive to others? Your brothers/sisters? Your mother/father? Your spouse?
10. Do you think your drinking/drug use is a problem? Why?

Table 8
Questionnaire for the Parents(s) of the Adolescent
Suspected of or Known to Be Abusing Drugs and/or Alcohol

1. Does your daughter/son spend many hours alone in his/her bedroom apparently doing nothing?
2. Does your son/daughter resist talking to you or persistently isolate himself/herself from the family?
3. Has your daughter's/son's taste in music had a dramatic change to hard rock music?
4. Has there been a definite change in your son's/daughter's attitude at school? With his/her friends? At home?
5. Has your daughter/son shown recent pronounced mood swings with increased irritability and angry outbursts?
6. Does your son/daughter always seem to be unhappy and less able to cope with frustration than he/she used to be?
7. Has your daughter's/son's personality changed from being a considerate and caring person to being selfish, unfriendly, and unsympathetic?
8. Does your son/daughter always seem to be confused or "spacey"?[a]
9. Have money or valuable articles recently disappeared from your home?[b]
10. Has your daughter/son begun to neglect household chores and homework?
11. Has there been a change in your son's/daughter's friends from age appropriate friends to older, "unacceptable" associates?[a]
12. Has there been a change in your daughter's/son's appearance (i.e.,sloppy dress and poor grooming and hygiene)?
13. Have there been excuses and alibis made, and has there been lying in order to avoid confrontation or not to get caught?[a]
14. Do you feel you have lost control of your son/daughter?[a]
15. Has your daughter/son begun lying in order to cover up sources of money and possessions?[b]
16. Have there been episodes of "ditching" or "skipping" school? Has your son/daughter lied to cover up bad report cards?[a]
17. Has there been stealing, shoplifting, or encounters with the police?[b]
18. Has your daughter/son become a "con artist"?
19. Have you noticed a marked increase in your son's/daughter's interest in drugs, drug literature, and the drug "culture"(i.e., clothing and accoutrements, paraphernalia, belt buckles, and T-shirts with a drug theme)?[b]
20. Has your daughter/son recently quit a sport or dropped out school clubs, social groups, stopped music lessons, quit the band or orchestra, or lost interest in a hobby?[a]
21. Has there been a deterioration of school performance, frequent truancy, or conflict with coaches or teachers?[b]

(continued)

Table 8 *(continued)*

22.	Do you feel your daughter/son has become untrustworthy, insincere, and distrustful ("paranoid")?[a]
23.	Has he/she become unpredictable or rebellious?
24.	Has your son/daughter been verbally abusive to you or your spouse?[a]
25.	Has your daughter/son been physically abusive to you or your spouse?[b]
26.	Has your son/daughter tried to introduce any of your other children to drugs or alcohol?[b]
27.	Has your daughter/son talked about suicide or running away?[b]
28.	Is your son/daughter more argumentative lately? Does he/she tend to blame others for his/her problems?
29.	Is there a paranoid flavor to all of your daughter's/son's relationships with adults, siblings, and authority figures?

[a]Strong indicator of problems and/or drug behavior.
[b]Very strong indicator of problems and/or drug behavior.

The Medical History

The review of systems during a routine visit may provide clues to drug abuse (*see* Table 9). Symptoms of allergic rhinitis and conjunctivitis may be associated with the use of alcohol, marijuana, and cocaine. Excessive sleeping, episodes of extreme hunger, chest pain, nipple tenderness, gynecomastia, or even galactorrhea may be seen with heavy use of marijuana, phenothiazine, or other drugs. Irritability and pronounced mood swings may be experienced by persons involved in the regular use of drugs, especially stimulants, barbiturates, and alcohol. Abdominal pain may be caused by the gastritis or pancreatitis associated with excessive alcohol use. "Hangovers" follow alcohol and barbiturate abuse, and frequently are observed and reported by parents. Constipation and secondary hemorrhoidal bleeding may result from chronic opiate or stimulant abuse. Weight loss and malnutrition, and in women irregular menstruation and amenorrhea are frequent complications of many kinds of abused drugs.

The Physical Examination and Laboratory Findings

The physical examination performed as part of a routine health maintenance visit usually discloses little or no findings of substance abuse. The reason is that most patients being seen for regular or routine visits, if abusing drugs, will be either experimenting or just beginning regular use.

Table 9
Symptoms and Signs to Be Considered in the Person
Who Is Highly Suspect of or Known to Be Abusing Substances

1. Central nervous system:
   A. Behavioral
      1. Acute/chronic depression
      2. Accident proneness
      3. Academic or work difficulties or failure
      4. Anxiety
   B. Neurologic/cognitive:
      1. Memory lapses and decreased short-term memory
      2. Tremor and/or difficulty with fine motor movements
      3. Distractibility and inability to concentrate
      4. Difficulty with time/space orientation
   C. Gastrointestinal:
      1. Abdominal pain/indigestion
      2. Weight loss
      3. Extreme hunger or anorexia
      4. Proctitis
   D. Skin:
      1. Skin abscesses or tracks
      2. Bruises (from injuries or injections)
      3. Poor nail and skin hygiene
   E. Respiratory:
      1. Cough and/or hoarseness
      2. Halitosis
   F. Cardiac:
      1. Hypertension
      2. Tachycardia/bradycardia
      3. Murmurs
      4. Palpitations/extrasystoles
   G. Musculoskeletal:
      1. Muscle weakness/flaccidity
      2. Muscle wasting
      3. Muscle cramps
   H. Genitourinary:
      1. Evidence of sexually transmitted disease
      2. Testicular enlargement/bogginess, or atrophy

(continued)

Table 9 *(continued)*

I. Eyes, nose and throat:
  1. Conjunctivitis
  2. Nystagmus(vertical or horizontal) blurred vision/diplopia
  3. Chronic rhinitis or discharge
  4. Epistaxis (recurrent)
  5. Nasal mucosal irritation or ulceration
  6. Hyperacusis/hypoacusis (conductive)
  7. Vertigo or dizziness

Tachycardia may reflect marijuana or stimulant (including cocaine) use. Abuse of stimulants, hallucinogens, and atropine-like drugs should be included in the differential diagnosis of weight loss and malnutrition, palpitations, cardiac dysrhythmias, and hypertension. Signs of allergic rhinitis, ulcerations of the nasal septum, or sinusitis may be caused by cocaine "snorting" (*see* Table 9).

The laboratory should *not* be used as a means of screening for drug use when patients are being seen for regular care. Screening should be done only when there are indications of substance abuse. Unless there are special circumstances, informed consent, should be obtained from the patient and the parent(s). One may inadvertently, during routine testing, discover proteinuria or an eosinophilia; these findings may be associated with opiate abuse. Other tests are listed in Table 10.

Laboratory evaluation for the known substance abuser must be more extensive and intended to identify organ system abnormalities resulting from chronic or extensive alcohol and other drug abuse. Analysis of both blood and urine should be done.

Immediate Intervention
Early Stages of Abuse

The early stages of abuse require individual counseling, and depending on the person's age, involvement with the parents, spouse, and family. Education and guidance by the physician is required, as well as exploration to determine any serious individual, family, or environmental factors that may predispose the patient to escalation to regular drug abuse. Stage 3 (regular use) is a stage that requires major intervention by a physician skilled in individual and family counseling or by a mental health professional. Persons

Table 10
Laboratory Tests to Identify Substances of Abuse
and Their Primary or Secondary Effects on Organ Systems

A. Hematologic
   1. Anemia/macrocytosis
   2. Eosinophilia
B. Metabolic function tests
   1. Liver function tests: SGOT(ALT), SGPT(AST), or GGT enzymes
   2. Electrolytes, BUN, Creatinine
C. Urinalysis:
   1. Proteinuria, hematuria
D. Toxicologic screen:
   1. Blood
   2. Urine
   3. Breast milk
E. Endocrine studies:
   1. Hypoglycemia
   2. Gonadotropins/prolactin
   3. Azospermia
   4. Testosterone
F. Serologic tests:
   1. VDRL
   2. Hepatitis screen
   3. HIV antibody
G. EKG
   1. Dysrhythmias

at this intermediate stage of involvement will continue to abuse alcohol and other drugs if the underlying individual, family, school, or job-related problems are not addressed. If outpatient counseling of the patient and family does not improve the situation, a residential treatment center will be required. Without this measure, the regular use of drugs to feel better may progress to an obsessive preoccupation (Stage 4). The abuser is often in emotional pain, and may for the first time be able and willing to ask for help. Intervention by a physician skilled in managing substance abuse problems may be successful. This would probably require intensive individual and family counseling sessions twice a week or more often, as well as involvement with Alcoholics

Anonymous or Narcotics Anonymous. As a rule, ongoing consultation with, or referral to a psychiatrist or psychologist is necessary. An alternative is to refer the patient to a community mental health clinic or drug program, which often provides counseling by recovered drug abusers who may succeed where more traditional therapists fail. In some instances, however, a residential treatment center may be the only way to separate the individual from the drug environment. Substance abusers are frequently depressed, and antidepressant therapy may be helpful. Such drugs must be prescribed in small amounts, only after a sufficiently long drug-free period and must be administered carefully by a professional who is mindful of the possibility that the individual in this stage of substance abuse is at a high risk of suicide.

Late Stages of Abuse

The physician seeing a drug-dependent person usually has been provided with some preliminary information by the spouse, parent(s), family member, or employer prior to the initial evaluation. It is crucial that the patient be accompanied to the initial visit by one of these persons or the one who arranged for the visit.

A person in an advanced stage of substance abuse is most often being seen primarily to document the abuse and to plan intervention. Unless the patient is himself/herself seeking help, the physician may be placed in a distasteful, adversarial position. The patient may not perceive the drug use as a problem, may be resentful, and may truly believe that the physician's involvement is an intrusion on his/her privacy and right to be "left alone." The patient often is sullen, belligerent, and at times openly hostile. Successful intervention for this patient requires great skill and patience. Some patients will acknowledge that there is justification for the visit and be relatively cooperative; others, although accepting the need for the visit, will test the physician with provocative posturing and statements. The patient must know that the physician can deal with the provocations, will be empathetic and understanding, and will remain in control of the clinical encounter. The physician must learn to "take the patient's wind out of the doctor's sails," allowing the person's angry barrage of hostile and derogatory comments to go by without becoming upset or responding in anger. This is not accomplished easily, and there are times when the patient must be confronted directly regarding his/her uncooperative and hostile behavior. This confrontation should be accomplished in a cool matter-of-fact manner using comments such as, "I realize you are angry and you certainly do not want to be here, but I wish you would consider my position. I have been asked to do a job, and I need your help to do it in the best way I know how." Depending on the patient's response, the visit may be continued or be terminated in an unemotional and calm manner. A return visit should be arranged, at which time the patient will hopefully have completed testing, accepted the physician as a possible resource, and adopted an improved attitude.

The patient will probably resist returning, giving assurances that there really is no problem and the substance abuse is nothing that he/she cannot handle. Initially, some patients may resist, but actually later comply if the physician insists that intervention is necessary and that a return visit is expected and anticipated.

Referral and Coordination of Care

Probably the most important and difficult responsibility of the primary care physician after determining which patient needs referral, is convincing the patient that there is a serious problem and that he/she needs help. Convincing a patient and his/her family that additional help is needed is often very difficult. There is often a strong element of denial, and when patients accept that there is a problem, they often feel that they can handle it on their own and refuse to accept the physician's recommendation. In all cases, it is necessary to involve the family in the referral process and to recommend or arrange future family counseling. No family member, spouse, or parent should be allowed to "sabotage" or undermine the referral or treatment program.

The later the stage of substance abuse, the more difficult a successful intervention will be. In the final stages of abuse (dependence), long-term hospitalization or residential treatment is required. The patient must be completely separated from his/her source of drugs and drug-using associates. This requires referral to a specialized residential drug and alcohol treatment program with highly structured activities, and one or more months of intensive, individual, and family group therapy. Consultation with a hospital social worker who is familiar with community resources may help in finding the best program within the family's means. Patients often refuse such hospitalization, and a court order for involuntary admission is very difficult to obtain once legal adulthood has been attained. Moreover, treatment is extremely expensive, often, not covered by insurance, and free or low-cost community resources are scarce and not always of high quality. Within an effective program, the prognosis for Stage 4 is favorable, but for Stage 5 ("burn-out"), it is poor. However, with appropriate and excellent treatment, many persons will overcome their dependence, but should always consider themselves *recovering* individuals.

Certain patients may be unable to accept the physician or treatment on any terms. In such situations, if the substance abuse is considered to be a major threat to the young person or his/her family, admission to a residential treatment center will have to be accomplished against his/her will: by subterfuge, court order, or even by force if necessary. It is paramount that the physician try to maintain the therapeutic alliance already established by avoiding a critical, authoritarian, or adversarial approach. Persuasion is preferred, but coercion or force may be necessary especially in life-threatening situations. By focusing on one aspect of the problem, such as deteriorating family relations or difficulties at school or work, the physician often can convince the patient of the need for help.

Family Support and Education, and Resources

The majority of primary care practitioners have not had advanced training in the treatment of chemical dependence, and therefore most often referral is necessary. For those in the advanced stages of abuse, a multidisciplinary treatment team is necessary. It is critical that the physician be knowledgeable of those mental health professionals in the community who are skilled in the treatment of substance abuse and know which facilities and drug treatment centers have high-quality programs. This information is usually available through local community mental health agencies or medical/psychiatric organizations. Other reliable sources of information include Alcoholics Anonymous, Alanon, Families Anonymous, Narcotics Anonymous, and national clearing houses, such as the National Clearinghouse for Alcohol and Drug Information (NCADI) at P.O. Box 2345, Rockville, MD 20852 (301-468-2600).[33] Referrals work best when the primary care physician has direct knowledge of the consultant and the drug abuse program, and can make a confident and enthusiastic recommendation to the patient and the family. Questions that are helpful in determining the quality of a program are found in Table 11.

Table 11
Questions to Determine the Quality of a Program and Facility

1. Does the program center around an expectation of total abstinence? Most experts in drug treatment agree that only programs requiring total abstinence have a proven success rate.
2. Does the program address the addictive process directly? Are there licensed drug counselors to supervise effective group confrontations and drug education experiences in the program?
3. Does the program have a family component that acknowledges the importance of parent involvement in treatment?
4. Does the program make adequate provisions for the fact that serious drug involvement is a chronic illness? Short-term programs that promise too much should be regarded with some suspicion, unless they are associated with followup programs that offer long-term support to the drug-free youth.

References

[1] I. J. Chasnoff, W. J. Burns, S. H. Schnoll, and K. A. Burnes (1985) Cocaine use in pregnancy. *N. Engl. J. Med.* **313,** 666–669.

[2] A. P. Streessguth, S. Landesman-Dwyer, J. C. Martin, and D. W. Smith (1980) Teratogenic effects of alcohol in human and laboratory animals. *Science* **209,** 35–361.

[3] D. A. Bateman and M. C. Heagarty (1989) Passive freebase cocaine ("crack") inhalation by infants and toddlers. *AJDC* **143,** 25–27.

[4] R. H. Schwartz, P. Peary, and D. Mistretta (1986) Intoxication of young children with marijuana: a form of amusement for "pot" smoking teenage girls. *AJDC* **140,** 326.

[5] L. D. Johnston, P. M. O'Malley, and J. G. Bachman. Drug use, drinking, and smoking: National survey results from high school, college, and young adult populations, 1975–1988. National Institute on Drug Abuse (NIDA).

[6] National Center for Health Statistics: Advance Report of Final Mortality Statistics, 1986. Monthly vital statistics report, 37(6)28, 1988.

[7] Surgeon General's Workshop on drunk driving; 1988 Proceedings US Department of Health and Human Services, (Public Health Service) Office of the Surgeon General, Rockville, MD, 1989.

[8] J. Bass, S. Gallagher, and K. Mehta (1985) Unintentional injuries among adolescents and young adults. *Pediatr. Clin. North Am.* **32,** 31–39.

[9] R. A. Goodman, J. A. Mercy, F. Loya, M. L. Rosenberg, J. G. Smith, N. H. Allen, L. Vargas, and R. Kalts (1986) Alcohol use and interpersonal violence:

alcohol detected in homicide victims. *Am. J. Pub. Health* **76,** 144–149.

[10] Sixth Special Report to Congress on Alcohol and Health. US Department of Health and Human Services, National Institute on Alcohol Abuse and Alcoholism, (DHHS publication no. (ADM) 87-1519), 1987, 21–23.

[11] L. D. Johnston, P. M. O'Malley, and J. G. Bachman National trends in drug use and related factors among American high school students and young adults, 1975–1986. National Institute of Drug Abuse, Rockville, MD, 1987.

[12] A. B. Lowenfels, and T. T. Miller (1984) Alcohol and trauma. *Ann. Emer. Med.* **13,** 1056–1059.

[13] K. L. Kumpfer. (1987) Special populations: Etiology and prevention of vulnerability to chemical dependence in children of substance abusers, in *Youth at Risk for Substance Abuse* (B. S. Brown and A. R. Mills eds.), National Institute on Drug Abuse, Rockville, MD (DHEW(ADM)87) p. 14.

[14] W. H. McGlothlin and L. J. West (1968) The marijuana problem: An overview. *Am. J. Psychiatry.* **125,** 370–378.

[15] R. Millman and E. Khuri (1981) Substance abuse: Clinical problems and perspectives, in *Adolescence and Substance Abuse* (Lowinson, Ruiz, eds.) pp. 739–751.

[16] Public Health Service, Office on Smoking and Health. Smoking and Health. A National Status Report. 1987.

[17] American Medical Association (1986) Health effects of smokeless tobacco. Council on Scientific Affairs and Health Applications of Smokeless Tobacco. Consensus Conference *JAMA* **255,** 1038–1048.

[18] M. J. Eckardt, T. C. Harford, C. T. Kaelber, E. S. Parker, L. S. Rosenthal, R. S. Ryback, G. C. Salmoiraghi, E. Vanderween, and K. R. Warren (1981) Health hazards associated with alcohol consumption. *JAMA* **246,** 648, 649.

[19] E. J. Khantzian (1988) The primary care therapist and patient needs in substance abuse treatment. *Am. J. Drug Alcohol Abuse* **14,** 159–167.

[20] S. K. Schonberg (1985) Perspective on the role of the pediatrician in the management of adolescent drug use. *Pediatrics in Review* **7,** 131.

[21] J. L. Schulman (1967) *Management of Emotional Disorders in Pediatric Practice.* Year Book Medical Publishers, Chicago.

[22] W. H. Missildine, ed. (Mar.–Apr. 1971) Feelings and their medical significance. *Ross Timesaver* **13,** 2.

[23] D. B. Kandel (1982) Epidemiological and psychosocial perspectives on adolescent drug use. *J. Am. Acad. Child Psychiatry* **21,** 328–347.

[24] C. Treece, and E. J. Khantzian (1986) Psychodynanic factors in the development of drug dependence. *Psychiatric Clinics of North America* **9,** 399–411.

[25] J. D. Hawkins, D. M. Lishuer, and L. F. Catalano (1985) Childhood predictors and the prevention of adolescent substance abuse, in *Etiology of Drug Abuse: Implications for Prevention* (C. L. Jones and R. J. Battjes, eds.) (USDHHS NIDA. DHHS (ADM)85–1335) Government Printing Office, 1985.

[26]J. Block, J. H. Block, and S. Keyes (1988) Longitudinally foretelling drug usage in adolescents: early childhood personality and environmental precursors. *Child Development* **59**, 336–355.

[27]D. W. Goodwin, F. Schulsinger, et. al. (1973) Alcohol problems in adoptees raised apart from alcoholic biologic parents. *Archives of General Psychiatry* **28**, 238–243.

[28]M. A. Schuckit, D. W. Goodwin, and G. Winokur (1972) A half-sibling study of alcoholism. *Am. J. Psychiatry* **128**, 1132–1136.

[29]D. W. Goodwin (1985) Alcoholism and genetics. *Arch. of Gen. Psychiatry* **42**, 171–174.

[30]G. S. Parcel (1982) The pediatrician's role in drug education. *Pediatr. Rev.* **4**, 144.

[31]D. B. Kandel (1978) *Longitudinal Research on Drug Use: Emipirical Findings and Methodological Issues* (John Wiley, New York).

[32]D. I. Macdonald (1984) *Drugs, Drinking, and Adolescents* (Chicago Year Book Medical Publishers, Chicago).

[33]*American Academy of Pediatrics Substance Abuse: A Guide for Health Professionals* (American Academy of Pediatrics, Elk Grove Village, IL) **198**, 72.

Using the DIS to Diagnose Drug and Alcohol Abuse

*The Effects of Language and Ethnic Status**

Robert E. Roberts and Howard M. Rhoades

Introduction

The purpose of this chapter is to present some findings on the effects of cultural background, specifically language and ethnic status, on the reliability and validity of the DIS. Our specific focus is on the ability of the DIS to correctly identify DSM-III diagnoses of drug abuse and alcohol abuse in different ethnic populations. The data are from a study of the influence of language, ethnic status, and acculturation on the operating characteristics of both clinical and nonclinical procedures for measuring psychological dysfunction.

The rationale for this research stems partly from a recognition that measurement issues remain a central problem in psychiatric research.[1-4] Much of the data in psychiatric epidemiology still is generated by procedures whose reliability and validity are not well-established. The principal effects of

*For reprints write to: Robert E. Roberts, Ph.D., Social Psychiatry Research Group, The University of Texas Health Science Center, P.O. Box 20186, Houston, Texas 77225.

Drug and Alcohol Abuse Prevention Ed: R. R. Watson ©1990 The Humana Press Inc.

these unresolved measurement problems are (1) classification errors that result in inaccurate estimates of incidence and prevalence, and (2) almost certain bias in observed associations between putative risk factors and psychiatric disorders. The problem is that the contexts under which these conditions are operant are not known and efficacious strategies for their resolution are not available. For example, little is known about the cross-cultural utility of many of these assessment procedures. This is true not only in cross-national comparisons, but also in intranational contexts, e.g., subgroups within American society that differ in terms of class, color, and culture.[5] One cultural group for whom little is known about the usefulness of these assessment procedures is the Mexican origin population. There is general consensus that this ethnic population represents a group that is socially, historically, demographically, and geographically unique.[6-11] Such a population is inherently intriguing, since it implies that there may be unique aspects to that group's illness experience as well.[12]

Research available on the reliability and validity of measures of psychological dysfunction in the Mexican origin population is sparse and the results often equivocal.[10,12,13] A major obstacle has been a lack of assessment procedures that are adequately translated and standardized with English and Spanish equivalency demonstrated.[14] In particular, an unresolved question in measuring psychological impairment of psychiatric morbidity in the Mexican origin population concerns the extent to which symptoms or disorders are manifested in a universal (etic) manner and to what extent in a culturally specific (emic) fashion.[15-17] With the exception of a few studies of folk medical syndromes, there is little evidence about whether and how Mexican cultural background shapes psychopathology in ways unique to this population.[14] Even less is known about how reliably or validly a given assessment procedure describes the experience of psychiatric disorder in this population. A case in point is the DIS.

The Diagnostic Interview Schedule

The DIS is a highly structured interview schedule designed to provide data that permit diagnostic categorization of subjects.[18,19] It can be administered by either lay interviews or mental health professionals. The instrument was developed originally as the core mental status assessment procedure for the Epidemiologic Catchment Area (ECA) research program, a multi-site collaborative study of over 18,000 subjects.[20] To date, a number of studies have been published that examine the operating characteristics of the DIS, either reliability, validity, or both.[18,19,21-32] In their review of much of this research, Erdman et al.[31] note that, thus far, the data indicate that the DIS in the hands of lay interviewers has proved to be comparable to other structured methods in terms of reliability. However, they note that the consistently poor agreement of the DIS with independent clinical diagnosis remains a cause for concern.

This observation is illustrated very well in three studies reported thus far, which have had as their focus the efficacy of the DIS with Black and Hispanic subjects. Hendricks et al.[22] compared the DIS to routine chart diagnoses for 46 adult Black patients in three diagnostic categories. Although the description of the methodology is somewhat scanty, the concordance between the DIS (administered by medical students and mental health clinicians in training) and medical record diagnosis was perfect for major depression (1.0), good for alcohol (.50), and poor for schizophrenia (.24), using the κ statistic. No data on test–retest reliability were presented. More importantly, the design was not comparative. That is, the operating characteristics of the DIS were not compared directly for Blacks and other ethno-cultural groups nor were direct comparisons made with the majority group.

Two studies of the reliability and validity of the DIS with Hispanics have been reported, one conducted in Los Angeles and the other in Puerto Rico. For the ECA survey in Los Angeles, the researchers translated the DIS into Spanish,[33] conducted a study of the test–retest reliability of the Spanish version and compared it with diagnoses made independently by clinicians to assess its concurrent validity.[24] The subjects were 151 Mexican-American outpatients. The κ values for the test–retest component of the study (overall) ranged from a high of .79 for antisocial personality to a low of .30 for dysthymia. κs were .56 for major depression, .63 for alcohol abuse, .54 for anxiety disorders, and .49 for phobias. There was considerably less agreement between DIS-generated diagnoses and those made by clinicians. κs ranged from a high of .60 for alcohol abuse to a low of .05 for dysthymia. κs were .58 for drug abuse, .34 for schizophrenia, .38 for major depression, .33 for anxiety disorders, and .29 for antisocial personality disorder. In fact, using criteria suggested by Landis and Koch,[34] the agreement between the DIS and independent clinical diagnoses was poor for 13 of 18 categories considered. Although the study by Burnam and her colleagues did not permit simultaneous assessment of the effects of language and ethnic status (no nonHispanics were included), there was no significant language effect noted among Hispanics. That is, the English and Spanish versions of the DIS demonstrated comparable operating characteristics.

In the other study of the reliability of the DIS and its concordance with clinical diagnoses among Hispanics, a modified version of the Spanish DIS used in Los Angeles was administered to 129 outpatients and 60 community residents in Puerto Rico.[30] The design was similar to that of Robins et al.[18] Comparison of the lay-administered DIS and the DIS administered by psychiatrists yielded κ values (test–retest) mostly in the moderate range (.4–.6); the mean for 14 diagnoses was .55, and the range was .27–.79. The κ for alcohol abuse was .48; for alcohol dependence it was .79. For several diagnoses, agreement was poor: somatization was .27 and dysthymia was .33, for example. Comparisons also were made between the lay-administered DIS and clinical diagnoses made by the psychiatrists, based on clinical assessments made after completion of the DIS. Concordance in this context was reduced. κs ranged from .23–.71 ($\bar{x}$ = .41). For a number of diagnoses, concordance was quite low: major depression (.26); dysthymia (.30); schizophrenia (.29); and manic episode (.37), as cases in point. For alcohol abuse, κ was .28; for alcohol dependence, .61. The data did not permit direct examination of the effects of either language or ethnocultural factors, since the design included only Puerto Ricans living on the island who were assessed only in Spanish.

Thus far, the available data suggest that the issue of the reliability and validity of the DIS in different ethnocultural contexts is unresolved. This is especially true in the case of the Mexican origin population. The results from the only study of this population to data raise serious questions about the reliability and validity of the DIS with subjects from groups whose cultural repertoires[35] regarding recognition, interpretation, and reporting of signs and symptoms of psychiatric disorder may differ from subjects drawn from the mainstream of American life. Based on their results, in fact, Burnam et al.[24] have urged more studies of the DIS in both English and Spanish. The data presented here are in response to that recommendation.

This chapter presents data comparing the test–retest reliability of the DIS administered by lay interviewers and the concordance of this assessment with independent clinical diagnosis. This chapter also contrasts the operating characteristics of the DIS between Anglos and persons of Mexican origin who were interviewed in English and/or Spanish. This study is the first to assess the effects of language and ethnic status directly in the same research design.

Procedures

Subjects

The study subjects consisted of patients admitted to San Antonio State Hospital and to the Bexar County Mental Health and Mental Retardation Substance Abuse Program (also in San Antonio) during the course of the research project. Those from the hospital were inpatients, and those from the substance abuse program were outpatients. To select the sample, the research staff, in consultation with the clinical staff, eliminated patients who were under the age of 18, who were not Anglo or Hispanic in origin, who were mentally retarded, who were too violent or incoherent to be interviewed, or who would not be available for at least two additional weeks, which was the minimal time interval required to complete the full assessment sequence. In general, all eligible Hispanics were included, and a one-in-three sample of Anglos was chosen. This fraction was selected to yield sufficient Anglos for comparison with the Hispanic groups. At the conclusion of the data collection phase (April, 1984–May, 1985), this strategy had yielded an eligible sample of 1060, of whom 322 (30.4%) refused to participate in the study and another 139 (13.1%) agreed to participate, but withdrew before completing the initial assessment. Thus, 56.5% of the eligible sample was assessed. Of these, 210 Anglos and 352 Hispanics provided data sufficient for analysis.

Measures

Ethnic background was assessed using two items. One inquired about the respondents' racial background (e.g., Black, not Hispanic; white, not Hispanic; Hispanic). The other inquired about cultural or ethnic background (e.g., Anglo-American, Afro-American, Cuban, Puerto Rican, Mexican American, Latin American, other Spanish, and so on) For the data reported here, persons of Mexican origin refer to those patients who reported that they were Mexican American, Chicano, or Mexican/Mexicano.

The core psychological assessment procedures were:

1. The Center for Epidemiologic Studies Depression Scale (CES-D);
2. The DSM-III Checklist developed by John Helzer and his associates at Washington University;[25] and

3. The DIS developed initially by Robins and her colleagues at Washington University with the support and collaboration of the Center for Epidemiologic Studies at the National Institute of Mental Health.[18]

Unlike its progenitors, such as the Schedule for Affective Disorders and Schizophrenia (SADS),[36] the DIS was developed primarily to be used by trained lay interviewers in community surveys, although it can be used by clinicians and in clinical settings as well. The DIS was designed to elicit data for most of the DSM-III adult diagnoses, the Feighner criteria diagnoses, and the Research Diagnostic Criteria (RDC) diagnoses on both a lifetime and current basis. Current disorder is defined for four time periods: the last 2 wk, the last month, the last 6 mo, and the last year. Each diagnosis is based on subjects meeting a minimum number of criteria, and since subjects need not meet all criteria, individuals may be assessed for the severity of each diagnosis by counting how many of the criteria they meet. Across diagnoses, severity may be determined by the number of different diagnoses present, the total number of symptoms, over how many years they have had the symptoms, as well as the degree of functional impairment. The DIS also ascertains the age at the last symptom, the age at which the first symptom appeared, and whether medical care was ever sought for symptoms of a disorder. The DIS was designed to reduce variation resulting from interviewer discretion to a minimum by making virtually all response categories close-ended and precoded, with explicit instructions (including a Probe Flow Chart). After the interviewer follows these explicit instructions, actual diagnosis is made by computer. Computer programs have been developed to provide diagnosis, age of onset and termination of syndromes, the total number of symptoms ever manifested, diagnosis with earliest onset, total number of lifetime diagnoses, and the number and types of current diagnoses.

Several versions of the DIS have been developed; we used Version 3. More specifically, we used the English and Spanish versions of the DIS used in the Los Angeles ECA project (Burnam et al., 1983). The UCLA group translated the DIS into Spanish using a rigorous forward and backward translation procedure.[33]

The diagnostic criterion measure was the standard DSM-III diagnosis recorded by clinicians using the DSM-III Checklist. The latter was chosen because it also was used in the UCLA study. The Checklist was developed to be used independent of any other assessment procedure. Helzer assisted us in training our clinical raters in the use of this instrument and provided ongoing consultation in its use. From a methodological perspective, it is believed that this instrument provided a more defensible procedure for establishing the validity of the diagnoses generated from the lay interviewer-administered DIS than routine clinical diagnosis. Also, from an operational point of view, it was not necessary to translate the checklist formally, since the clinicians were bilingual and the checklist is not an interview schedule, but a method of organizing and recording clinical observations. However, a standard Spanish translation of the key questions and criteria in each section of the Checklist was provided, so that the Spanish-speaking clinicians felt comfortable with the fact that all were using standard phrases and terminology in their psychiatric interviews. Informed consent and assessment of linguistic ability were obtained when patients were enrolled in the study. As soon as possible after the treatment team recorded the DSM-III diagnosis(es), the patients who provided consent were interviewed, usually within a few days. Within another 7–14 d, those subsamples of the T_1 interviewees, who were to be part of the test–retest reliability study, were reinterviewed. The interview instrument used at T_1 and T_2 was identical. Interviewers consisted of bilingual Mexican Americans. Interviewers and subjects were matched on gender and different interviewers were assigned to subjects at T_1 and T_2 to assure independent assessments.

The lay interviewers received a 1-wk didactic training session on the DIS and several additional weeks of subsequent review and practice using the DIS, with and without supervision. Training ceased when no instance of conjoint patient interviews (involving all lay interviewers) was less than 75% (that is, three out of four had to be in agreement on a specific diagnosis). The clinicians received a 2-d didactic session on the use of the DSM-III Checklist followed by several weeks of review and practice. Again, training halted when there was no instance of conjoint interviewers with less than 75% agreement on a specific diagnosis. Once data collection began, each completed DIS was reviewed by a supervisor with the interviewer to ensure information had been elicited and recorded correctly. Similarly, the DSM-III Checklists completed by the clinicians were reviewed by two senior psychiatrists, one on the faculty of the University of Texas Medical School in Houston and one (Hispanic) from the University of Texas counterpart in San Antonio.

Language proficiency in English and Spanish was assessed using the Bilingual Assessment Instrument (BAI) developed for this project by Edward Codina and Roberts (unpublished). This instrument is composed of three subtests reflecting three aspects of language use and takes 15–20 min to administer. The first section or subtest includes questions concerning preference for and use of English and Spanish. These 10 questions were selected from an acculturation section used in the DIS questionnaire. Scoring for this section consists of averaging the individual item scores for all applicable answers. This average score is then classified as:

1. Monolingual English;
2. English dominant;
3. Bilingual;
4. Spanish dominant; or
5. Monolingual Spanish.

The second subtest consists of a vocabulary test of 24 English words and 24 Spanish words. The administration procedure, scoring, and most of the words were adapted from the vocabulary subtests of the Wechsler Adult Intelligence Scale (WAIS)[37] and the Escala de Intelegencia Wechsler Para Adultos (EIWA).[38] In addition to the scoring procedure outlined in the WAIS and EIWA, these scores are converted to language category scores. This is done by obtaining the ratio of the English vocabulary score to the Spanish vocabulary score and then finding its equivalent language category score on a table developed specifically for this procedure. The last subtest records oral language production in each language. A sample of oral language is recorded from the subjects' descriptions of two photographs and their paraphrasing of two short paragraphs read to them. The scoring criteria for these language samples follows those outlined by Duncan and De Avila.[39] Again, the ratio of the English scores to the Spanish scores is converted into its equivalent language category. The final language category is determined by a similar language category score in at least two of the three subtests. Interrater reliability among the three language assessors was very high. There was 100% agreement on the final language category as well as for each subtest category. At the raw score level for each subtest, the reliability was greater than 85%. Only about 3% of the subjects could not complete an interview in their assigned language.

Analytic Design

In order to permit an assessment of the effects of language and ethnic status, as well as test–retest reliability and validity of the psychiatric instruments, the design specified that each patient receive two assessments.

Half of the respondents were assessed twice with the DIS and the other half were assessed a second time by clinicians (clinical psychologists and psychiatrists) who made an independent psychiatric evaluation in which their diagnosis was documented using the DSM-III Checklist. Based on the results of our language assessment procedure, patients of Mexican origin were classified as English dominant, Spanish dominant, or bilingual. Participants classified as English dominant were assessed in English, those classified as Spanish dominant were assessed in Spanish, and bilinguals were randomly assigned to either an English or Spanish language assessment at T_1. At T_2 bilinguals were randomly assigned again, 1/3 receiving the DIS in the same language twice, 1/3 receiving the DIS in the other language, and 1/3 receiving the DSM-III Checklist in the same language as the T_1 DIS. Based on language assessment and administration of the DIS assessment, the study generated 67 Spanish only, 57 English only, and 228 bilingual interviews at T_1. Of the latter, 116 (50.8%) were assessed initially in English and the remainder in Spanish.

Analyses involve two comparisons. The first focuses on test–retest reliability of the DIS across three groups: Anglos and two Mexican origin subgroups (English dominant or Spanish dominant). The second comparison examines concordance of the diagnoses generated by the lay-administered DIS and diagnoses made by the research clinicians using the DSM-III Checklist. As has been the case in other studies,[24,25] concordance is examined using lifetime diagnoses, i.e., the presence of a disorder now or at any time in the past. Data on concordance also focuses on three groups: Anglos and Mexican origin patients assessed either in English or in Spanish.

Concordance and test–retest for both alcohol and drug problems, defined according to DSM-III criteria are examined. Diagnoses of alcohol and drug abuse are examined. Specific symptoms, or criteria, that are used to determine whether a subject meets DSM-III diagnostic threshold for alcohol or drug abuse are also examined. Examples include, "Have you ever wanted to stop drinking but couldn't?, and, "Have you ever had withdrawal symptoms—that is, have you felt sick because you stopped or cut down on any of these drugs?

The κ statistic[40] is used as the primary estimator for test–retest reliability and concordance. κ is an index of chance-corrected agreement with the desirable property that it is asymptotically equivalent to the intraclass correlation coefficient. However, there are some patterns of data for which κ cannot be calculated. For example, if at the first interview each person responded "no" to a particular question, and then at the second interview some "yes" as well as "no" responses were given to the same question, κ cannot be calculated. Under this and similar conditions, the raw agreement rate is reported, expressed as a percentage.

Results

Demographic information regarding the study groups is presented in Table 1. Whereas the age distribution of subjects in the three groups appears similar, the distributions were found to differ statistically ($\chi^2 = 31.21$, $df = 6$, $p < .001$). Males outnumbered females in all groups: however, there were relatively more females in the Anglo group than in the two Mexican origin groups ($\chi^2 = 14.05$, $df = 2$, $p < .001$). The distribution of marital status in Anglo and Spanish interview groups differed ($\chi^2 - 27.73$, $df = 4$, $p < .001$) with a larger number of Anglo subjects having never been married (36.2% vs 19.1%) and a smaller number being currently married (18.6% vs 40.4%). The distribution of education level in the three groups was very different ($\chi^2 - 102.0$, $df = 4$, $p < .001$). Fifty-four percent of the Anglo group had completed 10–12 yr of school, whereas 63.7% of the Spanish interview group had completed less than 10 yr of school. The English interview, Mexican origin group education level fell between the other two groups.

Test–retest reliability coefficients for ten, nonexclusive, lifetime diagnoses from individuals interviewed twice using the DIS are presented in Table 2. Three measures were calculated for each diagnosis within each group: percent agreement, the ϕ statistic, and κ statistic. The ϕ and κ coefficients have approximately the same interpretation as the intraclass correlation. Percentage agreement is not chance corrected and is included, because in some instances (e.g., bipolar disorder) at least one mariginal frequency value was observed to be zero. Test–retest results were good for alcohol abuse across all three groups. Other diagnostic categories were found to exhibit lesser amounts of consistency across ratings.

For example, drug abuse was .54 in both Mexican origin groups, but .77 for the Anglos. Dysthymia, in the Spanish interview group, was the least reliable diagnosis observed in this sample ($\kappa = 0.12$). In general, diagnoses of depression, dysthymia, generalized anxiety, phobia, panic, and schizophrenia evidenced marginal to less than acceptable reliability in this sample. There were no consistent differences in reliability of diagnosis found among the Anglo and Hispanic groups.

Table 1
Percent Distributions of Demographic Variables
for Anglo and Hispanic Groups

Demographic characteristics	Anglo	Mexican origin Spanish interview	Mexican origin English interview
Age			
<29	32.4	20.1	33.1
30–44	42.4	39.7	48.5
45–59	21.4	26.8	14.8
>60	3.8	13.4	3.6
(n)	(210)	(179)	(169)
Gender			
Male	53.8	65.0	72.2
Female	46.2	35.0	27.8
(n)	(210)	(183)	(169)
Marital status			
Never married	36.2	19.1	32.5
Married	18.6	40.4	29.0
Not currently married or separated	45.2	40.5	38.5
(n)	(210)	(183)	(169)
Education (n y)			
0–9	14.7	63.7	36.6
10–12	54.4	32.5	43.0
>12	30.9	3.8	20.4
(n)	(204)	(157)	(142)

Differences between groups in concordance rates were observed when DIS diagnoses was compared to physicians' diagnoses. Table 3 presents base rates, sensitivity and specificity, κ, Yule's Y, and positive and negative predictive power indices for six diagnostic categories. For the diagnoses, major depressive disorders, dysthymia, and drug abuse, the concordance for the Anglo group was observed to be greater in magnitude than for one or both of the Mexican origin groups. For all affective disorders, there was a trend

Table 2
Reliability and Agreement of DIS Lifetime Diagnoses for Anglo and Hispanic Groups

		Group	
		Mexican origin	
DIS Diagnoses	Anglo, 102	Spanish interview, 87	English interview, 76
Major Depression			
% Agreement	78.43	86.21	86.84
ø	.32	.39	.39
K	.32	.38	.37
Dysthymia			
% Agreement	82.83	89.16	90.79
ø	.32	.12	.32
K	.31	.12	.31
Bipolar			
% Agreement	96.97	98.81	98.68
ø	.79	N/C[a]	N/C[a]
K	.79	N/C[a]	N/C[a]
Mania			
% Agreement	96.97	98.81	98.68
ø	.79	N/C[a]	N/C[a]
K	.78	N/C[a]	N/C[a]
Generalized anxiety			
% Agreement	84.04	89.33	89.74
ø	.56	.31	.44
K	.56	.18	.44
Phobia			
% Agreement	76.47	85.06	81.58
ø	.37	.49	.39
K	.35	.49	.39
Panic			
% Agreement	89.00	95.24	94.67
ø	.30	.49	.59
K	.29	.48	.57
Schizophrenia			
% Agreement	89.79	92.41	89.33
ø	.40	.63	.45
K	.39	.62	.44

(continued)

	Table 2 (continued)		
Alcohol abuse			
% Agreement	90.32	92.59	91.55
∅	.79	.85	.84
K	.79	.85	.83
Drug abuse			
% Agreement	91.18	93.10	88.16
∅	.77	.54	.54
K	.77	.53	.54

[a]N/C: Values are not calculable because of zero marginals.

toward much lower concordance in the English interview Mexican group. Overall, the concordance between diagnoses derived from the lay-administered DIS and those derived from the interview schedule administered by clinicians was low with the exception of alcohol abuse. κs for this diagnosis were .79 for Anglos, .46 for Mexican origin subjects assessed in English, and .69 for those interviewed in Spanish. κs for drug abuse, on the other hand, were much lower, .38 for Anglos and 0.02 and .03 for the two Mexican origin groups.

Burke,[41] based on the work of Landis and Koch,[34] classifies κ values greater than .75 as indicating excellent agreement, κs .40–.74 as indicating good agreement, and κs below .40 as poor agreement among raters. Using these criteria, concordance was poor for Mexican origin patients interviewed in English ($\bar{x} = .14$). For those Mexican origin patients interviewed in Spanish, concordance was poor to fair ($\bar{x} = .27$). By contrast, κs for the Anglo group were rather consistently higher ($\bar{x} = .38$), although still only fair overall. Comparison of the data on Anglos with those from nonBlack, nonHispanics in other studies indicates the results we obtained are quite similar to those reported by other researchers (generally in the .3–.4 range).

A subset of 11 symptoms taken from the Alcohol section of the DIS were examined for their test–retest reliability. κs were generally moderate to high in value as shown in Table 4. Mexican origin patients interviewed in English and Spanish had a comparable distribution of κ values, whereas the Anglo patients showed a slight increase in the number of high κ values. In general, test–retest reliability of responses to the Alcohol section of the DIS was very acceptable.

Table 3
Comparative Ability of DIS to Detect Clinical Diagnosis

Diagnosis	Measures	Anglo, 76	Mexican origin English Interview, 63	Mexican origin Spanish language, 55
Major depressive Disorder	Base rate	48.6	44.4	38.2
	Sensitivity	43.2	10.7	23.8
	Specificity	89.7	91.4	97.1
	K	0.33	0.02	0.24
	Yule's Y	0.44	0.06	0.53
	P.P.P.[a]	80.0	50.0	83.3
	N.P.P[b]	62.5	56.1	67.4
Dysthymia	Base rate	17.8	14.5	24.1
	Sensitivity	53.8	11.1	23.1
	Specificity	88.3	94.3	97.6
	K	0.41	0.07	0.27
	Yule's Y	0.50	0.18	0.55
	P.P.P.[a]	50.0	25.0	75.0
	N.P.P[b]	89.8	86.2	80.0
All affective	Base rate	72.4	50.8	38.2
	Sensitivity	51.1	25.0	33.3
	Specificity	83.9	87.1	94.1
	K	0.32	0.12	0.31
	Yule's Y	0.40	0.20	0.48
	P.P.P.[a]	82.1	66.7	77.8
	N.P.P[b]	54.2	52.9	69.6
Alcohol Abuse	Base rate	52.0	46.0	64.2
	Sensitivity	89.7	93.1	82.4
	Specificity	88.9	64.7	89.5
	K	0.79	0.56	0.69
	Yule's Y	0.79	0.67	0.73
	P.P.P.[a]	89.7	69.2	93.3
	N.P.P[b]	88.9	91.7	73.9
Drug Abuse	Base rate	22.4	12.7	5.5
	Sensitivity	88.2	75.0	66.7
	Specificity	64.4	32.7	44.2
	K	0.38	0.03	0.02

(continued)

Table 3 *(continued)*

	Yule's Y	0.57	0.09	0.11
	P.P.P.[a]	41.7	14.0	6.4
	N.P.P[b]	95.0	90.0	95.8
All Nonaffective	Base rate	89.0	96.7	94.3
	Sensitivity	80.0	65.5	74.0
	Specificity	50.0	50.0	66.7
	K	0.20	0.03	0.14
	Yule's Y	0.33	0.16	0.41
	P.P.P.[a]	92.9	97.4	97.4
	N.P.P[b]	23.5	4.8	13.3

[a]P.P.P. = Positive Predictive Power.
[b]N.P.P. = Negative Predictive Power.

Table 4
Number of Test–Retest Reliability Coefficients
Falling in Three Categories by Ethnicity and Language

	Anglo	Mexican origin	
		English	Spanish
Alcohol section of DIS			
$K < .40$	0	1	1
$K \geq .40$ and $< .75$	6	8	8
$K \geq .75$	5	2	2
Substance abuse section of DIS—			
Global Questions			
$K < .40$	0	0	7
$K \geq .40$ and $< .75$	3	3	2
$K \geq .75$	6	6	0
Substance Abuse Section of DIS —			
Five Drug Categories[a]			
$K < .40$	6–16%	1–3%	4–11%
$K \geq .40$ and $< .75$	19–50%	17–53%	8–22%
$K \geq .75$	13–34%	14–44%	25–67%

[a]Differing table entries per group are the result of K not being calculable in all instances. *See* text for discussion.

A similar examination of responses to specific questions in the Drug Abuse section of the DIS was also undertaken. For each question, a global response was elicited without regard to specific drugs. If the global response was positive, the question was repeated for a specific drug or drug classes. The results from nine questions in the drug abuse section are presented in the lower sections of Table 4. Test–retest reliability of the initial, nondrug specific questions was moderate to very high in the Anglo and Mexican origin patients interviewed in English. In contrast, κ values for the Mexican origin group interviewed in Spanish fell in the low range for seven questions and for no question did κ fall in the upper range.

When reliability of responses to five drugs or drug classes (marijuana, amphetamines, cocaine, heroin, inhalants) was assessed, a slightly different pattern emerged. As the percentages in the lowest section of Table 4 indicate, each of the three groups evidenced differing patterns of κ values. The differences between the Anglo and Mexican origin patients interviewed in English lies in the Anglo group's larger percentage of low κ values. The Mexican origin patients interviewed in Spanish had the greatest percentage of κ values falling in the high range and a moderate amount falling in the lowest range. This is a different pattern than that observed for the global questions. In general, the relative number of high, medium, and low κs was shifted downward for the Anglo and English interview groups, when compared to the responses of the global questions. The opposite was true for the Mexican origin group interviewed in Spanish. The differences may be the result of the reliabilities regarding specific drugs being based on a subset of those patients who responded to the global questions. That is, only those subjects who answered in the affirmative to the stem question were subsequently asked specific questions about drugs used and patterns of use.

The reliability of responses to questions about specific drugs tended to vary with the drug or class of drug. The reliabilities for questions concerning heroin and inhalants were uniformly skewed to the higher of the three categories for all three language/ethnic status groups. κ values for questions about marijuana, amphetamines, and cocaine were much more evenly distributed across the three categories for the three groups of patients. An example of reliability scores for five drugs or drug classes broken down by three language/ ethnic status groups is presented in Table 5. As can be seen, the pattern of reliability coefficients for marijuana, amphetamines, and cocaine is much more variable than for heroin and inhalants.

Table 5
Test–Retest Reliability Estimates for the DIS Question
"Have You Used Drugs So Much You Feel Dependent?"
in Three Ethnic/Language Groups

	Anglo	Mexican origin	
		English	Spanish
Global response	.95	.83	.20
to question	(49)	(43)	(32)
Marijuana/hashish	.66	.43	.38
	(30)	(24)	(19)
Amphetamines	.58	.92*	.36
	(29)	(12)	(9)
Cocaine	.26	.40	.80*
	(18)	(12)	(5)
Heroin	1.00	1.00	1.00
	(27)	(26)	(24)
Inhalents	.87*	.67*	1.00
	(8)	(3)	(4)

*Values are K coefficients with sample sizes in parenthesis except where denoted by an asterisk (*), indicating raw percent agreement because K could not be calculated.

Discussion

These analyses indicate several things regarding reliability and validity of the DIS. First, the instrument appears to have moderate-to-good test–retest reliability over a brief followup period for a number of diagnoses. In addition, there appears to be little systematic variation in test–retest reliability across major diagnostic categories among the ethnic-language groups compared. That is, the instrument appears to have comparable reliability when used with Anglo or Mexican origin subjects or in English or Spanish in the latter group. There was some variation across diagnostic categories, as can be expected, but none reached statistical significance. Test–retest reliability was quite high for major depression, and was also high for bipolar disorder, mania, alcohol abuse, and drug abuse. Test–retest reliability for the remaining diagnostic categories examined was considerably lower, particularly for dysthymia, phobic disorders, panic disorders, and generalized anxiety; a diagnosis of schizophrenia was only moderately reliable.

In terms of queries about specific drugs, there were differences in reliability across the three ethnic/language groups. However, the pattern observed is very difficult to interpret. On the one hand, when the drug queries examined are the initial probes concerning global drug use, the Spanish interview group had less reliable responses. On the other hand, when analyses focused on patterns of specific drug use, the reverse was observed. The straightforward explanation for these results is that the analyses of specific drug items is based on a subset of subjects. It appears that Anglos and Mexican origin patients interviewed in English were more reliable concerning global questions about drug use, but that the Spanish interview group was more reliable about specific drugs used. There is no obvious explanation of why this might be true, but clearly there appear to be possible ethnic or language effects that need to be explored further.

The other finding of note is that reports of use of heroin and inhalants were more reliable than for marijuana, amphetamines, or cocaine, across all three groups. Given the focus on cocaine use in contemporary America, these data suggest a note of caution in interpreting results of surveys that inquire about cocaine. Whether these findings hold for crack cocaine is unclear, since the DIS drug section was developed before crack cocaine had surfaced as a problem drug.

Second, the validity of the DIS, as measured by agreement between its DIS/DSM-III diagnoses and those made by clinicians using the DSM-III Checklist, was considerably less than desirable. For affective disorders, the problem is the low sensitivity of the lay-administered DIS vs clinician judgment. Clearly the clinicians judged more patients to have had a history of major depression, dysthymia, or other affective disorders than did the DIS. On the other hand, the DIS and the clinicians were in fairly good agreement for patients who did not have a history of affective disorders, i.e., specificity was reasonably good. By contrast, for all nonaffective disorders, and particularly for drug abuse, the sensitivity of the DIS was higher than its specificity. In fact, only alcohol abuse had adequate sensitivity and specificity when comparing the DIS and the clinicians. For two diagnoses (major depression and dysthymia), the results indicate that those Mexican origin patients interviewed in English by both lay interviewers and clinicians had very low diagnostic concordance. For a third diagnostic category—drug abuse—the κ values also indicate essentially no chance-corrected agreement between the DIS and clinician diagnosis when Mexican origin patients were assessed in English or in Spanish.

These results in general are congruent with those reported by other investigators concerning agreement between diagnoses generated by the lay-administered DIS and diagnoses made by clinicians. In this regard, the findings presented here strongly support the conclusions of Shrout, Spitzer, and Fleiss[4] and of Erdman et al.[31] that concordance between the DIS and clinical diagnosis is generally poor. Furthermore, this lack of agreement extends to use of Spanish-language versions of the DIS used with persons of Mexican origin. The results of our study and those of Burnam et al.,[24] indicate that concordance is as low or lower with Spanish-speaking persons of Mexican descent as with the general population, nor is this effect limited to this particular Hispanic population. The study by Canino et al.[30] also produced low concordance between lay-DIS and clinician diagnoses in Spanish among Puerto Ricans.

For example, in the three studies of Hispanic populations completed thus far, test–retest κs for alcohol abuse were .63, .48, .83, and .85. Only one study (ours) reported test–retest data for drug abuse ($\kappa = .53$ and .54). In terms of concordance between lay and clinician interviews, κs were .60, .28, .56, and .59 for alcohol, and .58, .02, and .03 for drug abuse. Clearly, the DIS does better diagnosing alcohol than drug problems.

Based on the evidence from our study, and that from other such studies of the operating characteristics of the DIS, what can be concluded about the usefulness of this particular psychiatric assessment procedure? At least two conclusions are warranted. First, there is good evidence that the DIS can provide a reasonably reliable method of generating data on psychiatric impairment, particularly in treatment populations. The evidence is less persuasive in regard to its reliability in community populations, primarily because few assessments of reliability have been carried out using subjects drawn from the general population.[27,30]

Second, the question of the validity of the DIS is unresolved. Evidence about validity of the DIS is of two types—direct and indirect. Direct evidence is available in the form of concordance between diagnoses made using the DIS and those made using other procedures, either diagnoses from medical records or diagnoses made independently by clinicians using some other method of recording and organizing information on psychiatric symptomatology. The bulk of the direct evidence, including that from this study, suggests that the DIS has low validity. As Spitzer[2] has noted, there is no gold standard in psychiatric diagnosis. Still, the standard of the scientific community vis-a-vis accuracy of diagnosis remains assessments by clinicians. Burnam et al.[24] compared lay-administered DIS and clinician diagnosis using a sample of Mexican origin outpatients and found κs ranging from .05 (dysthymia) to 0.60 (alcohol abuse), with an average of .32 for 15 diagnoses. Canino et al.[30] compared lay-administered DIS with clinician diagnoses using a sample of outpatients and community residents in Puerto Rico and reported κs ranging from .23 (obsessive-compulsive) to .71 (cognitive impairment), with a mean of .41 for 14 diagnoses. Robins et al.[19] examined chart diagnoses in relation to the DIS in a patient sample and found κs ranging from −.01 (phobia) to .40 (bipolar disorder), with an average of .22 for 10 diagnoses (presented in Erdman et al.[31] Helzer et al.[25] compared clinical diagnoses from a DSM-III Checklist to the DIS (in a sample of "cases" selected from a community sample) and found κs ranging from .12 (obsessive-compulsive disorder) to .63 (alcohol abuse/dependence), with an average of .30 (weighted; average of .40 unweighted). Anthony et al.[26] used the lay-DIS and an adapted Present State Examination administered by clinicians (PSE) in a community sample and found uniformly low κs— from −.02 (panic disorder) to .35 (alcohol abuse/dependence), with an average of .15 for eight diagnoses.

Thus far, the studies by Helzer et al.[32] and Anthony et al.[26] are the largest, most systematic attempts to assess the reliability and validity of the DIS. Data from these studies suggest that the DIS administered by lay interviewers yields different results, in some instance markedly different, than from examination by clinicians.

In her commentary on these two articles, Robins[42] identifies still another problem that involves issues of reliability and validity vis-a-vis the DIS. She notes that in the four ECA sites, which to that point had completed both waves of data collection, respondents in the second interview frequently failed to report symptoms that they reported in the first interview. Unpublished data from the ECA program (Charles E. Holzer, III, personal communication) indicate that this T_1-T_2 decay in prevalence may range from 10–20, depending upon the diagnostic category. As Robins correctly points out, psychiatric symptoms are not socially desirable, 80 few subjects should be expected to report symptoms they never had. Thus, the drop in lifetime prevalence observed in longitudinal studies probably indicates less validity at reinterview than at the initial assessment. The problem of response error in followup studies using the DIS further illustrated in a study by Pulver and Carpenter (1983). Their study had as its focus the feature of the DIS permitting estimates of lifetime prevalence of psychiatric disorders. Pulver and Carpenter[23] report that their data suggest that the DIS seriously underestimates the lifetime experience of psychotic symptoms. For example, a third of the patients with a well-documented episode of hospitalization for a psychotic illness was not identified by the DIS as ever having a history of psychotic illness. The DIS failed to elicit from 12–80% of seven specific symptom dimensions of psychotic illness. Additional evidence is provided by Schulberg and his colleagues,[28] who used the DIS in a multistage depression screening project in both primary medical and psychiatric settings. They, too, report low concordance of the DIS with diagnoses of depression by clinicians, both medical practitioners and psychiatric practitioners. For example, primary care providers diagnosed as depressed only 44% of the medical patients so diagnosed using the DIS ($9\kappa = .32$). In contrast, psychiatric providers assigned 164% more diagnoses of depression among mental patients than did the DIS ($\kappa = .10$).

Nor is the problem specific to the DIS. Bromet et al.[43] report poor test–retest reliability of the SADS over an 18-mo followup period. Only 38% of the subjects (all women) consistently reported RDC episodes of depression at both interviews. In fact, of those reporting a lifetime episode of major depression at T_1, only 48% reported a lifetime episode at T_2, a substantial decay in lifetime prevalence. Bromet et al.[43] found that, although clinical status during the 18-mo followup interval influenced reliability of SADS-RDC diagnoses, demographic, psychosocial, and interviewer characteristics did not. In general, those women who reported episodes of depression prior to T_1 and T_2 and who had not previously reported any episode, were more likely to have experienced psychiatric difficulties in the T_1–T_2 interval. Conversely, those women who reported lifetime episodes at T_1, but not at T_2, were less likely to have experienced difficulties in the T_1–T_2 interval. By way of confirmation, Aneshensel et al.[44] report finding a substantial decline in reports of lifetime episodes of depression in subsequent waves of a prospective study in Los Angeles. At T_1 and T_5, a depressive episode was described, and respondents were asked if they had ever had such an episode for a period of at least 2 wk. The overall error rate at T_5 was 24%; 86% of the error was failure of subjects at T_5 to report an episode reported at T_1. Those positive at both T_1 and T_5 comprised only 32% of those positive at either time.

What about indirect evidence concerning validity of the DIS? Robins[42] argues that there are three types of indirect evidence to suggest that the DIS is a reasonably accurate measure of psychiatric disorders:

1. The prevalence rates for various disorders are consistent across the five ECA sites and similar to those reported using the DIS in studies in West Germany, Peru, and Puerto Rico;
2. The ECA prevalence rates are consistent with those obtained by researchers in other countries using other, more comprehensive methods of ascertaining caseness;[45,46] and
3. Correlations of previously identified risk factors (gender, social class, and so on) with the DIS are in the expected directions suggesting that the DIS has construct validity.

There appears to be indirect evidence suggesting lack of validity as well. A recent commentary by Parker[47] raised questions regarding the validity of lifetime diagnoses. He examines three facets of the data on lifetime prevalence from the ECA studies—the high ratio of lifetime to 6-mo prevalence, discordance with previous estimates of lifetime morbidity, and the curvilinear assocation of lifetime prevalence with increasing age—and concludes that the weight of the evidence suggests substantial underestimates of lifetime prevalence using the DIS. Roberts[48] has examined data on Blacks and Hispanics from the ECA surveys, which also raise questions about the validity of the estimates of lifetime prevalence of depression. He notes that the lifetime rate of major depression in Los Angeles is almost twice as high for Anglos as for Hispanics, yet there is little difference in the 6-mo prevalence. Likewise, DIS surveys in Puerto Rico and in Los Angeles find little difference in the lifetime rates of major depression for Puerto Ricans and Mexican Americans, yet there is a twofold differential for Anglos. Blacks have higher rates of 6-mo prevalence than Whites, but lower rates of lifetime prevalence of major depression. The ratio between 6-mo and lifetime prevalence also seems problematic; the ratio of lifetime to 6-mo prevalence is very low, but lower yet for Blacks and Hispanics. Finally, there are dramatic differences across ECA sites, with particular references to Los Angeles. The lifetime prevalence of major depression for Anglos, Blacks, and Mexican Americans in Los Angeles is twice that found in other sites. By contrast, the 6-mo prevalence rates are much more concordant. It is difficult to imagine anything other than methodological artifact to account for true observed patterns.

Concluding Remarks

In the past decade, there has been a virtual explosion in the field of psychiatric epidemiology. The ECA studies, and the method of case ascertainment developed for these studies, the DIS, represent significant milestones during this period. Whereas the DIS in many respects represented a new approach to collecting data on psychiatric disorders in epidemiologic investigations, there have emerged serious questions about the operating characteristics of the procedure, particularly its agreement with independently derived diagnoses by clinicians. Burke[41] has summarized issues concerning research on the utility of the DIS as problems deriving from:

1. Nature of the examination;
2. Marginal cases;
3. Subject variance over time;
4. Criterion variance—assessment of inclusional items;
5. Criterion of symptoms or episodes;
6. Differential diagnosis—misallocation into specific categories; and
7. Inherent unreliability of assessments.

None of the studies conducted to date have examined any of these issues in detail, and certainly none of the studies have examined a broad subset of these issues within the same research design. In addition to Burke, at this point a number of authors[4,25,26,42] have discussed issues of reliability and validity of psychiatric assessment from the perspective of the DIS. The points raised by these researchers provide explicit guidelines for future research. In this regard, we concur in particular with Burke[41] that two types of studies are needed. The first type involves test–retest studies of reliability using both short and long followup intervals. The second type involves longitudinal studies to assess the relationship between diagnostic assessments and external criteria, such as subsequent course, response to treatment, and family history (*see also*[2]). To this is added a plea that such studies be carried out using both clinical and community samples, the latter have been notably underrepresented in studies of the operating characteristics of diagnostic procedures for psychiatric disorders.

Three other lines of investigation that may prove particularly informative should be noted: the issue of the reliability and validity of current vs lifetime diagnoses, reliability and validity in potentially problematic subgroups, such as the elderly, persons of lower socioeconomic status, and persons from nonEnglish and nonWestern cultural backgrounds; and the influence of social-psychological factors on reliability and validity of psychiatric assessments[43,44,48].

Regarding our findings on the possible effect of cultural background (language and ethnic status) on the reliability and validity of the DIS for assessing alcohol and drug use, this question clearly warrants further scrutiny, in both patient and community populations. To date, most of the information presented here on reliability and validity of substance use emanates from questionnaires rather than diagnostic interviews. Do these findings using the DIS hold for nondiagnostic procedures or, indeed, for other diagnostic interviews? Given recent studies,[49,50] a research strategy that incorporates a multitrait–multimethod approach might be particularly informative by permitting simultaneous assessment of ethnic status, language, socioeconomic status, and multiple measures of substance use derived using different data collection strategies.

Acknowledgments

This research was supported in part by grant No. MH 37294 from the National Institute of Mental Health, by grant No. DA 03948 from the National Institute of Drug Abuse, and by a grant from the Hogg Foundation for Mental Health. Robert E. Roberts was recipient of Research Scientist Development Award No. K02-MH00047 from NIMH during this research. Appreciation is expressed to Zhiying Wang, who provided assistance with analyses of the data.

References

[1] W. M. Grove, N. C. Andreasen, P. McDonald-Scott, M. B. Keller, and R. W. Shapiro (1981) Reliability studies of psychiatric diagnosis. *Arch. Gen. Psychiatry* **38**, 408–413.

[2] R. L. Spitzer (1983) Are clinicians still necessary? *Compr. Psychiatry* **24**, 399–411.

[3] M. M., Chang and T. G. Bidder (1985) Noncomparability of research results that are related psychiatric diagnosis. *Compr. Psychiatry* **26**, 195–207.

[4] P. E. Shrout, R. L. Spitzer, and J. L. Fleiss (1987) Quantification of agreement in psychiatric measurement revisited. *Arch. Gen. Psychiatry* **44**, 172–177.

[5] R. E. Roberts (1980) Reliability of the CES-D Scale in different ethnic contexts. *Psychiatry Research* **2**, 125–134.

[6]E. S. Levine and Padilla, A. M. (1980) Crossing cultures in Therapy: Pluralistic Counseling for the Hispanic. (Wadsworth, Inc., Belmont, CA).

[7]M. Ramirez, III. (1983) Psychology of the Americas: Mestizo perspective on Personality and Mental Health. (Pergamon, NY).

[8]J. L. Martinez and R. H. Mendoza, eds. (1984) *Chicano Psychology* (2nd ed.), Academic, Orlando, FL.

[9]R. de la Garza, F. Bean, C. Bonjean, R. Romo, and R. Alvarez (1985) *The Mexican American Experience: An Interdisciplinary Anthology* (University of Texas Press, Austin, Texas).

[10]R. C. Cervantes and F. G. Castro (1985) Stress, coping, and Mexican American mental health: A systematic review. *Hispanic Journal of Behavioral Science* 7(1), 1–73.

[11]W. A. Vega and M. R. Miranda, eds. (1985) Stress and Hispanic Mental Health: Relating Research to Service Delivery (DHHS Publication No. (ADM) 85–1410). US Government Printing Office, Washington, D.C.

[12]R. E. Roberts (1987) An epidemiologic perspective on the mental health of people of Mexican origin, in *Mental Health of the Mexican Origin Population of Texas: Proceedings of the Fifth Robert Lee Sutherlan Seminar* (R. Rodriquez and M. Coleman, eds.), Hogg Foundation for Mental Health. Austin, TX.

[13]R. E. Roberts and S. W. Vernon (1984) Minority status and psychological distress reexamined: The case of Mexican Americans, in (J. R. Greenley, ed.), *Research in Community and Mental Health*, vol. 4 JAI, Greenwich, CT, pp. 131–164.

[14]I. Cuellar and R. E. Roberts (1984) Psychological disorders among Chicanos, in *Chicano Psychology* (J. L. Martinez, Jr. and R. H. Mendoza eds.), 2nd ed., Orlando, FL, Academic, pp. 133–161.

[15]W. J. Lonner (1980) The search for psychological universals, in *Handbook of Cross-Cultural Psychology* (H. Triandis and W. Lambert eds.), vol. 1 Allyn and Bacon, Boston, pp. 139–159.

[16]J. W. Berry (1969) On cross-cultural comparability. *Int. J. Psychology* 4, 119–128.

[17]R. W., Brislin, W. J. Lonner, and R. M. Thorndike (1973) *Cross-Cultural Research Methods*, John Wiley, New York.

[18]L. N. Robins, J. E. Helzer, J. Croughan, and K. S. Ratcliff (1981) National Institute of Mental Health Diagnostic Interview Schedule: Its history, characteristics, and validity. *Arch. Gen. Psychiatry* 38, 381–389.

[19]L. N. Robins, J. E. Helzer, K. S. Ratcliff, and W. Sevfried (1982) Validity of the Diagnostic Interview Schedule, Version II: DSM-III diagnoses. *Psychol. Med.* 12, 855–870.

[20]W. E. Eaton and L. G. Kessler eds. (1985) Epidemiologic Field Methods in Psychiatry (Academic, Orlando, FL).

[21] V. Hesselbrock, J. Stabenau, M. Hesselbrock, P. Mirkin, and R. Meyer (1982) A comparison of two interview schedules: The Schedule for Affective Disorders and Schizophrenic-Lifetime and the NIMH Diagnostic Interview Schedule. *Arch. Gen. Psychiatry* **39,** 674–677.

[22] I. E., Hendricks, J. A. Bayton, J. I. Collins, C. B. Mathura, S. R. Macmillan, and T. A. Montgomery (1983) The NIMH Diagnostic Interview Schedule: A test of its validity in a population of black adults. *J. Natl. Med. Assoc.* **75,** 667–671.

[23] A. E. Pulver and W. T. Carpenter, Jr. (1983) Lifetime psychotic symptoms assessed with the DIS. *Schizophr. Bull.* **9,** 377–382.

[24] M. A., Burnam, M. Karno, R. L. Hough, J. Escobar, and A. B. Forsythe (1983) The Spanish diagnostic interview schedule: Reliability and comparison with clinical diagnoses. *Arch. Gen. Psychiatry* **40,** 1189–1196.

[25] J. E., Helzer, L. N. Robins, L. T., McEvoy, E. L., Spitznagel, R. K. Stoltzman, et al. (1985) A comparison of clinical and diagnostic interview schedule diagnoses. *Arch. Gen. Psychiatry* **42,** 657–666.

[26] J. C., Anthony, M. Folstein, A. J. Romanoski, M. R. Von Korff, G. R. Nestadt, et al. (1985) Comparison of the lay Diagnostic Interview Schedule and a standardized psychiatric diagnosis. *Arch. Gen. Psychiatry* **42,** 667–675.

[27] H. U. Wittchen, G. Semler, and I. vonZerssen (1985) Comparing ICD diagnoses with DSM-III and RDC using the Diagnostic Interview Schedule (Version II). *Arch. Gen. Psychiatry* **42,** 677–684.

[28] H. C. Schulberg, M. Saul, M. McClelland, M. Ganguhi, W. Christy, and R. Frank (1985) Assessing depression in primary medical and psychiatric practice. *Arch. Gen. Psychiatry* **42,** 1164–1170.

[29] J. T. Escobar, E. T. Randolph, J. Asamen, and M. Karno (1986) The NIMH-DIS in the assessment of DSM-III schizophrenia disorder. *Schizophr. Bull.* **12,** 187–194.

[30] G. J., Canino, H. R. Bird, P. E. Shrout, M. Rubio-Stipec, and M. Bravo (1987) The Spanish diagnostic interview schedule: Reliability and concordance with clinical diagnoses in Puerto Rico. *Arch. Gen. Psychiatry* **44,** 720–726.

[31] H. P. Erdman, M. H. Klein, J. H. Greist, S. M. Bass, J. K. Bires, and P. M. Machtinger (1987) A comparison of the Diagnostic Interview Schedule and clinical diagnosis. *Am. J. Psychiatry* **144,** 1477–1480.

[32] J. E., Helzer, E. L. Spitznagel, and L. McEvoy (1987) The predictive validity of lay diagnostic interview schedule diagnoses in the general population. *Arch. Gen. Psychiatry* **44,** 1069–1077.

[33] M. Karno, A. Burnam, J. I. Escobar, R. L. Hough, and W. W. Eaton (1983) Development of the Spanish Version of the National Institute of Mental Health Diagnostic Interview Schedule. *Arch. Gen. Psychiatry* **40,** 1183–1188.

[34] J. R. Landis and G. G. Koch (1977) The measurement of observer agreement for categorical data. *Biometrics* **33,** 671–679.

[35] A. Swidler (1986) Culture in action: Symbols and strategies. *Am. Sociol. Rev.* **51**, 273–286.
[36] J. Endicott and R. L. Spitzer (1978) A diagnostic interview. The schedule for affective disorders and schizophrenia. *Arch. Gen. Psychiatry* **35**, 837–844.
[37] D.Wechsler (1981) Wechsler Adult Intelligence Scale-revised. (Harcourt Brace Johanovich, NY).
[38] D. Wechsler, R. F. Green, and J. N. Martinez (1968) *Escala de Intellgencia Wechsler para Adultos.* (The Psychological Corporation, NY).
[39] S. C. Duncan and E. A. De Avila (1981) Scoring and interpretation manual for language assessment scales. San Rafael: Linguametrics Group.
[40] J. L. Fleiss (1981) *Statistical Methods for Rates and Proportions.* (John Wiley, NY).
[41] J. D. Burke (1986) Diagnostic categorization by the Diagnostic Interview Schedule (DIS): A comparison with other methods of assessment, in (J. E. Barrett and R. M. Rose, eds.), *Mental Disorders in the Community: Progress and Challenge* Guilford, NY, pp. 255–279.
[42] L. N. Robins (1985) Epidemiology: Reflections on testing the validity of psychiatric interviews. *Arch. Gen. Psychiatry* **42**, 918–924.
[43] E. Bromet, L. Dunn, M. Connell, M. Dew, and H. Schulberg (1986) Long-term reliability of diagnosing lifetime major depression in a community sample. *Arch. Gen. Psychiatry* **43**, 435–440.
[44] C. A., Aneshensel, A. L. Estrada, M. J. Hansell, and V. A. Clark (1987) Social psychological aspects of reporting behavior: Lifetime depressive episode reports. *J. Health Soc. Behav.* **28**, 232–246.
[45] T. Helgason (1964) Epidemiology of mental disorders in Iceland. *Acta Psychiatr. Scand.* 40 (supp 173), 1–258.
[46] O. Hagnell (1966) *Prospective Study of the Incidence of Mental Disorder.* Svenska. Bokforlaget., Lund, Sweden.
[47] G. Parker (1987) Are the lifetime prevalence estimates in the ECA Study accurate? *Psychol. Med.* **17**, 275–282.
[48] R. E. Roberts (1988) The epidemiology of depression in minorities, in *Research Perspectives on Depression and Suicide in Minorities* (P. Muehrer, ed.), National Institute of Mental Health, pp. 1–20.
[49] A. W. Stacy, K. F. Widaman, R. Hays, and M. R. DiMatteo (1985) Validity of self-reports of alcohol and other drug use: A multitrait-multimethod assessment. *J. Consult. Clin. Psychol.* **49**, 219–232.
[50] R. D. Hays, and G. J. Huba (1988) Reliability and validity of drug use items differing in the nature of their response options. *J. Consult Clin. Psychol.* **56**, 470–472.

Sensation Seeking, Marijuana Use, and Responses to Prevention Messages

Implications for Public Health Campaigns

Lewis Donohew, David M. Helm, Patricia Lawrence, and Milton J. Shatzer

Introduction

Research on public health campaigns has focused predominantly on use of the mass media to alter attitudes and behaviors of largely unsegmented mass audiences.[1,2] Little attention has been paid to evolving evidence about the nature of human information processing or to message response differences among individuals. Yet these two areas of research have wide-ranging implications for the design of prevention campaigns aimed at health-destructive behaviors, such as substance abuse, because it is apparent that they significantly affect audience responses to mass media messages.[3] Thus, an understanding of the effect of individual differences on message responses and of the impact of cognitive and affective processing on stimulus selection[4] can be instrumental in determining if health campaigns attract and hold the attention of target audiences for whom messages are specifically designed. Ultimately, it can determine if the campaigns succeed or fail. In this chapter, we report on an experimental study that takes these factors into account.

Individual Differences

Research on SS has found that levels of need for arousal vary across persons.[5-7] Zuckerman[8] has observed that:

> The high sensation seeker is receptive to novel stimuli; the low tends to reject them, preferring the more familiar and less complex. The high sensation seeker's optimal level of stimulation may depend on the levels set by the characteristic level of arousal produced by novel stimuli. Anything producing lower arousal levels may be boring.

Previous studies have indicated that persons with a high need for arousal tolerated, or even required, more stimulating message styles for attracting and holding their attention. For people who score high on Zuckerman's sensation-seeking scale (SSS), it has been assumed that the most likely state at any given point in time is one of *stimulus hunger,* and for those scoring low it is *stimulus satiation.* Thus, high ss most of the time would be in an *arousal-seeking* mode, and low ss would be in an *arousal-avoidance* mode.

Information Processing

This research on responses to messages drew upon an activation model of information exposure.[3] This model assumed that, under controlled processing, individuals make decisions in highly self-aware ways. Under automatic processing, behavior is somewhat routinized, overlearned through previous repetitions, and is guided by processes of which individuals are less cognizant.[9,10] A central assumption of the model involved "automatic" processing, in which individuals enter information exposure situations with the expectation of achieving or maintaining an optimal state of arousal (*see* Fig. 1). From this assumption, two propositions were deduced:

1. If the optimal level is achieved or maintained, individuals will continue exposure to the message; and
2. If the optimal level is not reached, or is exceeded, individuals will turn away from the message. Conditions under which this theory operates are:
   (a) that individuals vary in their levels of need for arousal;

Responses to Prevention Messages

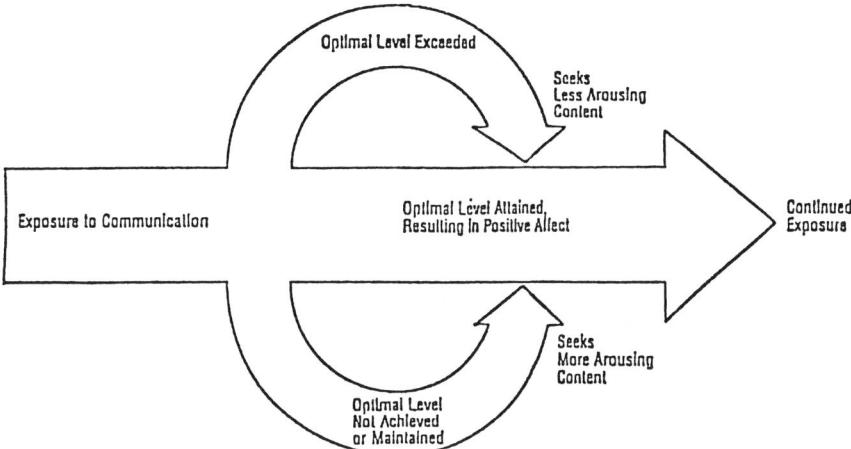

Fig. 1. An activation model of information exposure. Reprinted with permission from Lewis Donohew, Seth Finn, and William Christ (1988) "The nature of news" revisited: The roles of affect, schemas, and cognition, in *Communication, Social Cognition and Affect* (Lewis Donohew, H. Sypher, and E. T. Higgins, eds.), Erlbaum, Hillsdale, NJ, pp. 195–218.

(b) that discrepant information will generate more arousal than supportive information; and

(c) that high involvement in the topic will generate more arousal than low involvement.

Under conditions in which the topic is highly salient, however, the individual may switch to a more controlled processing state in which exposure is based on cognitive needs. As noted elsewhere, individuals may switch back and forth between responses guided primarily by arousal and those guided in controlled processing by their cognitions.[11] Although arousal needs appear to guide much of the exposure,[12–14] it has been observed that individuals "may choose to override these affective tugs for any of a number of reasons, such as desire to learn more about a topic of importance to them in which they perceive themselves to be deficient."[15]

The model was grounded in three established optimal level of arousal assumptions. First, behavioral efficiency increases as arousal increases to some optimal level and then decreases as the arousal level continues to increase.[16] Second, the more arousal potential a stimulus is perceived to have, the more attention will be paid to it.[17] Finally, up to a point, increasing attention will be accompanied by increasing pleasure, but beyond this point increasing attention will be accompanied by increasing displeasure.[18]

A test of the activation model involving differences in the arousal needs of subjects has demonstrated that persons with a high need for arousal tend to tolerate or even require stronger messages for attracting and holding their attention than do persons with a low need.[3] The findings from these studies offer a cognitive-affective alternative to the once widely accepted selective exposure hypothesis, which grew out of consistency theories based on cognition alone.

Under the activation model, decisions to avoid or continue exposure are a function of both arousal needs, of which the individual usually is only dimly aware and over which the individual has little control, and cognitive responses to the information content, where controlled processing is at work. Here, under conditions of extremely high arousal, both high sensation seekers (HSS) and low sensation seekers (LSS) are likely to avoid a message. One shortcoming of the activation model is that it is difficult to specify what is high arousal, because there is no parsimonious procedure for establishing individual arousal baselines. Thus, it is necessary to employ the probabilistic assumptions described under individual differences above.

Application to Health Campaigns

This chapter reports on an experimental study that took into account individual differences in arousal needs in the cognitive and affective processing of messages. The study addressed the message design aspect of public health campaigns by seeking to identify what types of individuals respond in what ways to what types of messages. More specifically, the study examined how teenagers respond to messages about the prevention of marijuana use. Of particular interest were the ss tendencies of the adolescents, their levels of marijuana use, and the design of the messages in terms of style and content.

Research has demonstrated that messages containing the same factual content can generate significantly different levels of attention and comprehension as a function of style.[19-23] However, these findings do not take into account individual differences in levels of need for arousal and do not cover topics directly involving the readers (such as decisions about drug use or nonuse). On topics directly pertaining to the readers or viewers of a message, increasing arousal-inducing elements of the message might be more effective

Responses to Prevention Messages 77

with one segment of the audience, but provide too much (or too little) stimulation for the other, causing those members to turn away.

The study reported here combined principal factors from two previous studies—arousal responses to message styles[19] and cognitive responses to message discrepancy-support characteristics.[3] In addition, the content of the message was about a behavior in which half of the subjects were directly involved (marijuana use), and it was concerned with a behavioral decision that the other half had confronted or were likely to confront at some time in the near future. Prior research suggested that HSS would have been more likely to prefer the narrative style message and LSS more likely to prefer the expository style. However, it was not known if, or how, direct involvement in the topic (through drug use) might confound those expectations. Thus the study was exploratory rather than predictive in nature, and relied upon the general pattern of findings to form a "nomological net" of plausible relationships,[24] rather than the testing of specific hypotheses.

In two of the groups, the combination of arousal and cognitive factors might be expected to reduce their willingness to attend to the message. HSS who use drugs might experience a level of arousal that is too high even for them as a result of their direct involvement in the matter and the discrepant information provided. On the other hand, LSS not using drugs might find the material irrelevant and thus failing to meet even their modest needs for arousal.

The other two groups (HSS nonusers and LSS users) contained more individuals whose attitudes were inconsistent with their behaviors. These groups might be expected to exercise a "cognitive override" and engage in controlled information processing. That is, HSS nonusers—those likely to be at higher risk in terms of potential marijuana use—and LSS users—whose drug use behaviors are beyond their normal levels of risk-taking as indicated by their SS profiles—might look to the messages for assistance on how to respond to the cross-pressures of their situations and prefer to continue exposure.

The following research questions were proposed:

1. Do individual differences in arousal needs and marijuana use make a difference in the way individuals respond to prevention messages about marijuana use?
2. Does the style in which the message is presented make a difference in preference for continued exposure to or comprehension of the message, or in attitude or behavioral changes toward marijuana?

3. Does the medium make a difference in exposure preferences, comprehension, attitude, or behavior change?

Method

Experimental Design

Effects of narrative and expository messages presented via print or video in a laboratory setting, were studied using a 2 × 2 × 2 × 2 analysis of variance design. Independent variables were:

1. Use of marijuana (nonuse or moderate);
2. Need for activation (high or low sensation seeking);
3. Message style (expository or narrative); and
4. Medium (print or video).

Dependent variables were:

1. Preferences for continued information exposure;
2. Skin conductance response (SCR);
3. Comprehension;
4. Attitude; and
5. Behavioral intention.

Independent Variables

Level of Marijuana Usage. A 60-item instrument based on the work of a NIDA committee on consequences of adolescent drug abuse was employed. However, the principal determinants for classifying subjects were questions involving current marijuana usage at either a low or moderate level.

Need for Activation. This variable was measured using Zuckerman's[7] (SSS), Form V. The 40-item scale* measures four factor analytically derived dimensions:

1. Thrill and adventure seeking;
2. Experience seeking;
3. Disinhibition; and
4. Boredom susceptibility.

---

*Three of the 40 items in the subscales concern drug use. The data for this study were analyzed with and without these items, and no significant differences in results were observed. The version reported here contains all the items in the original scale.

With the exception of the boredom susceptibility dimension, which has a reliability of .56, reliabilities of the component sections range from .68 to .88.

Messages. Experimental messages were based on the NIDA pamphlet, "For Kids Only: What You Should Know About Marijuana." Scripts of approximately the same length were written representing expository and narrative styles, the latter style having generated greater arousal in previous studies.[3]

Narrative messages presented the factual information in a more dramatic form without altering its fundamental information content. For the expository message, text taken directly from the pamphlet was used. The text was rewritten for the narrative message, presenting the factual information in a more active form but without altering its fundamental information content. For example, when presenting facts about the effects of marijuana use on one's driving ability, the expository text stated:

> Driving experiments show that marijuana affects a wide range of skills needed for safe driving—thinking and reflexes are slowed, making it hard for drivers to respond to sudden, unexpected events. Also, a driver's ability to stay in the lane through curves, to brake quickly, and to maintain speed and the proper distance between cars is affected. Research shows that these skills are impaired for at least 4–6 hours after smoking a single marijuana cigarette.

The narrative message reads:

> Did you know that just one joint reduces your coordination skills for at least four to six hours? If you drive a car, you'll have trouble staying in your lane through curves. Braking quickly will be a problem. You'll also have trouble maintaining the proper speed and the right distance from other cars.

Color illustrations taken from the NIDA pamphlet were used in both the video and the print conditions. Videotapes were narrated off-camera by a professional announcer. Bound booklets were prepared for the print condition.

Media. For the print condition, messages were presented in pamphlet form. For the TV condition, subjects watched a videotaped version of the message.

Dependent Variables

Information Exposure Preferences. In both media conditions, the prevention message was interrupted by a message that read, "STOP. Please open the Yellow Booklet and follow directions." Preference for continued exposure to the message was measured on a seven-point scale ranging from "yes" to "no." Subjects were asked to circle one of the numbers near the word that described their response to the question, "Would you like to continue with this message?" The procedure was designed to meet criticisms of selective exposure research in which subjects merely had been asked to indicate what they would watch or read from lists of topics.

Arousal. Skin conductance response (SCR) measured autonomic activity as an indicator of activation and arousal in response to an external stimulus.[25] The computation of SCR scores for use in data analysis involved the average of differences between tonic and phasic changes sampled at intervals of one-fifth of a second, following a procedure recommended by Venables and Christie.[26]*

Comprehension. Comprehension was measured by a multiple-choice questionnaire which included an assessment of prior knowledge gained from exposure to the message. The test was based on measurement tools devised by Graesser et al.[20] and Thorndyke.[23] Questions measured what reading theorists refer to as active knowledge (that involving actions, events, methods, plans, goals, reasons, and processes) and static knowledge (that involving actors, objects, locations, times, quantities, and attributes).

Attitude and Behavioral Intention. Attitude was measured by a semantic differential scale using four sets of bipolar adjectives. A similar measure with one set of bipolar adjectives representing the estimated probability of smoking marijuana in the next month was employed to indicate behavioral intention.** Each individual's attitude score was obtained by summing across

---

*In the procedure used here, subjects were fitted with silver-silver chloride electrodes on the palm of one hand, and a small amount of electricity involving a constant voltage circuit was run across the palm before and during exposure to stimulus materials. Changes in SCR were recorded using a Beckman R411 Dynograph Recorder and digitized through use of an IBM/AT, a Data Acquisition and Control Adapter (digitizer), and a LabTech Notebook software package, which acted as the executive driver for the digitizer. SCR was measured in microsiemens, a unit of analysis that represents the reciprocal of microohms of skin resistance.

**The bipolar adjectives used in the attitude index represent four of the most commonly used adjectives that represent the evaluative (attitude) dimension of the scale.[26,27] Loadings of these adjectives on the evaluative factor consistently have been reported at .79 or higher (For example, see.[27])

the four seven-point scales and averaging. Changes in attitude and behavioral intention were determined by using difference scores from before and after administrations of the items during the experimental procedure.

Sample

Subjects for the study were selected on the basis of responses to a survey conducted among 906 persons of high school age in a city of about 200,000 population. The survey contained selected demographic indicators, Zuckerman's (1978) SSS, Form V, and a NIDA instrument on drug use behaviors and attitudes. Subjects for the laboratory study were selected on the basis of their responses to the questionnaires.

In preparation for administering the screening protocols, the instruments were explained, and respondents were assured that responses would be anonymous. Participants were administered drug use and need for activation instruments. Subjects were divided into nonuser and moderate user groups and then further subdivided at the median on need for activation scores. This produced four subject pools:

1. Nonuser LSS;
2. Nonuser HSS;
3. Moderate user LSS; and
4. Moderate user HSS.

Four sets of 10 male and 10 female subjects were randomly selected from each of the four pools and assigned to each of the two message conditions and each of the two media conditions. Each cell included approximately equal distributions of ages. About 10% of the subjects in each cell were black. No significant differences were found in responses by sex, age, or ethnic group on drug use.

Procedure

A total of 342 subjects meeting selection criteria participated in the experimental study, conducted at the university's communication research laboratory. Each subject was paid $10, and transportation was provided when needed. Subjects were brought into the laboratory in groups of six to eight and were told that the study concerned evaluation of drug abuse prevention messages. No effort was made to group subjects arbitrarily according to the experimental design. Instead, those in the video condition and those in the print condition were scheduled according to the message style randomly assigned to them. While in the laboratory, each subject was seated at a carrel partitioned for privacy. Subjects were observable to the researchers through a one-way curtained mirror.

Results

It is clear from this study that individual differences in need for sensation and in prior drug use play a major role in responses to prevention messages about drug use, both in who is likely to attend to prevention messages in a public campaign and in the effects these messages have on personal attitudes and behavioral intentions. Levels of sensation seeking were significantly involved in interactions or as main effects in analyses across four of the five dependent measures and approached significance on the fifth. Message style was involved in four of the measures and drug use in three.

The study also indicated that, not only the message style, but also the types of media in which messages will be presented should be taken into account in designing prevention campaigns involving health behaviors. Although each individual was exposed briefly (approx 3–5 min) to only one message, distinct message effects nonetheless emerged.

Exposure Preferences

In preference for exposure, significant interactions of sensation seeking by marijuana use [$F(1, 322) = 5.78; p < .02$] and message style by medium [$F(1, 322) = 6.16; p = .01$] were found (Figs. 2 and 3).

Subjects showing the greatest preference for the message were those for whom it was perhaps most relevant to their behavior: LSS users ($M = 5.48$) and HSS nonusers ($M = 5.28$), the two groups expressing more divided attitudes on drug use. The latter group might include the greatest at-risk subjects because of their SS needs.

LSS nonusers, those for whom the message was least relevant and who on the basis of both national and local statistics were least likely to use the drug, indicated the lowest preferences to continue with the message ($M = 4.97$). At the other end of the continuum, HSS users, those for whom the message was the most redundant with their existing level of knowledge and most discrepant with existing attitudes, also indicated a lower preference for the message ($M = 4.80$).

These interactions remain even when adjustments are made for covariance effects of prior attitude toward use of marijuana [$F(1, 322) = 6.62;$

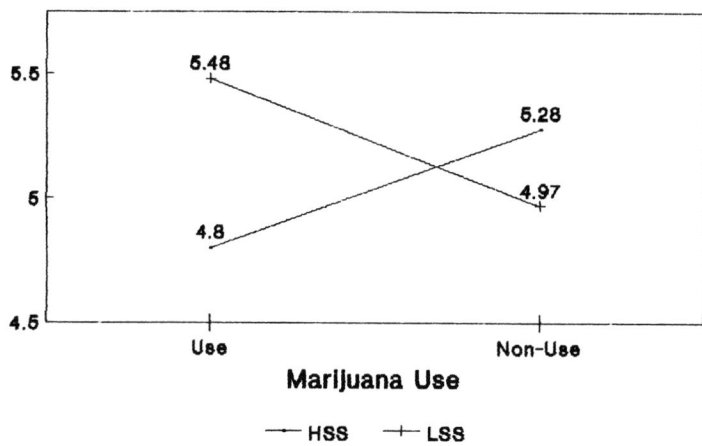

p=.017

Fig. 2. Interaction of use and ss on preference for continued exposure.

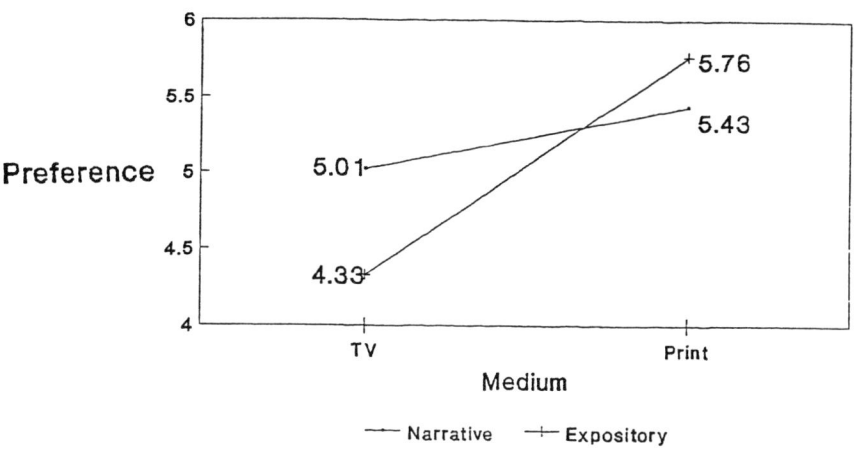

p=.014

Fig. 3. Interaction of message style and medium on preference for continued exposure.

$p = .01$]. Although the interaction between drug use and SS is not substantially affected when means are adjusted for prior attitude as a covariate, attitude nonetheless appears to play a role in message preferences.

The two cells in which preference to continue with the message was lowest—HSS users and LSS nonusers—also were those with the highest

Table 1
Drug Use Attitudes and Marijuana Use

	Premessage attitude		Postmessage attitude	
	Pro-use	Anti-use	Pro-use	Anti-use
LSS nonusers	3.6% (3)*	96.4% (80)	1.2% (1)	98.8% (82)
LSS users	67.6% (50)	32.4% (24)	48.6% (36)	51.4% (38)
HSS nonusers	20.7% (19)	79.3% (73)	8.7% (8)	91.3% (84)
HSS users	83.5% (66)	16.5% (13)	67.1% (53)	32.9% (26)

*Actual numbers reported in parentheses.

premessage percentages of attitude responses in a single direction. As shown in Table 1, 83.5% of HSS users held a promarijuana-use attitude and 96.4% of LSS nonusers reported an antimarijuana-use attitude. Thus, under conditions of certainty, the messages were least likely to hold attention.

Under conditions of doubt, however, this preference to continue was more likely. Among LSS users, 32.4% held attitudes counter to their behaviors as opposed to 16.5% of HSS users. In the group facing the higher risk of becoming users, i.e., the HSS nonusers, 20.7% indicated a favorable attitude toward use of marijuana as opposed to only 3.6% of LSS nonusers. Thus, under conditions in which there was conflict between attitudes and behaviors, preferences for continued exposure to the messages were highest, and it is those people who are more likely to be reached by prevention messages.

Which message is most likely to hold attention? As indicated in the message style by medium interaction, this depends on which medium delivers the message. In the print condition, the expository style of presentation generated the higher preference ($M = 5.76$) for message continuation. In the video condition, the narrative style was more preferred ($M = 5.01$).

Skin Conductance

With skin conductance as the dependent measure, a three-way interaction involving use, message style, and medium was observed [$F(1, 316) = 9.3; p = .002$]. This interaction was partitioned into two two-way tables. When the medium is video (Fig. 4), it is apparent that narrative style

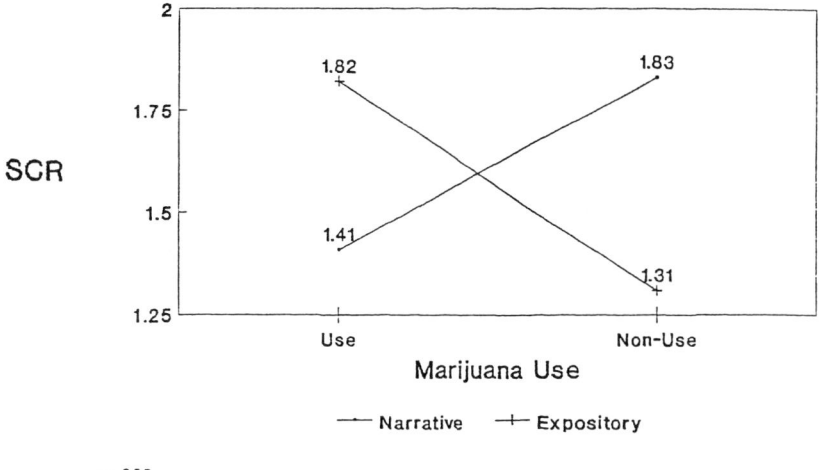

Fig. 4. Interaction of use and message style (via video) on SCR.

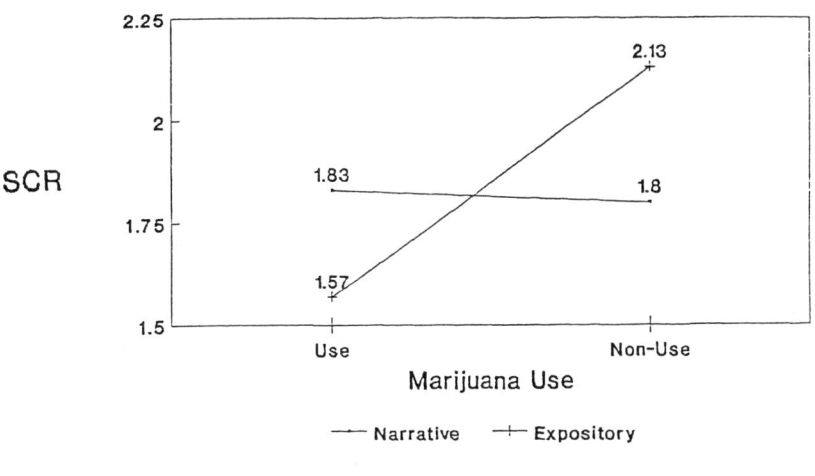

Fig. 5. Interaction of use and message style (via print) on SCR.

generates more arousal among nonusers ($M = 1.83$) and expository style more arousal among users ($M = 1.82$). When the medium is print, however (Fig. 5), the expository style generates more arousal with nonusers ($M = 2.13$) and the narrative style generates more arousal among users ($M = 1.83$).

A main effect of sensation seeking approached significance [F (1, 316) = 3.46; p = .064], with HSS showing higher SCRs (M = 1.83) than LSS (M = 1.59).

Comprehension

With message comprehension as the dependent variable and prior knowledge as a covariate, both SS and message style emerged as significant main effects. In the SS main effect [F (1, 302) = 5.77; p .02], HSS subjects had somewhat greater comprehension of the message (M = 9.68) than LSS subjects (M = 9.23). Among messages [F (1, 302) = 10.46; p = .001], those presented in a narrative style were better understood (M = 9.76) than those presented in an expository style (M = 9.15). There were no differences in comprehension level by medium.

Attitudes

Effects on attitudes were evaluated in two ways: first through an assessment of factors related to attitudes prior to presentation of the message, and then by adding a repeated measures factor (pre- vs postmessage attitude) into the design.

The initial analysis indicated significant main effects of use [F (1, 312) = 552; p .01] and SS [F (1, 312) = 42.2; p .01]. As would be expected, users were considerably more favorable (M = 2.01). It was also found that HSS were more favorable (3.82) than LSS (3.02).

In the repeated-measures analysis, the new variable of attitude change was found to interact with use [F (1, 312) = 3.94; p = .048]. As indicated in Fig. 6, both users and nonusers reported less favorable attitudes toward marijuana following exposure to the message. Users (M = 4.82) showed a greater drop (M = 4.21) than nonusers (from M = 2.01 to M = 1.69), although the small change in the latter may be a function of a ceiling effect. There was little room for nonusers to move.

Although these results may reflect a response to the message that is only temporary, they tend to be consistent with message style preferences. An indication of the validity of these findings is that changes among both users and nonusers were in a direction of reduced support for marijuana use.

Behavioral Intention

Behavioral intention was evaluated in the same manner as attitudes: first by analysis of factors related to premessage attitudes and then through introduction of a pre- vs postmessage behavioral intentions factor. As in the

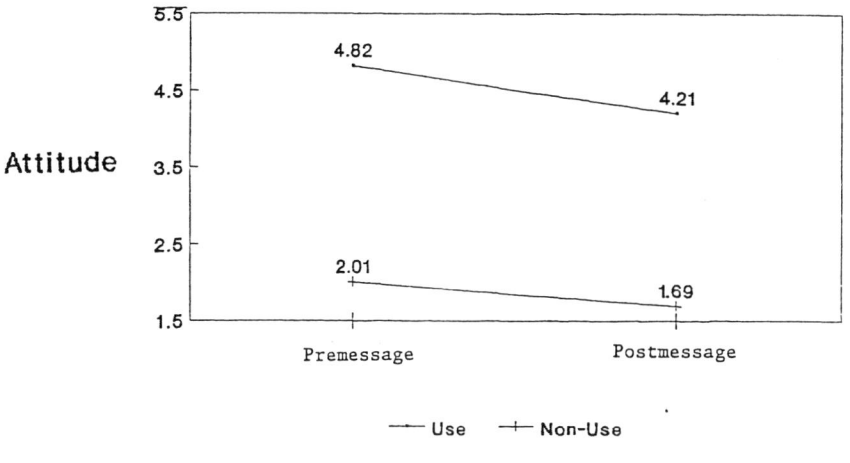

p=.048

Fig. 6. Interaction of use and attitude, pre- and post-message exposure.

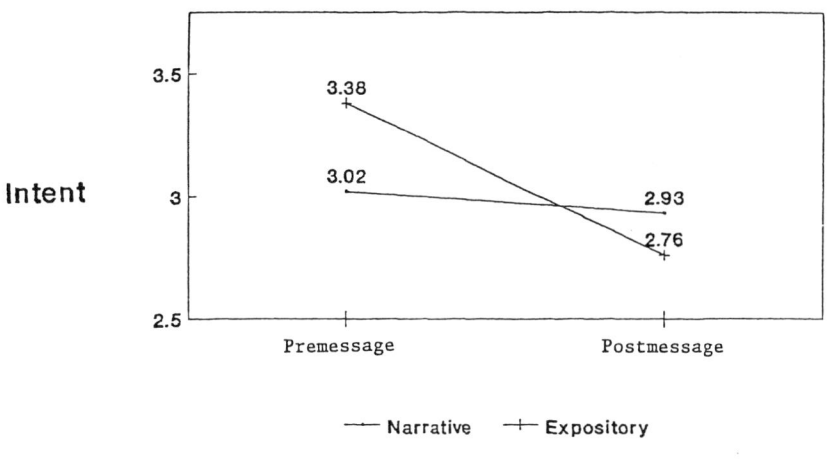

p=.009

Fig. 7. Interaction of use and behavioral intention, pre- and post-message exposure.

previous section, main effects of use [$F(1, 323) = 529; p$ .01] and sensation seeking [$F(1, 323) = 25.2; p$ .01] emerged. Again as would be expected, users ($M = 4.94$) expressed substantially greater intentions to use marijuana in the next 30 d than did nonusers ($M = 1.45$). HSS ($M = 3.55$) also expressed greater intentions than LSS ($M = 2.84$).

In the repeated measures analysis, a message style by intent change interaction was observed [F (1, 323) = 6.89; p .01] (see Fig. 7). Here, substantial changes occurred between premessage (M = 3.38) and postmessage (M = 2.76) responses to expository messages. There was very little change from premessage (M = 3.02) to postmessage (M = 2.93) responses to narrative messages.

A note of caution is in order here, however, considering that a single televised or printed message was presented only once in each of these conditions, unaccompanied by repetitions and other elements found to be important in public health campaigns, changes in behavioral intentions between prior intentions and postmessage intentions were not expected and perhaps should be considered unstable.

Discussion

Three principal research questions were posed by this chapter:

1. Do individual differences in SS and marijuana use affect the way high school students respond to antimarijuana messages;
2. Does the message style—expository or narrative—make a difference in preference for continued exposure to or comprehension of those styles of messages; and
3. Does the medium—print or video—account for differences in preferences for continued exposure to communication?

These are reviewed below.

In response to the first question, both SS and drug use affected responses. On preferences for continued exposure they interacted, with HSS nonusers and LSS users preferring continued exposure significantly more than HSS users and LSS nonusers.

In the beginning of this chapter, empirical support was cited for the proposition that persons with higher needs for sensation will tend to seek stronger sources of stimulation—including drugs—and those with lower needs will tend to seek weaker sources. In such a situation, it is plausible that the HSS nonuser is in a position of greater risk to become a marijuana user than the LSS nonuser and is more likely to be in a state of conflict about marijuana use. Similarly, the LSS user is likely to be experiencing conflict over engaging in a behavior that involves an uncharacteristic level of risk-taking. Thus, the finding in this study that the two groups do, indeed, contain a substantial number of subjects for whom their marijuana use or nonuse is counterattitudinal lends support to the general expectations of this study.

Responses to marijuana prevention messages also are consistent with these expectations. In the preference for continued exposure portion of this study, one of the findings was a classic crossover interaction between SS and use, with LSS users and HSS nonusers preferring to expose themselves to the messages. Overall, HSS comprehended the messages better than LSS and experienced greater arousal. On both attitudes and behavioral intentions, premessage positions were strongly related to SS and drug use, but attitudes became less favorable among users following exposure to the message.

In response to questions two and three, except on comprehension, message styles had different effects in different media. When presented by video, narrative styles generated greater preferences for continued exposure and greater arousal responses (SCRs) among nonusers, with expository messages generating greater arousal among users. When presented in print, expository messages elicited greater preferences for continued exposure and greater arousal responses among nonusers, with narrative messages generating more arousal among users. Narrative styles were comprehended better in both print and video conditions. It is something of a surprise that the expository messages bring about more change in behavioral intentions.

Implications for Drug Abuse Prevention Campaigns

These results take on more meaning when considered in the context of a drug abuse prevention campaign employing the mass media. The findings are particularly pertinent when the objective of the mass media portion of the campaign is to bring audiences into situations where interpersonal contact can be initiated. This latter might involve, for example, motivating audiences to call a hotline for further information or to take part in a workshop.

Pragmatically, on the first basic hurdle of maintaining attention, as represented in this instance by the measure of preference, the prevention messages reached a prime target audience. That is, those presumed to be most vulnerable to using marijuana (HSS nonusers) and those whose behaviors were (for many) counterattitudinal (LSS nonusers), are prime prospects for conversion to nonusers. Among LSS nonusers, the prevention messages were largely redundant, given the low sensation seeking nonusers' strong antiuse attitudes, and would have been reinforcing, at best. Thus, in a public health campaign employing these messages and these media, only the HSS users would have been left to be reached. Although, overall, HSS users showed the lowest for continuing exposure to the messages, their indicated choices were messages presented in a narrative style in both the print and video conditions. Further study is needed on ways to reach this group. New messages developed on the basis of formative research with HSS and LSS are currently being tested, and the preliminary results are excellent.

Unlike experimental studies, in actual public campaigns attainment of each stage is a prerequisite for the next. Only those who have paid attention to the messages and then understood them will be affected, regardless of the persuasive qualities of the messages. Thus, this study has its greatest implications for the two prime target groups described earlier. In a public campaign using the messages and media employed in this experiment, these are the persons who would be most likely to expose themselves often enough to campaign appeals to be affected by them. Although continued reinforcement is desirable, the approach most likely to yield results would be to target those already in a state of conflict—seeking to reinforce those most at risk and to convert those most likely to reduce or stop marijuana use.

As noted above, what types of messages will work best with these target groups was not clearly determined. The narrative style of messages generated greater preferences in the video condition and greater comprehension in both print and video conditions. However, expository messages brought about greater preferences for continued exposure in the print condition.

Before theories of information processing can be adapted to develop a predictive theory of drug abuse prevention that permits design of better-targeted interventions, more must be known about the relationships among the various motivating forces. For example, if need for sensation is such a powerful force for drug abuse—for which there is mounting evidence—how does one account for the demonstrated effects of environmental forces? One of the most consistent findings in the substance use literature is the effect of peer influence. It is plausible that individuals with high SS needs will tend to have similar interests and be members of the same peer group. It also is plausible that both social and biological forces are operating in a two-way causal fashion, in effect "causing" each other in a reinforcing spiral. A longitudinal study has just been indicated to examine interactions of both biological and behavioral antecedents of drug use over time.

On the basis of what is known at this point from the studies reported here and from the work of others, it appears that individuals with high needs for sensation are very likely to experiment with drugs and some of them will eventually become drug abusers—unless external sources of influence, such as peer group, family, religious, or others, intervene to influence them to abstain or divert their attention to other sources of stimulation. These individuals are likely to require not only effective messages, but also community or school-based programs involving activities offering exciting prosocial alternatives to drug use that meet their needs for sensation. As a corollary, it also appears likely that individuals with lower needs for sensation are unlikely to become drug users unless they are pressured into doing so by peers or other social forces. Such individuals may need only occasional moderate reinforcement from messages offered through the mass media, peers, or both.

It is necessary to target messages according to the subject's sensation seeking level and to more precisely determine the types of messages that are effective at various levels. A two-pronged approach employing both affect and cognition presently is being studied, with sensation value of messages being manipulated through use of scene changes, pace, music, and movement. Further research also is needed on the types of appeals or programs of activities that high-risk subjects might find to be satisfying prosocial alternatives to drug abuse.

Acknowledgment

This research was carried out under Grant No. DA03462 from the National Institute on Drug Abuse to the University of Kentucky and Lewis Donohew, principal investigator.

References

[1] B. Flay, D. DiTecco, and R. Schlegel (1980) Mass media in health promotion: An analysis using an extended information-processing model. *Health Educ. Q.* 7, 127–147.

[2] B. Flay (1986) Mass media and smoking cessation. Paper presented at the annual meeting of the International Communication Association, Chicago, IL.

[3] L. Donohew, P. Palmgreen, and J. Duncan (1980) An activation model of information exposure. *Communication Monographs* 47, 295–303.

[4] J. Bryant and D. Zillmann (1984) Using television to alleviate boredom and stress: Selective exposure as a function of induced excitational states. *Journal of Broadcasting* 28, 1–20.

[5] P. Pearson (1970) Relationships between global and specified measures of novelty-seeking. *J. Consult. Clin. Psychol.* 37, 23–30.

[6] P. Pearson (1971) Differential relationships of four forms of novelty experiencing. *J. Consult. Clin. Psychol.* 37, 323–330.

[7]M. Zuckerman (1978) Biological bases of sensation seeking, impulsivity and anxiety (Erlbaum, Hillsdale, NJ).

[8]M. Zuckerman (1988) Behavior and biology: Research on sensation seeking and reactions to the media, *Communication, Social Cognition, and Affect* (L. Donohew, H. Sypher, and T. Higgins, eds.), Erlbaum, Hillsdale, NJ, pp. 173–194.

[9]E. Langer (1980) Rethinking the role of thought in social interaction, in *New Directions in Attribution Research* (H. Harvey, W. Ickes, R. Kidd, eds.), vol 2, Erlbaum, Hillsdale, NJ, pp. 35–38.

[10]R. Schank and R. Abelson (1977) *Scripts, Plans, Goals, and Understanding: An Inquiry into Human Knowledge Structures.* Erlbaum, Hillsdale, NJ.

[11]J. Franklin, L. Donohew, V. Dhoundiyal, and P. Cook (1988) Attention and our ancient past: The scaly thumb of the reptile. *American Behavioral Scientist* 31, 312–326.

[12]S. Finn (1983) An information theory approach to reader enjoyment of print journalism. *Dissertation Abstracts International* 43, 2481A–24482A.

[13]S. Finn (1984) Unpredictability as a correlate of reader enjoyment of news articles. *Journalism Quarterly* 62, 9334–9345.

[14]S. Finn (1984) Information-theoretic measures of reader enjoyment. *Written Communication* 2, 358–376.

[15]L. Donohew, S. Finn, and W. Christ (1988) "The nature of news" revisited: The roles of affect, schemas, and cognition, in *Communication, Social Cognition, and Affect* (L. Donohew, H. Sypher, and T. Higgins, eds.), Erlbaum, Hillsdale, NJ, pp.195–218.

[16]J. Cacioppo and R. Petty (1983) Foundations of social psychophysiology, in *Social Psychophysiology: A Sourcebook* (J. Cacioppo, R. Petty, eds.), Guilford, NY, pp. 3–36.

[17]C. Martindale (1981) *Cognition and Consciousness.* Homewood, (Dorsey, IL).

[18]D. Berlyne (1971) *Aesthetics and Psychobiology.* Appleton-Century-Crofts, NY.

[19]L. Donohew (1981) Arousal and effective responses to writing styles. *Journal of Applied Communication Research* 9, 109–119.

[20]A. Graesser, M. Higginbotham, S. E. Robertson, and W. Smith (1978) A natural inquiry into the National Enquirer: Self-induced vs task-induced reading comprehension. *Discourse Processes* 1, 355–372.

[21]G. Green (1979) Organization, goals, and comprehensibility in narratives: Newswriting—a case study (Technical Report No. 132). Center for the Study of Reading. University of Illinois, Urbana, IL.

[22]G. Rarick (1967) Field experiments in newspaper item readership. University of Oregon, School of Journalism, Eugene, OR.

[23]P. Thorndyke (1979) Knowledge acquisition from newspaper stories. *Discourse Processes* 2, 95–112.

[24]L. J. Cronbach and P. E. Meehl (1955) Construct validity in psychological tests. *Psychol. Bull.* **52,** 281–302.

[25]R. Petty and J. Cacioppo (1983) The role of bodily responses in attitude measurement and change, in *Social Psychophysiology: A Sourcebook* (J. Cacioppo and R. Petty, eds.), Guilford, NY, pp. 51–101.

[26]P. Venables and M.Christie (1980) Electrodermal activity, in *Techniques in Psychophysiology* (I. Martin and P. Venables, eds.), Wiley, NY, pp. 4–67.

[27]S. Fisher and R. Botto, (eds.) Marijuana attitude scale, in *Drug Abuse Instrument Handbook* (A. Nehemkis, M. A. Macari, D. J. Lettieri, eds.), National Institute on Drug Abuse, undated, Rockville, MD, pp. 234, 272.

[28]C. Osgood, G. Suci, and P. Tannenbaum (1957) *The measurement of meaning.* University of Illinois Press, Urbana, IL.

Evaluation of Girls Clubs of America's Friendly PEERsuasion Program™

Monitoring Program Implementation

Marcia R. Chaiken

Prologue

Thirteen-year-old Kamameesha's eager voice rang out and joined the chorus of the other girls repeating, "Yes ma'am! I did! I did!" Her enthusiastic response brought her from a sitting position on the floor of the school room to her knees.

"That's wonderful!," a young woman replied, her warm smile directed at each of the enthusiastic adolescent girls seated on the floor with her. "Please tell us, Kamameesh. How did you use the refusal skills we practiced last week?"

Kamameesha smiled and then looked self-conscious and serious as she sank back and sat on her heels. "My boyfriend wanted me to drink beer," she said, her eyes fixed on the young woman's face, "but I said, uh-uh." Her head shook vigorously from side to side.

"Good for you, Kamameesha! Did you identify the problem?" the young woman urged.

"Yes, ma'am, I told him we're not supposed to drink and that drinking is no good for us."

"That's right, Kamameesha," the woman smiled and then turned to the other girls. "Kamameesha identified the problem." The other girls nodded and Kamameesha proudly smiled. "And how about the consequences, Kamameesha? Did you talk about the consequences?" the young woman continued in a soft, but compelling voice.

Kamameesha smiled even more proudly, "Yes, ma'am. I told him I was in big trouble if my grandmother found out."

"Wonderful, Kamameesha. And then what happened?" prompted the young woman.

Kamameesha frowned and put her hands on her hips. "I did everything you told us, ma'am. I said uh-uh, it's wrong, it's trouble, and he kept saying to drink and I kept saying uh-uh, and so I punched him real hard in the stomach."

The other girls looked delighted. The young woman looked less than delighted. "You really tried hard, didn't you, Kamameesha," she said approvingly, "but do you think there was something else you could have done, something you could do next time other than hit him?"

Kamameesha looked stern and shook her head no. "No ma'am, he's my boyfriend. When he wants something he just won't listen to me and I just have to hit him."

Kamameesha is one of 127 girls who participated in a federally funded experimental drug abuse prevention program provided by Girls Club Inc. of Birmingham staff in the fall of 1988 and the spring of 1989.

Introduction

Faced with growing public concern about substance abuse among US youth, in 1986 Congress allocated funds through the Office for Substance Abuse Prevention for increasing the numbers of effective prevention programs. The Girls Clubs of America Inc. received a grant for developing and evaluating a prevention program targeting youngsters who are at high risk for using drugs. The program is based on the combination of two prototypical programs previously implemented at the Girls Club in Arlington, Texas, for preventing alcohol and drug abuse. The curriculum was modified to prevent the initial use of a wide range of substances; it also was redesigned to be more relevant for girls of color. The new program, Friendly PEERsuasion was implemented by Girls Clubs' staff in Arlington and four other sites: Birmingham, Alabama; Pinellas County, Florida; Rapid City, South Dakota; and Worcester, Massachusetts.

The program essentially consists of three basic components:

- Outreach to early adolescent girls at high risk for substance abuse;
- Training high-risk girls to provide substance abuse prevention activities to younger children; and
- Providing an opportunity for girls who have received training (PEERsuaders) to plan and lead substance abuse prevention activities for younger children (PEERsuadeMes).

Underlying Friendly PEERsuasion is the theory that girls who are prepared to teach other children not to use substances would be less at risk of using these substances themselves. More particularly, through a process of "anticipatory socialization" (seeing themselves as future leaders), the girls trained by Girls Clubs staff to be PEERsuaders would be more likely to identify with the values and norms expressed by the staff than girls who had not undergone the training. As in all Girls Clubs programs, the fundamental purpose is to build girls' capacity to become adults who are responsible, confident, economically independent, and personally fulfilled.

The more specific goals were to increase the probability of the girls' spending time outside the program context with youngsters who were not abusing substances and, over time, to decrease the probability of the girls' participating in substance abuse.

The program primarily consisted of 14 biweekly sessions, approximately one hour long, of PEERsuader training for 6th, 7th, and 8th grade girls. During the 14 sessions, the girls carried out activities designed to improve their leadership and communication skills, heighten their awareness of choices they are making and their consequences for the future, provide them with realistic methods and resources for resisting peer pressure and dealing with stress, and teach them about physical, social and psychological effects of substance abuse (including smoking, drinking, and the use of over-the-counter, prescribed, and illicit drugs).

To achieve these ends, the curriculum was designed to focus on one specific objective each session, and to build on the skills and information as the program progressed from earlier sessions to later sessions. For example, the first sessions focused on building communication skills. Later, these skills were drawn on as the girls carried out role-playing and other activities requiring verbal articulation.

To design the curriculum activities, the staff drew on their extensive knowledge of the likes and dislikes of adolescent girls. For example, none of the activities required sitting still for long periods of time, many of the activities involved working together in small groups, tasks requiring motor coordination were relatively easy for the girls to perform yet not "babyish," and many activities provided an opportunity for giggles. Although all activities were heuristic devices, the girls thought of them as games or arts and crafts; however, each game or craft was integrated with or followed by a discussion of what could be learned.

For example, in the session on media pressure, the girls created a large collage of magazine advertisements of people smoking and drinking. As they cut and pasted the pictures, they discussed the intent of the advertisers in presenting the picture. "What do the advertisers want you to think from that picture?" the leader asked one girl.

"They want you to think you have to drink to have fun," was the immediate response.

"You're so right," the leader said. "That is what they want you to think! But do you think that's so? Do you have to drink to have fun?"

"No! You don't have to drink to have fun!" the girl replied indignantly. "We're having fun right now."

At the end of the 14 sessions, the girls graduated as PEERsuaders. Graduates met for approximately five hours to plan activities for teaching younger children not to abuse substances; these were most often variations on activities they had carried out in PEERsuader training that emphasized communications, stress management, peer pressure, and effects of harmful substances. The PEERsuaders, in teams of two or three, led small groups of younger children through the activities they had planned in sessions lasting approximately 30 minutes. After the teams had finished teaching, the adult leaders debriefed the girls about their teaching experiences.

This report provides information about the evaluation of the implementation of the PEERsuader training program. The methods used to evaluate the program are described and the results of evaluation in one site are provided. More specifically, the report addresses the following issues:

- How was the program implemented, and was it implemented as designed?
- Were girls at high risk of using drugs involved in the program?
- Did the girls like the program?
- Where there any indications that the girls learned from the program?

The Challenge of Program Evaluation

One of the basic challenges of program evaluation is to measure program input objectively, as well as outcome and impact. To know whether or not a program "worked," one must first know whether or not the program was implemented as designed and whether it reached the population for whom it was designed. A fundamental obstacle to measuring program input is the reluctance of program providers to divert resources needed for implementing the program to activities required for systematic evaluation. Another common barrier is the difficulty program staff have in articulating in clear terms what activities are to be involved in the program; for example, the generic term "counseling" may be used and encompass a host of interactions.

Typically, if program implementation is measured at all objectively, it is measured in terms of duration (the length of time participants were in the program), intensity (the frequency of participation), and broad characteristics of participants (for example, sex, age, and race). More commonly, subjective variables are used to assess program delivery; for example, occasional on-site observation by supervisory staff is used to monitor and evaluate program activities.

The Girls Clubs of America's Friendly PEERsuasion Program presented an excellent opportunity for attempting to meet the challenge of designing more objective measures of program input. The Office for Substance Abuse Prevention provided needed resources for implementing the substance abuse prevention program in five sites and evaluating the program in one site. Girls Clubs of America includes both research and program directors who have been involved in carefully designed evaluations of other programs, and who were sincerely interested in systematic monitoring and evaluation of Friendly PEERsuasion. Program staff have long-term experience in designing detailed curricula and training local staff to carry out all details of curricula. Also, one of the criteria used to select the sites to implement the program initially was willingness on the part of the local staff to cooperate with the evaluation.

The primary evaluation site was Birmingham, Alabama. Birmingham was selected because of the relatively large numbers of potentially "high-risk" girls they were able to recruit for the program ($N = 127$). (The girls were recruited in two schools in areas where knowledgeable practitioners indicated that drug abuse and sales were serious problems.) Although just Birmingham information is presented in this report, data were collected in three other sites as well; funds from the William T. Grant Foundation will allow analysis of data from the other sites in the near future.

In the following sections, the implementation of the program in Birmingham is described on the bases of on-site observations conducted during the fall of 1988. The system for monitoring program implementation on an ongoing basis in all sites is then discussed, and the data collected in Birmingham using this system are presented. Finally, the next steps for program implementation and evaluation are discussed.

The Organizational Context of the Program in Birmingham

Girls Club Inc. of Birmingham celebrated its 50th anniversary in 1988. Originally located in a single building used as a safe place away from home for working girls, at the time of its anniversary celebration, the Girls Club was operating from three different locations in the city. Until relatively recently, girls came to the Clubs for programs. The Clubs' Directors and staff were concerned that girls from some economically depressed areas in the city were not coming to the Clubs because of transportation problems and because their parents were not taking the initiative to enroll them in programs. In 1986, an Outreach Program was organized to serve these girls. Friendly PEERsuasion became one of the outreach programs.

All Club programs operate under the supervision of the Executive Director, who reports to the Executive Committee and the Board of Directors. The Executive Director takes primary responsibility for financial development and public relations. She is served by the Director of Program Operations, who in turn supervises the Directors of the three Clubs and the Outreach Director.

The Friendly PEERsuasion Coordinator formally provides a liaison between the PEERsuasion program staff leaders and the Outreach Coordinator. Actually, the Outreach Director, the Friendly PEERsuasion Coordinator, and one of the Club Directors were all involved in leading PEERsuasion groups. The cross-cutting roles appeared to be the source of a minor degree of consternation about division of responsibilities. However, as discussed below, the organization of the program appeared to function well.

Physical Context of the Program

Friendly PEERsuasion operates from the Club located in a downtown area of Birmingham in close proximity to the government center, financial buildings, and luxury clubs and hotels. The Girls Club building, a two-story immaculately maintained modern structure, shares the block with a large church and a bank parking lot. Although a complex of low-cost houses is on the opposite side of the street and girls from this area do participate in Club activities, many of the girls who participate are driven by their parents from less proximate and more economically advantaged neighborhoods. In 1988, almost 30% of Club members were white and approximately 66% were from families with annual incomes of over $20,000.

In order to reach the girls at highest risk of substance abuse, the PEERsuasion program staff arranged with the Birmingham Board of Education and neighborhood school administrators to provide the program to students in two (kindergarten through 8th grade) schools in economically disadvantaged areas in the city. The two schools involved in the program evaluation are relatively old, stark, utilitarian buildings—typical of the architecturally graceless brick structures constructed around the country during the "baby boom era" to serve a rapidly growing population of children. The interiors, the wide halls with scuffed floors, the school office with high counters separating the secretaries' desks from the waiting area, and the neutral tone walls and high windows would evoke childhood memories of spelling bees and report cards from generations of Americans educated in public schools.

Working in classrooms and other meeting space during school hours, the Girls Club staff tried to arrive 10–15 minutes before the PEERsuaders appeared, and quickly rearranged furniture, hung posters, and laid out project materials. By the time the girls entered the room, a special, more club-like environment had been created, and the visual focus of attention was group activity rather than academic instruction. The specific arrangement of furniture and materials reflected the physical features of the room and the preferences of the staff. For example, one of the groups met in the school auditorium, and the staff member preferred to sit on the floor with the girls. She created a special place for activities by pushing a large portable chalkboard up against the stage area, arranging materials on the floor of the stage, and hanging posters on the side of the chalkboard facing the stage. Another staff member, who met with the girls in a classroom, preferred to sit in chairs.

She rearranged seats in a circle for discussions and role-playing, moved other chairs around a table with project materials for "hands-on" creative activities, and taped posters over the chalkboard.

The ability to arrive in the school rooms and quickly arrange materials for the program curriculum was obviously contingent on prior organization of necessary materials. This prior organization took place at the downtown Girls Club building. The PEERsuasion Program director had simplified coordination of curriculum materials using a row of cardboard boxes lined up against a wall in her office. One box was earmarked for each of the PEERsuasion groups; nonperishable materials for each curriculum activity scheduled during the week were provided in the boxes for each group. Perishable materials (apples, crackers, and other foods) were added to the materials on the day of instruction. Other boxes were designated for the return of materials, such as attendance forms. Patterns for materials that the staff members duplicated in preparing for each session, such as poster board jigsaw puzzles, hung on the wall near a box of necessary construction materials.

The staff members each had a PEERsuader carrying case or bag in which they had further organized materials used on an ongoing basis; for example, a drawstring bag containing blank slips of paper and one marked "research assistant" (used to select a girl who would administer the evaluation protocols at the end of the session). The staff members also added to their kits materials they had asked the girls to bring to the next session, such as pictures from magazines.

The Girls Club Friendly PEERsuasion Staff

The most overt characteristics the Girls Club Friendly PEERsuasion staff appeared to share were enthusiasm for their work with adolescent girls in general, enthusiasm for their involvement in Friendly PEERsuasion in particular, a keen sense of humor about the challenges adolescents can present, and a level of interest in the girls that far exceeded the delivery of the program.

They were keenly aware of disadvantageous home situations, such as lack of adult supervision, poverty, and illiteracy. They realized that, given the limited time they had with the girls, they could only begin to make a difference in the girls' lives. But they hoped to establish a relationship with the girls that would be possible to continue through other programs. Some provided a personal resource on whom the girls could call outside the program setting. For example, during one session concentrating on leaving situations in which other youngsters were using drugs, one girl commented that she would have no one to pick her up if she wanted to leave someone else's house in the middle of the night. The leader asked whether an aunt, or cousin, or friend might be available. In response to, "No ma'am, nobody," the leader suggested the girl call her home if the situation arose.

Aside from their attitudes toward their work and the girls (and all being women), the leaders were a relatively heterogeneous group. The staff included both blacks and whites, women from relatively wealthy families and others who grew up relatively poor, relatively young childless women and others who had adolescent children of their own. Their highest educational degrees ranged from high-school diplomas to Masters' Degrees (*see* Table 1). Few had a long-term association with the Girls Club and several were hired from other youth organizations specifically for the PEERsuasion program. As discussed above, each had her own style of program delivery. However, the training sessions provided by the Girls Clubs of America National Resource Center set an interactional tone for the program that appeared to be carried to the implementation sites and seemed similar from session to session.

The Interactional Context of the Program

The tone set for the program by the Girls Clubs of America's national project staff and the context local staff members work at maintaining was typically orderly, voluntary, verbally responsive, supportive, and cooperative. Three recurrent training sessions for staff implementing the program were held in 1988 and 1989. Every moment of the training sessions was planned in advance with the goal of imparting a wealth of details about program implementation—yet time and activities were structured to create a warm feeling of camaraderie among the participants, to provide the opportunity to criticize program session plan details constructively, and to generate enthusiastic participation.

So enticing were the training activities that a young research assistant assigned to take notes on training procedures continually forgot her role and joined the Girls Clubs staff rehearsals of program sessions. Also, so effective were the plans for building *esprit de corps* that, late one evening (after attending training sessions from early in the morning until dinner), this group of women from diverse backgrounds sat, roaring with laughter,

Table 1
Girls Club of Birmingham, Inc.
Background Characteristics of the Friendly PEERsuasion Staff
1988–1989, $n = 9$[a]

	Average	Range
Number of y on Girls Club Staff	.85	0–3.5
Number of y teaching adolescent girls	7.22	1–23
Number of y of post-high-school education[b]	3.55	0–6
Number of academic courses on substance abuse in past 5 y	.66	0–5
Number of other courses on substance abuse In past 5 years[c]	1.88	1–4
Importance of Friendly PEERsuasion compared to other Girls Clubs programs (scale of –2 to +2)	1.77	0–2

[a]Data collected September, 1988.
[b]Estimated from highest degree.
[c]Includes training for Friendly PEERsuasion.

as they traded confidences of common experiences of having been adolescent girls in America. This spirit of the program appeared to take hold in Birmingham.

In part, in Birmingham, orderliness also was established by the management of materials and time. The display of activity accoutrements, especially snacks, visibly interested the girls and piqued their curiosity. Questions such as, "What are they for?" and "When are we going to get them?" provided an opportunity for the staff member to tell arriving girls briefly about the order of the session. Furthermore, the prearrangement of materials signaled to the girls that the staff member was ready to begin. When time was too tight to finish laying out the equipment before the first girls arrived, involving them in the process of organizing and arranging appeared to accomplish the same purpose.

Usually, in most Girls Clubs programs other than Friendly PEERsuasion, the leaders have a self-selected group of girls with whom to work and receive more or less instant feedback from them about their enjoyment of the program. Several staff members commented, "Our girls vote with their feet. If they don't like an activity they leave."

Since, in Birmingham, Friendly PEERsuasion was implemented in schools during school hours, participation was semi-voluntary. If a girl absolutely did not want to participate in an activity, as long as she did not disrupt the other girls' activities, she could sit passively and not participate; however, she could not simply leave the room until her next scheduled class. Girls who did not want to continue participation at the end of the session were allowed to withdraw entirely from the program. (Program withdrawal was a rare occurrence; except for a couple of girls, withdrawal was the result of leaving the school because of family relocation.)

Generally, no matter why a girl suddenly decided she did not want to participate, the staff were able to smooth the path for continued involvement—or the activities were too enticing to remain passive. For example:

> Phileeppa arrived for the session with a very sullen look on her face. She tossed her books on the floor with a loud slam, slumped down in a chair with her legs stretched out in front of her and her arms crossed tightly across her chest, and scowled. The session leader came over and quietly spoke to her but Phileeppa merely scowled more fiercely and refused to respond. Once the session was under way, the leader tried several times to involve her with no success.
>
> Perhaps partial success could be attributed to the leader's efforts since at one point Phileeppa responded with a refusal that appeared to be based on lesson materials in an earlier session. "Leave me be," said Phileeppa, "I've been feeling a lot of stress. And you keep on me, make me feel more stress."
>
> As part of the session plans, two girls were acting out situations in which they were refusing peer invitations to smoke or drink; one girl was the "trouble-maker" the other the "PEERsuader." Phileeppa's posture and expression indicated that she was paying close attention and enjoying the scene. When the two girls concluded the scenario, the staff member asked for a volunteer to play the "trouble-maker" for the next situation. Phileeppa immediately jumped up and volunteered, was selected, and played her part very realistically.

Since Girls Clubs staff are used to working primarily with volunteers, the natural "trouble-makers" present a cause for concern. One leader confided that she wished she had a way of selecting just the girls who really wanted to be in the program. However, other leaders indicated that the girls most difficult to involve were precisely those most in need of the prevention program. Their concerns were focused more on the relatively short periods of time they had with the girls compared to the time they thought was actually required to establish a close working relationship. "If only I could be here after school hours so the girls could come and discuss anything they wanted to discuss," wished one leader.

Fortunately, the vast majority of the girls appeared to enjoy totally the activities, the "time-out" period from the usual school setting, and perhaps most of all the great interest and support provided by the Girls Clubs staff. From the time most enthusiastically entered the room until they reluctantly left, almost all girls focused their attention on the staff leader. Both before and after the planned activities, the leaders discussed events and topics that appeared to be very important in their lives, such as school report cards to be passed out at the end of the day, boyfriends, new babies in the family, and sports injuries. Also the girls responded vigorously to questions, offering little confidences, such as, "I know I'm going to get good grades on subjects, but I'm going to get a really bad grade for conduct in English, and is my mother going to be mad."

Establishing a positive and constructive forum for discussing topics that are important to the girls appeared to enhance the ability to carry out planned activities constructively. Many activities involved a process of using games or crafts to heighten the girls' awareness of situations conducive to substance abuse and then to discuss constructive ways of dealing with the situation.

For example, one curriculum activity involved tossing a hank of yarn from girl to girl as the tossers called out an event that creates stress; for example, "I really hate it when [my] sister lies to my mother about me." Each girl who caught the yarn held onto a strand as she tossed it to another participant—creating a tangled web. After each girl had a couple of turns, the staff member led a discussion about ways of cutting through stress, while using a pair of shears to cut through one strand in the tangle each time the girls suggested a constructive response to stress.

In addition to real-life events the girls presented during activities, the leaders were also aware of other predicaments the girls had confided, and could use them to help the girls to realize the more general concepts under discussion. For example, "When your mother gets angry about your grade in conduct how do you feel? Mad?" "Uh huh." "Stress?" "Right." "What do you think is a good way of cutting through that stress?"

All participation in activities was commented on by the leaders in a highly positive manner. ("That's real good, Keeona." "You did just great, Natalee.") And the common complaint by the girls in response to new activities, "I can't do that," almost universally was met on the part of the leaders by, "Sure you can; I know you can."

"We say that," explained one of the leaders, "because we mean it. Many adults tell girls that they are capable, but they [the adults] really don't believe they are capable. We're working with lessons that have been written for these girls ... activities they can do. So we can honestly say, 'I know you can do it.'"

The girls appeared to respond to the approval and confidence of the leaders with touchingly naive delight. As soon as they finished completing an activity, they turned to the leaders for anticipated compliments, and when they received them, they smiled shyly or broadly depending on the girl and some almost seemed to bask in the praise. They consciously or unconsciously imitated the leaders. When they carried out leadership activities, it was evident from the change in their natural tones and carriage that they were emulating the Girls Clubs staff.

For example, the girls who were PEERsuader Research Assistants sounded much like the Girls Clubs staff when they collected the Activity Checklists. They politely encouraged the girls to complete their sheets, and they provided positive comments to the girls for having returned the completed forms. Although there were frequent lapses, such as "Stupid, you forgot your name!" these more natural interactions helped highlight the more complimentary learned behaviors.

The School Context

Working within the schools rather than in the Club had both positive and negative ramifications for program implementation. The primary difficulties appeared to be the result of both operational and philosophical differences.

Operational differences appeared to be based in the fluid nature of the student population. The Girls Clubs staff typically planned programs far in advance of actual delivery. To plan resources and staff time for Friendly PEERsuasion, they had hoped to pin down during the summer their schedule for program delivery and the actual numbers of girls who would participate in the program in the fall. The school staff, however, knew from experience that plans made for class assignments before the youngsters actually arrived in the fall would be impossible to keep; they had virtually no way of knowing until the day school started who would be in their school population. The Girls Clubs staff were unhappy with what they interpreted as unresponsiveness on the part of the school staff. The school staff, on the other hand, felt that the Girls Clubs staff were making unreasonable demands that could not be met.

The essential philosophical conflict was rooted in differences in educational priorities. The Girls Club staff placed highest priority on comprehensive life skills, such as learning to make informed decisions and learning to set and achieve realistic goals; the Birmingham Schools stressed basic testable academic skills, such as reading and math.

The school staff considered Friendly PEERsuasion an important enrichment activity, yet were unwilling to allow the Girls Club to implement the program during times slotted for academic subjects. The Girls Club staff were willing to comply with these restrictions, yet realistically knew they could not compete with such activities as band for the attention of girls who had little or no contact with Club activities in the past. By scheduling the program for time allocated to nonacademic subjects that did not hold great appeal for the girls, such as gym class, the problem was resolved to the satisfaction of the school authorities, the girls, and for the most part the Girls Club staff. (There was some concern among the national staff, since sports are an integral part of Girls Clubs of America's program.)

Working around the academic class time and other activities required great flexibility on the part of the Girls Clubs staff. Leaders who taught more than one session at a school had to drive back and forth across the city several times in one day and set up for the same activities twice. On several occasions, leaders arrived at the schools and prepared to begin the session, only to find that a special program, such as a class in computer use, had been slotted for their scheduled PEERsuader time. Also, although most teachers tried their best to send the girls off to their next class on time, tardiness was a problem about which most leaders complained. The Girls Clubs staff tended to attribute tardiness to dislike of the program on the part of some of the teachers.

Although only very favorable remarks about the program and the Girls Club staff were provided by teachers and other school staff during site-visits, it was entirely possible that teachers who did not offer opinions resented the staff delivering the program. To gain permission to deliver the program in the schools, Girls Club staff briefed the Board of Education, the Superintendent of Schools, and principals about the program; however, the teachers were not provided with an opportunity to learn about the program before it was initiated. Since they knew little or nothing about the program, it was quite possible that some of the teachers viewed the Girls Club staff as outsiders competing for scarce time and resources.

The problems engendered by implementing the program in the schools appeared to be offset by the advantages. The primary reason the staff recruited girls in the schools was to involve high-risk girls who were not likely to become involved in Club activities spontaneously. According to the school staff, many of the girls in the program were at high risk. Housing projects close to the schools were characterized as places where drugs were frequently sold, and students in high schools in the same school districts were thought to have a high rate of substance abuse.

Moreover, the Girls Clubs staff suggested that, by working in the schools, they were generating good publicity for Club programs among the educators and the students. Judging from the high regard paid to Girls Clubs by educators and the actions of the students, they were correct. Principals and teachers alike indicated that Friendly PEERsuasion was a program they valued, since substance abuse was an extremely difficult problem faced by their students every day. They were acutely aware that simplistic measures failed to prevent drug use and they praised the Girls Club staff for their sustained effort.

The Community Context

The need for a sustained effort for preventing substance abuse among the city's youngsters appeared to be a view held by practitioners in many Birmingham agencies responsible for dealing with youth. Other educators, police officers, administrators of other youth organizations, and clergy all spoke of the pressing need to provide prevention programs that realistically addressed the problem. "You can't just tell them to say no," was an often repeated phrase, and most made it clear that, although the Girls Club's efforts were desirable and appreciated, Friendly PEERsuasion was but one of several approaches being implemented in Birmingham to combat drug abuse.

Birmingham in many ways is still trying to compensate for the negative publicity generated during the era of violent resistance to the civil rights movement. Both Black and white residents were quick to point out that the old days of deep racial schism and conservative reactions are gone. Many of Birmingham's problems including drug abuse are being dealt with in a progressive manner characteristic of the dynamism of the "New South."

The Birmingham Police Department was involved in two new antidrug programs sponsored by the federal government. The DUF (Drug Use Forecasting) Program screens arrestees for recent drug abuse using new technologies for urinalysis. The Department also started implementing the DARE (Drug Abuse Resistance Education) Program in the 6th grade in several schools and planned to enlarge the program to encompass all Birmingham schools. (The program had not yet begun in the schools in which the PEERsuasion program was operating in the fall of 1988.) The DARE program is similar to one component of Friendly PEERsuasion. Taught in classrooms by specially trained police officers, the program uses a combination of drug education and role-playing to provide youngsters with skills to resist peer pressure to use drugs.

In addition to the Girls Club and Birmingham Police, Aletheia House, a local United Way sponsored organization, also is providing in-school drug prevention programs. The Aletheia House staff, who also are involved in running a 12-bed treatment facility for young addicts and a day treatment center for addicted women, have been recruited from other Birmingham agencies serving high-risk youth. The staff includes a former police officer, a former juvenile probation officer, a therapist, and a former teacher. According to the Aletheia House director, the diverse backgrounds of the staff provide an opportunity for maintaining informal coordination with other agencies involved in antidrug abuse programs. The in-school program is provided for seventh graders in four contiguous counties; the primary goal is "increasing responsible decision making" and, more specifically, providing practical approaches for dealing with substances most likely to be abused. According to a survey of the seventh graders conducted by Aletheia House, these substances are alcohol, marijuana, and inhalants —particularly liquid paper.

Given the growing number of drug prevention programs being provided in the schools, the Birmingham Board of Education has established the position of Coordinator of Drug Abuse Programs. The Coordinator has primary responsibility for facilitating the integration of programs, such as Friendly PEERsuasion and DARE, into the school schedules. Additionally, she reviews drug abuse prevention materials, and provides information about the materials and additional resources to principals and teachers. She also arranges for special programs such as Free by Choice, a project involving inmates telling high school students about the wrong choices that led to their criminal behavior and resulting incarceration.

Recognizing that programs provided during school hours are only a partial remedy for preventing drug abuse among high-risk youngsters, the Board of Education also has established an extended day program. This Community School Program operates after school hours until 6:00 PM and involves "latch-key" children enrolled in grades up to the eighth grade. Located in 14 schools throughout the city, in addition to the Girls Club, the Director of Community Education and the Coordinators at the local levels call on such other outside organizations as the Camp Fire and Boy Scouts to provide programs. The mission of the Community School program is to target and involve youth at highest risk of problems, such as teen pregnancy, dropping out of school, and substance abuse.

The Superintendent of Birmingham Schools, the coordinators of the in-school and after-school programs, the police officers involved in the DARE program, and the directors of the youth organizations, including the Girls Club, all tended to see the efforts of their individual organizations as part of a comprehensive city-wide effort to reduce drug abuse. Naturally, the staff in each organization felt that their own efforts were in some ways superior to the programs of the other organizations. At times, discussions about competition for scarce resources, such as funding, resulted in some acerbic remarks about each other's organizational capabilities. However, the spirit of cooperation among organizations serving Birmingham youth was remarkable.

In the next sections, details of the results of this cooperation are presented. First, the system used to monitor the program on an ongoing basis is described and the analyses of the data are discussed. The results of the data analysis are then given. Those who are more interested in the program than evaluation methods may wish to skip to the section on the overview of data analysis results.

Components of the Monitoring System

In designing a system for monitoring the implementation of the Girls Clubs of America's Friendly PEERsuasion Program, the goals were to collect a rich base of data for analysis while placing minimal burden on the staff providing the program. To do so, traditional and relatively innovative methods for evaluating program implementation were incorporated. In addition to the on-site observations presented above, the program also was monitored on-site by the national Girls Clubs of America program staff. Attendance was taken at all sessions. Information about age, race, and ethnicity of participants was collected at the time they signed up for the program using self-administered questionnaires.

In addition to information traditionally collected about participant characteristics, it was possible to collect more confidential information using an anonymous questionnaire primarily designed for impact analysis. By using methods designed to assure the girls of confidentiality, a preprogram questionnaire was administered to all girls (who then were randomly assigned to the fall and spring programs). In addition to questions concerning substance abuse, the girls also were asked about eligibility for the school free lunch program, siblings who were school dropouts, sexual activity, and "latch-key" status.

The initial plan was to collect the more sensitive information from parents and guardians using mail-back questionnaires sent home with the girls along with information about the program and evaluation and informed consent forms. (Informed consent forms were returned to the local Clubs by the girls). Several methods were used to increase the numbers of these questionnaires completed and returned, including Spanish translations for Hispanic parents, the use of self-addressed envelopes that did not require postage, and assurances of confidentiality. However, the Girls Clubs local staff, who have had long-time experience with obtaining information from parents or guardians, suggested that a high return rate would be uncertain. Therefore, additional questions were added to the preprogram questionnaire.

Actually, the number of parent/guardian questionnaires returned was relatively high (approximately 70% return in Birmingham). However, since essentially the same data had been obtained by using the preprogram questionnaires completed by all 127 girls who enrolled for the program, the preprogram questionnaires presented a better source for determining the characteristics of the girls in the program.

Other components of the monitoring system were designed to incorporate the following features:

- *Ongoing collection of data about implementation of specific program activities*—in addition to occasional on-site observations, session-by-session information was collected about activities carried out and participants' reactions to these activities.
- *Quantitative measures* that could be used to compare program sessions and program participants, and in the future, program sites other than Birmingham. For example, numbers of designed activities carried out during each session.
- *Simple data collection procedures* that could be used by people already on site as opposed to prohibitively high-cost ongoing data collection by research staff.
- *Data uncontaminated by the program staff's natural wish to "look good"*— data on program implementation collected by the agencies being evaluated may be biased in favor of the agency; therefore, information about program implementation was also collected from program participants. Additionally, during site visits, information was obtained from persons cooperating with and peripheral to the program.

- *Methods for determining the quality of the data collected*—checks on data quality are always necessary in carrying out all types of research. Tests of quality are even more important for data collected without the direct supervision of trained researchers. As described below, information from the program participants was collected that provided a check on the quality of the data they provided.
- *Ongoing data entry and analysis procedures* that could be used to inform the Girls Clubs of America national staff about serious problems with program implementation if they arose. Tabular information periodically was sent to the Girls Clubs of America for review of program implementation.

Data Collection Forms Used on an Ongoing Basis

To collect data about implementation of specific activities integral to the Friendly PEERsuasion curriculum, two types of forms were designed to be filled out at the end of each of the 14 program sessions, PEERsuader Participation Sheets and Activity Checklists. These forms were provided in a kit of evaluation materials sent to the Girls Club of Birmingham (and the three other Clubs involved in the program's evaluation) several weeks before the program was implemented in the summer of 1988, the fall of 1988, and the spring of 1989. Since girls participating in each site were divided into small groups led by different Girls Clubs staff members, separate evaluation kit materials were provided for each group. *See* Figs. 1 and 2 for example forms. The evaluation kits also contained pre addressed postage-prepaid envelopes for returning completed forms to the research staff. (Other materials used for impact evaluation were also included in the kits.)

PEERsuader Participation Sheets were designed to be completed by the Girls Club staff session leaders. They were used to collect the following information for each session.

- Participants' names (a master sheet containing names of the girls in each group was prepared by the leader after the first meeting; 14 photocopies were made—one for each session);
- Participants' absence or presence;
- If absent, reason for absence;
- Participants' arrival on time or tardy;
- Participants' departure before or at end of the session; and
- Participants' attitude toward the session on a scale of 1–10.

Activity Checklists were designed to be completed by the program participants. They were used to collect information about:

YOUR NAME _____ YOUR BIRTHDATE _____
          First   Middle   Last   Month Day Year
GIRLS CLUB _____ BRANCH _____ LEADER'S NAME _____

Activity Checklist
Lesson 1
(Communication Skills)

Please put today's date here _____ and then circle Yes or No for each question.

(1) We played with a ball or a balloon.
    Yes   No
    If you circled yes: Was it fun?   Yes   No
                          Did you learn from it?   Yes   No

(2) We made posters.
    Yes   No
    If you circled yes: Was it fun?   Yes   No
                          Did you learn from it?   Yes   No

(3) We learned about how to listen.
    Yes   No
    If you circled yes: Was it fun?   Yes   No
                          Did you learn from it?   Yes   No

(4) We talked on toy phones.
    Yes   No
    If you circled yes: Was it fun?   Yes   No
                          Did you learn from it?   Yes   No

(5) We practiced saying what we mean.
    Yes   No
    If you circled yes: Was it fun?   Yes   No
                          Did you learn from it?   Yes   No

(6) We worked in small groups of girls.
    Yes   No
    If you circled yes: Was it fun?   Yes   No
                          Did you learn from it?   Yes   No

(7) We talked about being Peersuaders.
    Yes   No
    If you circled yes: Was it fun?   Yes   No
                          Did you learn from it?   Yes   No

DID YOU WRITE YOUR FIRST AND LAST NAME AT THE TOP OF THE PAGE?

Fig. 1. Activity checklist (reduced size sample)

PeerSuader Participation Sheet
(Please complete at END of each session)

Club _____ Branch _____ Leader _____ Date __/__/__

Lesson Number _____ Lesson Name _____

Girls' Names

Last First Middle (Nickname) Circle ABSENT or PRESENT

1. _____
   1. ABSENT: (if so, circle one reason) a. sick b. school detention
                                          c. other d. family needs
                                          e. other f. unknown
   2. PRESENT: If so, did she arrive late? (circle answer) no yes
                       Did she leave early? (circle answer) no yes
   3. Attitude During Today's Activities (circle one number)
   very hostile   bored   very positive
   0   1   2   3   4   5   6   7   8   9   10

2. _____
   1. ABSENT: (if so, circle one reason) a. sick b. school detention
                                          c. other d. family needs
                                          e. other f. unknown
   2. PRESENT: If so, did she arrive late? (circle answer) no yes
                       Did she leave early? (circle answer) no yes
   3. Attitude During Today's Activities (circle one number)
   very hostile   bored   very positive
   0   1   2   3   4   5   6   7   8   9   10

3. _____
   1. ABSENT: (if so, circle one reason) a. sick b. school detention
                                          c. other d. family needs
                                          e. other f. unknown
   2. PRESENT: If so, did she arrive late? (circle answer) no yes
                       Did she leave early? (circle answer) no yes
   3. Attitude During Today's Activities (circle one number)
   very hostile   bored   very positive
   0   1   2   3   4   5   6   7   8   9   10

4. _____
   1. ABSENT: (if so, circle one reason) a. sick b. school detention
                                          c. other d. family needs
                                          e. other f. unknown
   2. PRESENT: If so, did she arrive late? (circle answer) no yes
                       Did she leave early? (circle answer) no yes
   3. Attitude During Today's Activities (circle one number)
   very hostile   bored   very positive
   0   1   2   3   4   5   6   7   8   9   10

Fig. 2. PEERsuader participation sheet (reduced size sample).

- Name of session leader;
- Whether or not activities specified in the curriculum had been carried out;
- Whether or not the girl liked each activity she did; and
- Whether or not the girl thought she learned from each activity she did.

To check on the quality of the data collected from the girls, each sheet contained an activity that was not actually designed as part of the session. If a girl reported doing a "fake" activity, the other data she provided for that session were not considered reliable.

Using the Data Collection Forms

To be sure that program delivery and evaluation methods were consistent at all sites, the Girls Clubs of America National Resource Center staff held training sessions for the local Clubs' staff members involved in the PEERsuader program several weeks before each round of program delivery. In addition to actually carrying out the activities designed for the program, the local staff were thoroughly briefed on the evaluation design and data collection procedures. At the first training session, draft protocols were presented to the local staff, and their reactions to the instruments were requested. The final protocols reflected their comments and the results of pretests conducted at a Girls Club serving a population similar to the girls recruited for the PEERsuasion program.

The PEERsuader Fact Sheets and Activity Checklists simply required circling words or numbers to complete the forms. The girls were able to complete their forms in under five minutes. The leaders' forms required an initial period of approximately 30 minutes for printing the names of the girls in their group on a master PEERsuader Participation Sheet and photocopying 14 copies, one for each session. Once the copies were made, the sheet for each session could be completed at the same time the girls completed their Activity Checklists. PEERsuader participation forms completed by the leaders were mailed back to the research staff in the preaddressed envelopes provided in the evaluation kits; each return envelope was labeled with the name and sequential number of each of the 14 sessions and information that identified each group.

Leaders were not allowed to see the Activity Checklists before or after they were completed by the girls. Activity Checklists were provided in the evaluation kits in sealed envelopes clearly labeled for each session. A PEERsuader was selected at the beginning of each session and given the responsibility for the completion of the Activity Checklists; she also was given a badge provided in the evaluation kit designating her as the "PEERsuader Research Assistant" worn throughout the session. The PEERsuader Research Assistant opened the sealed envelope containing the Checklists at the end of the session, passed out the forms with pencils also included in the evaluation kit, collected the forms and pencils, placed the forms in the sealed envelope addressed to "The Researchers," and placed the envelope in the outgoing mail.

As the completed forms were received, data were keyboarded using a pre-formatted data entry file created for each participant. (*See* Fig. 3 for an example of a data entry file.) Separate files were maintained for summer, fall, and spring participants. Data for each girl for each session were entered from the PEERsuader Participation Sheets using preassigned codes. Data for each girl for each session from Activity Checklists were recorded by counting and entering:

- The number of activities the girl circled having done during the session;
- The number of activities the girl indicated she "liked"; and
- the number of activities for which the girl indicated she "learned something."

Additionally, if the girl circled having "done" the "fake" activity, a code "1" was entered for that lesson in the data entry file.

Analyzing the Data

All data analysis was conducted using the statistical software SPSS-PC. Data about participant characteristics were obtained from the preprogram questionnaire, and analyzed for the fall and spring participants together.

Data obtained from PEERsuader Participation Sheets and Activity Checklists were analyzed soon after the conclusion of the fall program to allow feedback to the Girls Clubs for the spring cycle. Analogous data collected during the spring program were analyzed after the girls had finished the 14 sessions.

Three types of variables were created about participation and activities.
- Variables concerning individual participation for all sessions:
  - ∞ The number of sessions attended
  - ∞ The number of times tardy
  - ∞ The number of times left early
  - ∞ Average attitude (as evaluated by the lesson leader) for all sessions
  - ∞ Percent of activities listed on all Activity Checklists that the girl said she liked (based on the number she reported doing)

```
Fact form NAME - first 10 letters                              CLUB/              BIRTHDATE
LAST         FIRST        MIDDLE          NICKNAME            BRANCH             MO  DAY  YR  AGE
01 DOExxxxxx JANExxxxxx xxxxxxxxxxxx     xxxxxxxxxxx            xx                xx   xx  xx   xx
RACE       LATCHKEY       FREE LUNCH
02  xx xx xx    xx              xx
PeerSuader Participation Sheet                                          Activity Checklist
LESSON 0–INFO FROM LEADER                                               INFO FROM GIRL:
LEADERID   PRESENT?   WHYNOT?   TARDY   LEFT   ATTITUDE                 NDID   NLIKED    NLEARNED   DID60X
03   05       1          x        1      0        10                     5       5          4         x

LESSON 1–INFO FROM LEADER                                               INFO FROM GIRL:
LEADERID   PRESENT?   WHYNOT?   TARDY   LEFT   ATTITUDE                 NDID   NLIKED    NLEARNED   DID10X
04   05       1          x        0      0        10                     4       5          4         x

LESSON 2–INFO FROM LEADER                                               INFO FROM GIRL:
LEADERID   PRESENT?   WHYNOT?   TARDY   LEFT   ATTITUDE                 NDID   NLIKED    NLEARNED   DID20X
05   05       0          F        x      x        xx                     x       x          x         x

LESSON 3–INFO FROM LEADER                                               INFO FROM GIRL:
LEADERID   PRESENT?   WHYNOT?   TARDY   LEFT   ATTITUDE                 NDID   NLIKED    NLEARNED   DID30X
06   05       0          C        x      x        xx                     x       x          x         x

LESSON 4–INFO FROM LEADER                                               INFO FROM GIRL:
LEADERID   PRESENT?   WHYNOT?   TARDY   LEFT   ATTITUDE                 NDID   NLIKED    NLEARNED   DID40X
07   05       1          x        1      0        07                     x       4          2         x

LESSON 5–INFO FROM LEADER                                               INFO FROM GIRL:
LEADERID   PRESENT?   WHYNOT?   TARDY   LEFT   ATTITUDE                 NDID   NLIKED    NLEARNED   DID50X
08   05       1          x        1      0        09                     5       5          5         x

LESSON 6–INFO FROM LEADER                                               INFO FROM GIRL:
LEADERID   PRESENT?   WHYNOT?   TARDY   LEFT   ATTITUDE                 NDID   NLIKED    NLEARNED   DID60X
09   05       1          x        1      0        09                     7       7          7         1
```

LESSON 7–INFO FROM LEADER				INFO FROM GIRL:			
LEADERID	PRESENT?	WHYNOT?	TARDY	LEFT	ATTITUDE	NDID	NLIKED	NLEARNED	DID70X
10 05	1	x	0	0	08	7	7	7	1
LESSON 8–INFO FROM LEADER				INFO FROM GIRL:			
LEADERID	PRESENT?	WHYNOT?	TARDY	LEFT	ATTITUDE	NDID	NLIKED	NLEARNED	DID80X
11 05	1	x	0	0	08	x	x	x	x
LESSON 9–INFO FROM LEADER				INFO FROM GIRL:			
LEADERID	PRESENT?	WHYNOT?	TARDY	LEFT	ATTITUDE	NDID	NLIKED	NLEARNED	DID90X
12 05	1	x	0	0	06	4	4	4	x
LESSON 10–INFO FROM LEADER				INFO FROM GIRL:			
LEADERID	PRESENT?	WHYNOT?	TARDY	LEFT	ATTITUDE	NDID	NLIKED	NLEARNED	DID10X
13 05	1	x	1	0	08	5	5	5	x
LESSON 11–INFO FROM LEADER				INFO FROM GIRL:			
LEADERID	PRESENT?	WHYNOT?	TARDY	LEFT	ATTITUDE	NDID	NLIKED	NLEARNED	DID11X
14 05	1	x	1	0	08	6	6	6	x
LESSON 12–INFO FROM LEADER				INFO FROM GIRL:			
LEADERID	PRESENT?	WHYNOT?	TARDY	LEFT	ATTITUDE	NDID	NLIKED	NLEARNED	DID12X
15 05	1	x	1	0	08	5	5	5	x
LESSON 13–INFO FROM LEADER				INFO FROM GIRL:			
LEADERID	PRESENT?	WHYNOT?	TARDY	LEFT	ATTITUDE	NDID	NLIKED	NLEARNED	DID13X
16 05	1	x	0	0	10	5	5	5	x

Fig. 3. Sample data entry form.

- Percent of activities listed on all Activity Checklists from which the girl reported learning (based on the number she reported doing).
- Variables concerning participation and reactions to activities for each of the 14 sessions:
  - The percent of girls enrolled who were present at the session
  - The percent of girls present at the session who were tardy
  - The percent of girls present at the session who left early
  - The average attitude of the girls attending the session as evaluated by the session leader
  - The percent of girls who completed all (valid) activities listed on the Activity Checklist
  - The percent of girls who completed all but one (valid) activity listed on the Activity Checklist
  - The average percent of session activities listed on the Activity Checklists that the girls liked
  - The average percent of session activities listed on the Activity Checklists from which the girls said they learned.
- Variables indicating that the data provided by a girl about a particular session were questionable (she reported doing a "fake activity").

Responses provided by girls who reported doing fake activities during a specific session were excluded from analysis of data for that session. For example, the number of activities reported carried out during Lesson 1 is excluded for a girl who on Activity Checklist—Lesson 1 circled "yes" for the fake activity (Item 4. We talked on toy phones). The percentage of girls who completed all activities is based on the total of girls who attended the session and who did not report fake activities.

The percentage of girls who reported doing fake activities in each session ranged from 0–24% (*see* Table 2). Approximately half the girls in both the fall and the spring sessions reported doing a fake activity at least once (54% in the fall; 53% in the spring). However, only one girl in the fall and one girl in the spring reported doing fake activities in one-half or more of the 14 sessions.

The Girls Clubs staff reported that the girls appeared to take their evaluation activities very seriously. They were anxious at the beginning of each session to see who would be selected as the PEERsuader Research Assistant and insisted that everyone "get a turn." Also according to the staff, the PEERsuader Research Assistants frequently were a source for reminding the leader to provide the envelope with the forms at the end of the session. These reports were validated by on-site observations. The girls' role in evaluation appeared to be part of a continual learning process involving emulation and identification with the Girls Club staff.

Table 2
Friendly PEERsuasion Program: Birmingham
Participants Who Reported Doing "Fake" Activities for Each Session[a]

Session	Fall participants, n = 49		Spring participants, n = 78	
	Number who reported "fake" activities	Among girls present, % who "did fake"	Number who reported "fake" activities	Among girls present, % who "did fake"
0 We are PEERsuaders	0	0	8	10.3
1 Communication skills	0	0	3	3.8
2 What am I saying	1	2.3	7	9.0
3 Stress and me	1	2.0	2	2.6
4 Stress management	2	4.3	3	3.8
5 I make my own choices	5	11.4	12	15.4
6 Media and peer pressure	10	23.8	6	7.7
7 Intro to substance abuse	2	4.7	2	2.6
8 Alcohol	6	12.2	10	12.8
9 Prescription/over-the-counter drugs	2	4.9	4	5.1
10 Other dangerous drugs	2	5.0	2	2.6
11 Dependency and resources	0	0	2	2.6
12 Tie-up	0	0	1	1.3
13 Celebration	1	2.3	3	3.8

[a]Sources: PEERsuader Participation Sheets (0–13); Activity Checklists (0–13).

Overview of Data Analysis Results

With a few exceptions discussed below, the on-site observations were supported by analyses of the data collected using the preprogram questionnaire and the Activity Checklists and PEERsuader Participation Sheets for all fall and spring sessions. More specifically:

- By recruiting girls in the schools, Birmingham Girls Club was able to involve girls at high risk of using harmful substances;
- Very good cooperation and institutional arrangements appeared to have been achieved. All sessions met regularly. Attendance was high, and although tardiness appeared to be a recurring problem, once the girls arrived for a session they were not likely to be called away until the session was over;
- The girls appeared to enjoy the program greatly;
- The girls appeared to be actively learning;
- The staff appeared to have established good rapport with the girls;
- The curriculum was being delivered as planned for the most part; however, not all activities designed for the program were completed.

Characteristics of the Girls

Participants had many of the same characteristics of youngsters found in past research to be at high risk for using harmful substances (see Table 3). They all were minority group members (Black or mixed-racial) from relatively poor families; 89% qualified for a free lunch at school. Although 97% of the girls were age 15 or younger, 14% were already sexually active. Twenty-five percent of girls who were age 12 or younger usually had no adult supervising them at home after school.

A relatively high number of girls reported substance abuse among older people surrounding them. Almost half of the girls had mothers who smoked (44%), and among girls who had older siblings, 11% had a sibling who smoked marijuana. Nine percent reported having a person at home "who drinks a lot." Obviously, illicit drugs were readily available in their neighborhoods, since 30% of the girls reported having seen someone selling drugs near their home during the summer of 1988.

All girls involved in the program were attending school and therefore were less likely than dropouts to become involved in substance abuse. However, if their siblings' behavior was an indication of their future behavior, a relatively large number would eventually dropout. Among girls with older siblings, 23% reported that a sister or brother stopped going to school before graduating from high school.

Session Attendance

All groups met in the schools on a regular basis. Although the leaders reported occasional problems of sessions being canceled by school administrators, they were allowed to schedule make-up sessions; all groups com-

Table 3
Characteristics of Girls Involved
in the Birmingham Friendly PEERsuasion Program[a]
Fall 1988–Spring 1989, n = 127

	Percent respondents
Race/ethnicity (categories are not mutually exclusive)	
Black	94
Puerto Rican	01
White	02
Chicana	01
Unknown	04
Qualify for free lunch at school	89
Sexually active during summer 1988	14
Older siblings who dropped out of school before high school graduation (among girls who have older siblings)	23
Sibling who smokes marijuana (among girls who have an older sibling)	11
Mother who smokes	44
Adult at home "who takes alot of drugs"	06
Person at home "who drinks alot"	09
Saw someone selling drugs near home	30
Latchkey (among girls 12 or younger)	25

[a]Source: Preprogram questionnaire.

pleted the 14 sessions designed as part of the curriculum. Attendance at the sessions was high. On the average, the girls attended over 12 of the 14 sessions (*see* Tables 4 and 5). During most sessions, 90% or more of the girls were present (*see* Tables 6 and 7).

Considering that the girls appeared to be at relatively high risk of becoming school dropouts, the in-school program attendance rates were surprisingly high. It is conceivable that the girls were actually attending school at higher rates than usual because they looked forward to participating in the program; however, since data on school attendance were not collected or analyzed, this hypothesis could not be tested.

The dismay expressed by the leaders about difficulties with tardiness was congruent with the finding that, during the fall session, on the average the girls arrived late for over two sessions (*see* Table 4). However, although tardiness still appeared to be a problem in the spring, the teachers

Table 4
Friendly PEERsuasion Program
Attendance and Participation of Birmingham Fall Participants
$n = 49$, for 14 Sessions[a]

	Average	SD	Mode	Range
Number of sessions attended	12.37	2.5	13	2–14
Times tardy	2.08	1.4	2	0–6
Times left early	0.31	0.6	0	0–3
Average attitude (for all sessions) (scale of 1–10)	8.6	0.6	–	6.9–9.8
Percent activities liked	94.8	16.1	100	15.5–100
Percent activities learned something	85.4	28.2	100	0–100

[a]Sources: PEERsuader Participation Sheets (0–13); Activity Checklists (0–13).

Table 5
Friendly PEERsuasion Program
Attendance and Participation of Birmingham Spring Participants
$n = 78$, for 14 Sessions[a]

	Average	SD	Mode	Range
Number of sessions attended	12.26	1.9	14	6–14
Times tardy	1.85	1.7	1	0–9
Times left early	0.86	1.8	0	0–8
Average attitude (for all sessions) (scale of 1–10)	8.2	0.6	–	6.5–9.2
Percent activities liked	93.8	12.9	100	32.2–100
Percent activities learned something	86.8	22.6	100	0–100

[a]Sources: PEERsuader Participation Sheets (0–13); Activity Checklists (0–13).

obviously tried even harder to send the girls off to the program on time; on the average, the girls were late in the spring for under two sessions (*see* Table 5). Unfortunately, as discussed below, the late arrival of the girls appeared to curtail the number of program activities that could be carried out in each session.

Disruption of program implementation because of calling out the girls for other school activities did not appear to be a significant problem in the fall (*see* Tables 4 and 6). In close to two-thirds of all fall sessions, none of the girls left early. The need to leave early appeared to emerge as

Table 6
Friendly PEERsuasion Program: Birmingham Fall, 1988
($N = 49$) Participants' Attendance, Participation, and Response to Activities for Each Session[a]

Session	Percent present	Percent tardy	Percent left early	Average attitude	Average percent activities liked	Average percent activities learned something
0 We are PEERsuaders	100	0	0	8.4	90	84
1 Communication skills	94	47	0	8.7	96	83
2 What am I saying	90	10	0	8.8	94	74
3 Stress and me	94	17	0	8.4	94	74
4 Stress management	94	43	11	8.3	94	82
5 I make my own choices	90	5	2	8.7	96	88
6 Media and peer pressure	86	5	0	8.7	93	85
7 Intro to substance abuse	88	45	8	8.5	95	87
8 Alcohol	90	2	0	9.5	98	89
9 Prescription/over-the-counter drugs	83	18	5	8.5	91	86
10 Other dangerous drugs	82	6	0	8.3	92	83
11 Dependency and resources	82	24	0	8.3	94	83
12 Tie-up	79	13	0	8.2	96	90
13 Celebration	90	0	3	9.7	95	90

[a]Sources: PEERsuader Participation Sheets (0–13); Activity Checklists (0–13).

Table 7
Friendly PEERsuasion Program: Birmingham Spring, 1989
(N = 78) Participants' Attendance, Participation, and Response to Activities for Each Session[a]

Session	Percent present	Percent tardy	Percent left early	Average attitude	Average percent activities liked	Average percent activities learned something
0 We are PEERsuaders	96	28	0	8.0	89	78
1 Communication skills	90	13	0	8.5	96	91
2 What am I saying	90	17	0	8.7	93	76
3 Stress and me	92	6	0	8.4	92	86
4 Stress management	90	11	7	7.9	93	85
5 I make my own choices	90	3	10	8.0	97	90
6 Media and peer pressure	82	31	14	7.9	96	89
7 Intro to substance abuse	82	24	8	7.9	95	88
8 Alcohol	81	2	11	8.7	97	89
9 Prescription/over-the-counter drugs	91	13	13	7.8	96	91
10 Other dangerous drugs	80	42	8	7.6	94	90
11 Dependency and resources	84	8	10	7.8	93	93
12 Tie-up	91	17	6	8.4	95	90
13 Celebration	92	0	11	9.3	95	89

[a]Sources: PEERsuader Participation Sheets (0–13); Activity Checklists (0–13).

more of a problem toward the end of the spring cycle (see Table 7), perhaps because of the number of special school events that traditionally occur in the spring. However, even during the spring semester, on the average, the girls left early on less than one occasion (see Table 5).

Program providers who are "guests" in a host organization must always reach an accommodative relationship with regular staff members who have control over participants' schedules. Otherwise, program implementation is vulnerable to subtle forms of sabotage. Given their ability to implement all sessions, the high rates of attendance they achieved, and the minimal disruption to sessions they experienced once they were under way, the Girls Club staff appeared to have brought about good cooperative relationships with the school staff.

Participants' Reactions

The enthusiastic participation of the girls noted during site visits was also reflected in their self-reports on the Activity Checklists (see Tables 4, 5, 6, and 7). The fall girls on the average reported liking almost 95% of the activities they did; the spring girls were only slightly less enthusiastic and reported liking an average of almost 94% of activities. The session in both the spring and fall for which the girls appeared to have least enthusiasm was the very first session. Quite possibly, as many adolescents in new situations, the girls were suspicious and prepared *not* to like the program, but even in the very beginning, the girls reported enjoying at least 89% of the activities.

The session the girls appeared to like most was a session during which the girls acted out different roles at a party at which pretend "drinks" were being served. Example roles included someone who drank too much and threw up, someone who drank too much and became depressed and cried, and someone who did not drink at all and tried to deal with the alcohol-related problems of the other girls. After the "party," the girls discussed each role in terms including physical effects of alcohol, reasons for drinking, refusal skills, and what might have happened if boys had been at the party.

It is notable that, at the training session in which the local Girls Clubs staff carried out the activities to be implemented in their communities, they also appeared to take delight in playing the party roles; at a meeting at a later date they reminisced about the "party." At least in this case, the leaders' level of enthusiasm at training sessions appears to be a good indicator of the future enthusiasm of the girls.

It is also notable that, when implementing the plans for this session (and other sessions), the leaders increased the relevance for the girls in their community by incorporating local variations on the primary theme. For example, rather than using simulated bottles of liquor at the "party," at one site the girls pretended to be drinking punch spiked with liquor. Probably, the leaders' attention to local realism helped heighten the girls' enjoyment.

The girls were more likely to report enjoying activities than learning something from them (*see* Tables 4–7). Even so, the fall participants reported learning something from an average of slightly over 85% of the activities completed, and the spring participants reported learning from an average of 87%. The session for which the girls were least likely to report learning in both the fall and the spring was a session designed to improve oral communication. Although the girls reported liking such activities as giving each other explicit directions for making peanut butter and jelly sandwiches, many did not feel as if they learned anything. Possibly the girls saw the exercise as teaching them how to make sandwiches—a skill they already had. Or perhaps the simplicity of the activity prevented participants from seeing the exercise as a device for improving positive communication skills.

The session during which the fall girls reported maximum learning was the last session, in which lessons from all sessions were reviewed and plans for teaching the younger children were begun. The spring participants, on the other hand, indicated that they learned most from a session in which they learned about resources for dealing with chemical dependency. Since these are simply immediate self-reports of learning, it is not possible to tell from these data which activities actually had a lasting heuristic effect.

In addition to the girls' reports of liking and learning from the program, the leaders indicated on the PEERsuader Participation Sheets that the girls' attitude was, for the most part, very positive (*see* Tables 4–7). On a scale of 0 (very hostile) to 10 (very positive), the leaders evaluated the girls' average attitude for all sessions in the spring and fall between 8–9. According to the leaders' evaluations, none of the girls appeared to be consistently hostile; however, many were consistently positive. The excellent rapport between the leaders and the girls observed on site in the middle of the fall session apparently also was established in the spring, and both sessions seemed to end on a high note; the average attitude for the last session in the spring and fall was close to perfect.

Table 8
Friendly PEERsuasion Program: Birmingham Fall, 1988
Participants' Reports of Having Completed Activities Specified
in Curriculum for Each Session[a]

Session	Percent who completed all activities[b]	Percent who completed all but one activity[b]
0 We are PEERsuaders	53	81
1 Communication skills	64	96
2 What am I saying	59	81
3 Stress and me	61	86
4 Stress management	68	98
5 I make my own choices	39	82
6 Media and peer pressure	29	52
7 Intro to substance abuse	35	85
8 Alcohol	72	97
9 Prescription/ over-the-counter drugs	24	65
10 Other dangerous drugs	3	23
11 Dependency and resources	24	55
12 Tie-up	61	92
13 Celebration	60	95

[a]Sources: Activity Checklists (0–13).
[b]Excludes girls who included fake activity.

Problems with Implementation

Although the Girls Club staff were able to carry out all sessions in a very positive manner, some of the activities originally designed as part of the curriculum were not carried out by the girls (*see* Tables 8 and 9). Part of the difficulty with implementing the total lesson plan obviously was time constraints exacerbated by the need to fit the program into a relatively inflexible school schedule; the curriculum was developed as 60-minute sessions, but school periods lasted only 45 minutes. Further, leaders could not keep the girls one minute past the end of the period allotted to the program. Too, tardiness on the part of participants shortened the time for activities, and evaluation activities took about five minutes from the class period.

Yet, perhaps ironically, implementation of planned activities also seemed to be the result of the success of the program. In the fall, the girls

Table 9
Friendly PEERsuasion Program: Birmingham Spring, 1989
Participants' Reports of Having Completed Activities Specified
in Curriculum for Each Session[a]

Session	Percent who completed all activities[b]	Percent who completed all but one activity[b]
0 We are PEERsuaders	12	70
1 Communication skills	44	75
2 What am I saying	56	81
3 Stress and me	66	89
4 Stress management	73	95
5 I make my own choices	30	86
6 Media and peer pressure	59	82
7 Intro to substance abuse	28	88
8 Alcohol	65	91
9 Prescription/ over-the-counter drugs	18	60
10 Other dangerous drugs	4	24
11 Dependency and resources	27	76
12 Tie-up	64	91
13 Celebration	48	77

[a]Sources: Activity Checklists (0–13).
[b]Excludes girls who included fake activity.

appeared to be completing fewer activities in some of the sessions that they enjoyed most (compare Tables 6 and 8); for example in Session 6, the girls liked on an average of 96% of the activities they did, but only 35% of the girls completed all activities. This raised the suspicion that the leaders were having difficulty disengaging the girls from the activities they were enjoying and redirecting their attention to the next planned activity. When asked by the national program director, the local staff members confirmed this impression. Given the difficulties of increasing program time in the schools and the obvious desire to maintain the enthusiasm of the girls, the most practical solution is to fine tune the curriculum in the future. If components thought to be essential could be carried out before or as part of the activities the girls enjoy the most, there would be less need to be concerned about time constraints.

Next Steps

Except for a few minor problems, the process of implementing Friendly PEERsuasion in Birmingham schools has been carried out by the Girls Club staff in an exemplary manner. All people involved are proud of the program and relatively confident about its success. Success however needs also to be measured in terms of the program's effect on the participants.

In addition to cooperating in the collection of data discussed in this report, the Girls Clubs staff and school administrators also cooperated in a study designed to measure program impact. Girls who initially enrolled in the program were randomly assigned to participate in the fall and spring cycles. Questionnaires were administered before random assignment, after fall participants completed PEERsuader training, after Christmas vacation but before the spring cycle began, and at a reunion in late spring after the spring cycle was completed. Self-report data were collected about attitudes toward use of harmful substances; interactions with peers who were smoking, drinking, or using drugs; and the girls' own participation in these behaviors. Survival rate analyses were used to compare the behaviors of the girls assigned to the fall program with those of the girls assigned to the spring over time.

Results from the analyses of these data indicate that the program did have a significant, although not dramatic, effect on participants' behavior. The methods for determining program impact and the results of the analysis will be provided in future reports. Meanwhile, the national Girls Clubs of America staff has refined the curriculum and produced materials for implementing the program in Clubs throughout the nation. Ideally, implementation will proceed as fruitfully as it did in Birmingham, Alabama.

Acknowledgments

The development and utilization of methods for evaluating the implementation of Friendly PEERsuasion benefited greatly from the cooperation of many practitioners and researchers.

The Girls Clubs of America national staff involved in the program contributed many suggestions for protocol development, prepared the evaluation kits sent out to the Clubs, arranged for meetings to train local staff cooperating in the evaluation, and provided oversight for the design and implementation of the evaluation methods. In particular, Dr. Heather Johnston Nicholson, Research Director, Jane Quinn, Program Director, and Dolores Wisdom, Director of Friendly PEERsuasion, greatly facilitated the evaluation.

Birmingham Girls Club staff assumed major responsibility for implementing data collection methods designed for the study. Without their cooperation we could not have carried out this evaluation. All spent hours organizing, distributing, collecting, and mailing back evaluation protocols. They graciously provided the opportunity to observe the program in action and to discuss their reactions. We especially would like to thank Sandra McMillian, Executive Director, Wanda Minor, Director of Program Operations; Jennie Paulding, Outreach Director; Penny Southward, Friendly PEERsuasion Coordinator; Angela Eakins, Brenda Curry, and Priscilla Davis.

Birmingham Board of Education members who took time from their busy schedules to discuss the implementation of substance abuse prevention programs are Dr. Cleveland Hammonds, Superintendent, Birmingham City Schools; Peggy Sparks, Director, Community Education; Beverly Dickson, Drug Education Coordinator. Other Birmingham educators and practitioners who provided valuable information include: Mrs. Purifoy, Principal, Hill School; Willie Sheppard, Principal, Washington School; Lieutenant Julius W. Walker, Director of Training, Birmingham Police Department; and Chris Retain, Aletheia House.

Girls Clubs of America National Resource Center staff who devoted many hours to producing evaluation kits and to entering data are Lisa Barnes, Susan Ellis, Beth Pitzer, Tiffany Pitzer, and Pat Taylor. Research Assistants at Abt Associates Inc. provided support throughout the evaluation including revising protocols, keeping logs of completed data collection instruments, and coding and entering data; they are Sarah Hechtman, Melissa Weissberg, and Linda Skudlark.

My colleagues Peter Finn and Joan Mullen provided appreciated advice for carrying out this study. Finally, I would like to thank the Birmingham program participants. The information they provided have helped us understand more about implementing substance abuse prevention programs for high-risk young women.

Alcohol Use Among LDS and Other Groups Teaching Abstinence

Rick D. Hawks

Introduction

The Church of Jesus Christ of Latter-day Saints (LDS), also known as the "Mormons," teaches abstinence from alcohol as a religious tenet. This chapter examines the special issues involved in the etiology, prevention and treatment of alcohol abuse among the LDS population. Myth and scarcity of accurate information concerning abstinence-teaching populations have precluded the building of a theoretical alcohol-use model. Such a model would provide valuable information for strategies that produce population-specific prevention and treatment interventions. Some experts[1] suggest that population-specific strategies might eliminate alcohol abuse problems for a given population.

The primary purpose of this chapter is to provide data for future researchers in constructing an alcohol use model for LDS and similar abstinence-teaching populations. It becomes clear that a prevention specialist and a therapist who are aware of those factors that maintain abstinence or, conversely, use and abuse in certain populations would have an advantage in planning prevention or treatment strategies for such groups.

Most members of a society receive a religious identification at birth, even though their parents may have no formal affiliation or involvement with a church. This religious identification usually provides an individual with a frame of reference for viewing the universe that often offers sociological controls for the use of alcohol. Nominal religious affiliation has been found to reduce an individual's identification with another given belief system and be useful in predicting that individual's drinking behavior.[2] In the following pages, the focus is on the influence affiliation with the LDS religion has on its members' alcohol use patterns.

Review of Related Research

Alcohol Use Patterns

Alcohol Use Continuum

In nonabstinence-teaching populations, behaviors that are often secondary to or related to the actual use of alcohol cause most of the problems for the individual or those around them (e.g., driving drunk, fighting). Alcohol use itself is typically accepted and might even be encouraged. In Fig. 1, the various levels of alcohol use ranging from abstinence to addictive use for a nonabstinence-teaching population can be identified. The "abstinence" group members are one rather small segment of the entire population.

In LDS and other abstinence-teaching populations, the alcohol using behavior *itself* causes most of the initial and ongoing problems. A member of an abstinence-teaching religion cannot consume any amount of alcohol harmlessly. Even small amounts of alcohol generate negative social and interpersonal consequences. Members of the LDS Church who drink alcohol, even in moderation, restrict themselves from full participation in worship services of the organization.[3] Such a phenomenon makes each use of alcohol among the LDS "problematic."

Several researchers have identified the LDS population as having the highest percentage of persons abstaining from alcohol compared to nonabstinence-teaching religious populations.[4-9] Within an abstinence-teaching model, the "abstinence" subgroup makes up the largest proportion of the alcohol use continuum. An LDS continuum of alcohol use and abuse is depicted in Fig. 2.

The high frequency of LDS abstainers might best be explained by Thorner's[10] concept of "counter anxiety." Thorner suggests that churches teaching abstinence develop an attitude regarding the use of alcohol that

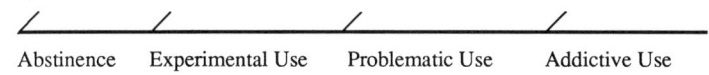

Fig. 1. Alcohol use continuum for a nonabstinence-teaching population.

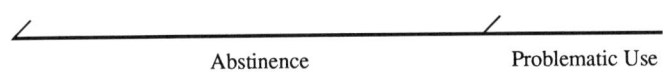

Fig. 2. Alcohol use continuum for an abstinence-teaching population.

tends to arouse sufficient anxiety to make sobriety norms become protected and stable. This pattern is very similar to the Alcoholics Anonymous attitude toward drinking. Thorner's counter-anxiety theory could also account for the delayed first use of alcohol reported by LDS alcohol users.

Age of First Use of Alcohol. Hawks[11] conducted a secondary analysis of the *Utah Incidence and Prevalence Survey,* collected by the Utah State Division of Alcoholism and Drug Abuse. The research sample included over 2700 respondents and was considered representative of the LDS population within the state of Utah. A statistical significant difference between the age of first use among LDS and nonabstinence-teaching populations was identified. A smaller percentage of LDS persons (40.4%) first used alcohol at age 15 or younger compared to a larger percentage of nonabstinence-teaching persons (46.5%). On the other hand, a larger percentage of LDS persons (39.1%) first used alcohol at age 16–18 compared to a smaller percentage of nonabstinence-teaching persons (34.5%). The late onset of "alcohol first use" by LDS alcohol users was reported by Hawks as being the result of several factors:

1. Positive family relationships that seem to occur among LDS families
2. A high level of agreement with the LDS religious abstinence-teaching tenet
3. The higher amount of stress that was measured among LDS than NonLDS persons during adolescence and a possible attempt to reduce that stress by alcohol use.

Based on the same research sample, Hawks[11] concluded that LDS adolescents in Utah exhibited additional unique characteristics. LDS adolescents were not as likely as nonabstinence-teaching adolescents to obtain their alcohol from "parents" or "brother or sister," but LDS adolescents were more likely than nonabstinence-teaching youth to obtain their alcohol from "friends." LDS adolescents were not as likely as nonabstinence-teaching adolescents to consume their alcohol at "home." LDS adolescents were more likely than nonabstinence-teaching youth to consume their alcohol in "nontraditional locations." The source and likely location to consume alcohol for LDS adolescents tended to be different than for other religious and nonreligious populations.

Paradoxical Alcohol Use

Research Perspectives

One principal characteristic of LDS alcohol use has been named by researchers[12,13] as "paradoxical alcohol use." That is, a large percentage of members from an abstinence-teaching religion are found not to consume alcohol. However, the small percentage that do report alcohol use tend to experience consequences associated with heavier drinking more frequently than do members of nonabstinence-teaching populations. Paradoxical alcohol use has been theorized to occur because of the norm qualities associated with abstinence. Mizruchi and Perrucci[14] reviewed the research in considering the norm qualities of abstinence and the differential effects upon deviant behavior. Abstaining Protestants and LDS were given significant attention in their review. They concluded that "predominantly proscriptive [abstinence-teaching] norms are more likely than predominantly prescriptive norms to lead to extreme degrees of pathological reactions when deviation occurs."[15]

Four characteristics of abstinence-teaching norms have been identified.[14] First, abstinence-teaching norms are inflexible. Alcohol use is defined as either compliant or deviant. Second, abstinence-teaching norms have no elaboration; that is, there are no rituals or embellishment associated with alcohol use. Third, abstinence-teaching norms are widespread in nature, focusing on the negative implications specific to the act of alcohol use applying to any and all contexts. Fourth, abstinence-teaching norms tend not to converge with other norms in the larger system that do accept alcohol use under certain conditions. In general, it would appear that the LDS population predisposes their deviant members to greater pathological reactions and, consequently, their religious structure to greater strain because of the characteristics of abstinence-teaching norms.

Bales' "Ritual Drinking" Theory. At the core of theories discussing paradoxical alcohol use patterns is Bales's[16] research. Bales postulated that cultures or social structures influence the rate of alcoholism in three ways:

1. The *functional alternative hypothesis*, where the culture provides alternative mechanisms for relief of tension
2. The *normative hypothesis*, where there are culturally supported attitudes toward drinking and intoxication that determine whether alcohol will be used as a means for relieving stress and tension
3. The *stress hypothesis*, where there are sociostructural factors that create stress and inner tension for members of a particular group or society.

Bales studied cultural differences in rates of alcoholism among Jewish and Irish people, and concluded that the extensive integration of drinking in the rituals of Orthodox Judaism was responsible for the absence (or low rate) of abusive drinking among Jews. Bales[16] suggested that this "ritual" attitude toward drinking adopted by the Jews led to a decrease in anxiety about drinking for personal reasons and thus precluded the development of alcoholism among Jewish people.

Normative Hypothesis. Blacker,[17] elaborating on Bales' theory, hypothesized after reviewing related literature that both prescriptive norms (how to drink) as well as proscriptive norms (how not to drink) were needed to maintain a low rate of alcoholism. Other researchers have agreed with Blacker's hypothesis and identified members "...of the ascetic [abstinence-teaching] Protestant groups-Mormons [LDS], Methodists, and the like— who drink and become alcoholic because there are no prescriptive norms."[18] Absence of a prescriptive drinking norm has been an influential characteristic unique to abstinence-teaching populations.

Preston[19] studied two communities within different socio-cultural regions of a southern state. Five hundred and sixteen adolescents were the focus of the study. The various religious denominations in the study were categorized into three types. Type I consisted of churches whose official policy was opposed to any consumption of alcohol and made alcohol use a moral issue. Type II consisted of churches that advocated personal temperance, but moderate use of alcohol was not considered sin. Type III consisted of churches that did not oppose the temperate use of alcohol. The LDS were listed as belonging with Type I churches along with the Baptists, Methhodists, and Church of Christ members. Preston's data supported the paradoxical use of alcohol associated with Type I churches. Preston found that coming from an abstinence-teaching background may not cause an individual to become an alcoholic, but if such an individual chose to use alcohol, the "...transition from an abstainer to a social drinker may be exceedingly difficult."[20]

Straus and Bacon,[21] for example, studied alcohol use patterns in college students. In order to sample the suspected diverse drinking patterns among various religious groups, questionnaires were administered to 16,300 students from 27 colleges representing metropolitan as well as rural areas. Brigham Young University, an LDS church owned and operated university, was included in the survey to ensure the existence of an LDS population. Similar measures were taken by the researchers to ensure the representation of other church groups within the sample.

The findings of the Straus and Bacon study[4] reported that 94% of Jewish males considered themselves users of alcoholic beverages, compared to only 54% of LDS males. However, for those males who drank to extremes, the opposite relationship appeared. Eighty-eight percent of the LDS males who drank reported themselves as having been "tight," 74% having been "drunk," and 40% having passed out. The Jews reported a lower percentage within each of the respective categories with 67% having been tight, 45% having been drunk, and 15% having passed out. The researchers went on to suggest that, if alcohol use was embraced by the LDS group, variation must be the rule since there were no norms. Therefore, extreme drinking was likely, since the behavior itself represented rejection of social rules. Straus and Bacon utilized "tight" as the first level of alcohol consumption, similar in meaning to intoxication, and followed in severity by being drunk and passing out. As part of the survey, students could have responded in more than one category, since the higher category of "passing out" would necessarily include the two lower categories.

Straus and Bacon also concluded that LDS male and female students who drink tend to experience a higher rating on a social complications scale than Catholics, Jews, and Protestants. The social complications scale contained such questions as the loss of friends and damage to friendships related to alcohol use. According to Straus and Bacon, the LDS intoxication and complication scales analyzed together suggested a reaction pattern. Those students who broke away from restrictions of their religious sanctions seemed inclined to react in a more dramatic, perhaps rebellious, manner than students whose drinking involved less rejection of their group.

Additional research using, in part or in whole, the Straus and Bacon's 1953 data was completed.[12,22] Snyder[22] performed a study using LDS and Jews in the research sample. The purpose of the study was to examine the cultural influences of drinking and sobriety. In addition to using data from the Straus and Bacon research sample, he obtained 73 interviews with a random sample of New Haven Jewish men and 644 questionnaires with male

Jewish college students. Snyder added to Straus and Bacon's observations that LDS alcohol users had no generally practiced norm of drinking. However, there was nonetheless, an implicit significance placed on abstinence. The emphasis on abstinence created an expectancy of extremes, namely, that drinking was necessarily utilitarian or hedonistic. The interpretation of the data was that drinking for members of the LDS church appeared to be for pleasure and drunkenness rather than being social or ceremonial. Snyder went on to say that LDS persons "divorce the act of drinking entirely from the contexts and symbolism (e.g., family, church, and religious community) which are primary sources of social control."[23]

Moss and Janzen[24] studied drinking patterns of Native Americans. The sample included 1811 heads of households in 20 Indian communities located on reservations in 10 states. Five percent of the sample identified themselves as LDS. Moss and Janzen observed various types of drinkers. Significantly more of the Catholics who used alcohol "seldom get drunk" than "never get drunk" or "always get drunk." Conversely, among LDS users of alcohol, significantly more of them "always get drunk" or "frequently get drunk" than "never get drunk" and "seldom get drunk." The authors explained the difference by using terminology similar to what other writers have observed with paradoxical drinking.

Smith[25] completed a study of approximately 5000 sociology students from the University of Washington, University of Utah, and Brigham Young University. About 2500 of the participants in the study identified themselves as LDS. The students responded to a questionnaire about how often they had ever or presently did drink to the point of drunkenness. Groups that disdained the use of alcohol, such as the LDS, seemed to experience drunkenness because of their inexperience with alcohol and their feelings of rebelliousness and adventure. The researchers concluded that "people who allow themselves to get drunk might be expected to be novices in the use of alcohol, [or] unhappy people trying to escape from reality... ."[26] Such feelings were theorized to prompt the LDS alcohol user to go "all the way."

Albrecht[27] reviewed geographic differences in the consumption of alcohol across the US. He reported that Utah ranked 50th in terms of per capita alcohol consumption, is 41st in terms of the total number of alcoholics, and is just 35th in rate of alcoholism. Albrecht estimated state prevalence and prevalence rates for alcoholics based on Cirrhosis mortality using the Jellinek Formula. When Albrecht made a regional comparison and calclated the rate of alcoholism (number of alcoholics per 100,000 population), Utah's rate was higher than that for the states of Arizona, Idaho, Montana, and Wyoming.

In explaining the higher frequency of alcoholism for Utah, Albrecht identified the high concentration of LDS Church members as a contributing factor. He suggested that, in absence of additional research, the comparative data on per capita consumption and alcoholism rates provide some support for a paradoxical alcohol use contention.

Hypothetical Examples

In a professional journal, Bacon[28] discussed four examples of social situations that influence alcohol problems, one of which depicted the LDS culture. An example was given of an LDS woman 45 years old who was an average participant in the community and who developed emotional problems. He concluded that she was unlikely to adopt the use of alcohol to alleviate her problems. For her there are positive moral, religious, and family group values attached to abstinence from alcohol. If alcohol use did occur, it would be similar to smashing altars or tearing up *Book of Mormons*. The woman would be more likely to adopt excessive eating, gambling, prescription drug use, or compulsive work habits.

On the other hand, Bacon stated, the young LDS male who is rebellious and opposed to the controls of parents and Church would find the use of alcohol to be advantageous. Unequipped with rules, models, sanctioning agents, realistic knowledge, and appropriate restraints or directions, but fully equipped with rebelliousness, many guilt feelings, and anxieties, this youth is probably an excellent prospect for alcoholism. With present changes in sex role identity, similar behaviors might be becoming more acceptable for young LDS females as well. A summary of available research on LDS drinkers and the existence of paradoxical drinking is displayed in Table 1.

Healthy LDS Alcohol Users

Hawks[11] conducted a secondary analysis of the *Utah Incidence and Prevalence Survey*, collected by the Utah State Division of Alcoholism and Drug Abuse in 1982. The research sample was considered representative of the LDS population within the state of Utah. Hawks noted, that, among the Utah LDS sample, when alcohol use did occur, an LDS subgroup of adolescents tended to use alcohol on fewer occasions than nonabstinence-teaching adolescents. In addition, when this LDS subgroup of adolescents did consume alcohol, they tended to use a similar quantity of alcohol (not a larger quantity as suggested by paradoxical drinking) on a typical day as did nonabstinence-teaching adolescents.

Table 1
Review of Research Studies Including Members of the LDS Church
and Discussing Paradoxical Drinking

Study (year)	Reference number	Description	Paradoxical drinking
Straus & Bacon (1953)	(21)	16,747 college students 778 LDS drinkers	+
Jones* (1957)	(6)	8507 high school-students 7238 LDS	0
Snyder (1958)	(22)	secondary analysis Straus & Bacon's Data	+
Skolnick (1958)	(12)	secondary analysis Straus & Bacon's Data	+
Smith (1969)	(26)	5000 college Sociology students-2500 LDS	+
Preston* (1969)	(19)	516 junior and high school students-LDS collapsed with other religions	+
Moss and Janzen (1980)	(24)	1811 Native American family heads-90 LDS	+
Utah I. & P. (1985)	(29)	Over 5000 3621 LDS	0
Albrecht (1985)	(27)	Per capita alcohol and estimation of alcoholics-50 states	+
Hawks* (1987)	(11)	Secondary analysis Utah I & P Survey 528-LDS adolescents	+

"+" indicates support of paradoxical drinking, "O" indicates no mention of Paradoxical Drinking, and "*" identifies adolescent studies.

In the same study Hawks expanded the research population to include the Utah "adult" survey respondents as well. He concluded that there was a statistical trend for a subgroup of LDS persons, both young and old, to consume a smaller quantity of alcohol than nonabstinence-teaching persons on occasions that drinking did occur. This would suggest that in addition to a subpopulation of "paradoxical" alcohol users, a subpopulation of conservative healthier LDS alcohol users also exists. It appeared from the Utah survey that the healthy LDS alcohol using subpopulations seemed to be larger than the paradoxical, heavy alcohol using subpopulation.

Hawks[11] concluded that the healthy LDS alcohol users tended to conform with their religious teachings of moderation even when using alcohol. They demonstrated their compliance by drinking smaller amounts and upon fewer occasions than their NonLDS counterparts. Additionally, a high rate of experimentation may have contributed to the healthy LDS alcohol using population. Supplementary research must be conducted to duplicate the findings concerning the existence of healthy LDS alcohol users.

The Effects of Religiosity

Snyder[22] extended Bales' theory by suggesting that Jewish ceremonies and rituals were not only forms for the expression of religious ideas and sentiments, but were also mechanisms that transmitted and sustained basic Jewish cultural values. According to Snyder,[30] one ethnocentric Jewish idea is that sobriety is a Jewish virtue, and that drunkenness is a Gentile vice. Snyder[22] suggested that Orthodox Judaism, which provides strong reinforcement for sobriety, precludes the development of alcoholism, whereas situations in which the transmission of Jewish culture is disrupted result in an increased rate of alcoholism. In short, Snyder reported that the rate of intoxication among Jews increased with a decrease in orthodoxy. Reports of intoxication were significantly rarer among students who reported an orthodox affiliation. The results of several other studies[31-33] also found an inverse relationship between religious orthodoxy and frequency of drinking among Jews.

A term found in the literature that is similar in nature to "orthodoxy" is "religiosity." Low religiosity has been shown to be positively related to alcohol use among adolescents in general[34-37] and among adolescents in Utah, a state predominantly LDS.[38-40] When focusing specifically on a national LDS adolescent sample, an inverse association between religiosity and drug use was much stronger for the LDS than for any other religious denomination, including Baptists, other Protestants, Catholics, Jewish, and groups with no religious affiliation.[41] A similar inverse relationship between religiosity and alcohol use was also found among the LDS adult population.[42-45]

In summary, Greeley et al.[46] concluded from their research that ethnic and religious drinking subcultures were relatively consistent in withstanding the changes in American drinking values in regard to their relationship to drinking problems. Flasher and Maisto,[47] after a comprehensive review of the literature, further resolved that increased orthodoxy within any religion "might" provide a viable deterrent against alcoholism.

Prevention Implications

The influences of various religious norms are particularly relevant to the prevention strategies of alcohol abuse. A generally accepted goal of alcohol prevention (for adults at least) is directed toward educating the general public about responsible drinking behavior.[48] That is, one should use alcohol in moderation and without adversely affecting oneself or others vs irresponsible drinking or alcoholism. Such a goal requires the acceptance of teaching "responsible drinking." Some experts[49-51] have extended the discussion to include "responsible marijuana use." Those authorities report that to control the use of alcohol and marijuana through preaching "abstinence" based on the "evils" of alcohol and marijuana use would undoubtedly be rejected and likely unsuccessful.

In October 1967, the National Cooperative Commission on Alcohol published its report [52] entitled *Alcohol Problems: A Report to the Nation*. The report recommended that those immunizing cultural effects (e.g., Jewish orthodox practice) should be extracted from the low alcoholism groups and fused into the new national alcohol policy. Simultaneously, those pathological effects found in the high-level alcoholism groups, such as the LDS, would be eliminated. This has sometimes been referred to as "making everyone a Jewish drinker."[53]

Based on negative implications associated with paradoxical alcohol use, the commission made several proposals. The commission wanted to reduce the emotionalism associated with responsible use of alcohol, such as feelings of guilt, conflict, and anxiety. The recommendations were made that organized churches, recreational groups, or athletic groups assist young people to adapt themselves realistically to a predominantly drinking society. Such steps as lowering the drinking age to 18 and making alcohol available at youth functions were among the suggestions.

Since 1967, the negative implications of paradoxical drinking have lessened. For example, legal drinking ages have tended to increase across America. Nevertheless, the ongoing proposal of preventing alcoholism by encouraging the responsible use of alcohol has negative implications for members of an abstinence-teaching population. They believe that abstinence from "all" alcohol is the only acceptable norm. LDS and other abstinence-teaching populations, by definition, cannot accept the fundamental premise used in most alcohol abuse prevention strategies. Therefore, it would appear that a new and different prevention model would be necessary to reduce alcohol use and alcohol-related problems effectively among LDS and other abstinence-teaching populations. Furthermore, it would seem that prevention strategies that would be effective for the nonabstinence-teaching population would likely not be as effective for LDS and other abstinence-teaching populations.

"Just Say No" Campaign

Bachman, O'Malley, and Johnston conducted a survey entitled *Monitoring the Future: A Continuing Study of the Lifestyles and Values of Youth* under the direction of N.I.D.A. (National Institute of Drug Abuse) from 1979–1981, before they listed Latter-day Saints (LDS) as a unique religious denomination. Hawks[9] completed a secondary analysis of trends using the *Monitoring the Future* data base. He noted that there appeared to be a general lack of decline in alcohol use frequencies among the LDS subgroup from 1982–1986 when LDS trends were compared to the Other Religions (nonabstinence-teaching religions), No Religion, and American Seniors in general. The nonabstinence-teaching adolescent populations identified a general 1 or 2% decline in alcohol use, which has been viewed as significant. The LDS population exhibited no significant decline in alcohol use frequencies of "lifetime," "annual," and "monthly" from 1982–1986. Hawks[9] concluded that the factors that might have influenced LDS youth to reduce alcohol use appeared to be separate from those factors that have successfully reduced alcohol use in nonabstinence-teaching populations.

One explanation of the lack of LDS decline in alcohol use might be that those LDS seniors who may have been influenced by public abstinence campaigns, such as "Just Say No," have already been influenced by religious campaigns. Additionally, the relatively small percentage of LDS youth who do report alcohol use does not allow statistically much freedom to fluctuate as do other groups of seniors. This suggests that the results obtained in the Hawks study are, at least in part, an artifact of the small percentage of LDS alcohol users.

Physiological Factors

During the assessment of the alcohol abuser, the examiner frequently will inquire concerning the family's background to determine if a family history of substance abuse exists. If there is a history of alcoholism or substance abuse in the parents or grandparents of the individual being evaluated, then physical predisposition to the condition is usually assumed. When this occurs, the therapist frequently passes this information on to patients and those around them. The information is given so the patients will know that they are perhaps more prone to developing alcohol and drug abuse problems than others.

Typically, however, the three or possibly four generations of abstinence from alcohol found in an LDS patient's lineage are often overlooked and viewed as insignificant information. Such a response would suggest that the genetic predisposition toward addiction only has significance in the "use" direction. This would additionally assume that several generations of abstinence has no influence upon a first-generation user of alcohol either genetically or sociologically. One noted alcohol expert suggested that this is not the case.

Royce[54] stated that one theory why "dry" sects, such as the LDS, tend to have the highest per capita rates of alcoholism is because they lack physiological immunity. The physiological immunity is present because of selective breeding with one another. In other words, abstinence-teaching populations might have a genetic predisposition towards a limited capacity to metabolize alcohol because of the many generations of intermarriages where alcohol use has never or rarely occurred. If such is the case, then the first generation of alcohol users from an abstinence-teaching population might have a genetic risk towards alcoholism.

LDS–Tailored Alcohol Services

The establishment of LDS-tailored resources has been based on the assumption that members of the LDS population who use alcohol require unique services separate from or in addition to traditional alcohol treatment programs. At least two LDS-tailored alcohol abuse programs have demonstrated some effectiveness.[55-57] Perhaps the most successful LDS-tailored program has been S.A.V.E., which was discussed by Hawks and Buckner[58] and Little.[59] S.A.V.E. was incorporated by LDS community leaders as a private nonprofit corporation and patterned after Alcoholics Anonymous, but acknowledges and accepts the participants' religious affiliation.

Conclusions and Summary

It would be ideal to plan prevention and treatment for each individual after considering that person's specific needs. However, from a practical standpoint, this is nearly impossible. There are only a limited number of professionals, and there are many people who need help. Planning for specific populations is the next best approach. With the limited amount of funds available for prevention and treatment programs, it makes sense to target spending and researching efforts for populations who are either at high risk for developing alcohol problems and/or for populations where much can be learned about the prevention of alcohol abuse in general. The LDS population exhibits both characteristics. First, a certain subgroup of LDS alcohol users clearly are at more risk than the general population of drinkers for paradoxical or heavy alcohol use and related problems. Second, the large subgroup of abstinent LDS persons and the apparent subgroup of "healthy" alcohol users, if understood, would likely offer strategies for prevention and conservative alcohol use. In other words, making everyone an "LDS drinker" might be an appropriate goal as an abstinence alcohol use model is further developed and understood.

Several variables that appear to be unique to the LDS population were identified and discussed in this chapter. Those LDS variables were noted by this author as being different from the nonabstinence-teaching population of alcohol users. A prevention specialist or therapist dealing with an LDS alcohol user without acknowledging the apparent distinctive LDS attributes would likely be limited in effectiveness. A professional neglecting this responsibility would be similar to someone intervening with a teenage alcohol user without dealing with the developmental issues of adolescence or intervening with a Hispanic without accepting cross-cultural and language differences. Finally, to ask or imply that an LDS alcohol user must "stop going to church" or become "less active in that church" during treatment ignores the existence of the same psychosocial barrier that perhaps expedited the heavier drinking in the first place. To simply overlook and to set aside the religious issues limit an LDS alcohol user access to powerful resources that otherwise might be available in recovery. Additional research and model building must be completed to further evaluate and duplicate the conclusions of this chapter.

References

[1] G. Lawson and A. Lawson. (1989) *Alcohol and Substance Abuse in Special Populations.* Aspen, Rockville, MD.

[2] A. Beigel and S. Ghertner (1977) Toward a social model: An assessment of social factors which influence problem drinking and its treatment, in *Treatment and rehabilitation of the Chronic Alcoholic.* (B. Kissin and H. Begleiter, eds.) Plenum, NY, pp. 197–233.

[3] J. F. Smith (1976) *Teachings of the Prophet Joseph Smith* (Deseret Book, Salt Lake City, UT), p. 117.

[4] R. Straus and S. D. Bacon (1953) *Drinking in College* (Yale University, New Haven, CT).

[5] Charlotte Drug Education Center. Overview of key findings. [Record Number 11102] National clearing house for alcohol information, 1983.

[6] E. Jones (1957) *Student Drinking in the High Schools of Utah.* Unpub. doctoral dissertation, University of Utah, Salt Lake City, UT.

[7] J. F. Hoadley, B. C. Fuchs, and H. D. Holder (1984) The effect of alcohol beverage restrictions on consumption: A 25-Year longitudinal analysis. *Amer. J. of Drug Alcohol Abuse* **10**, 375–401.

[8] R. E. Johns (1981) Risk-factor-prevalence survey-Utah. *Morbidity and Mortality Weekly Report* **30**, 253–254, 259.

[9] R. D. Hawks (1989) Alcohol use trends among LDS high school seniors in America from 1982–1986. *J. Assoc. Mormon Counselors and Psychotherapists (AMCAP)* Brigham Young University, Provo, UT, **15**, 43–51.

[10] I. Thorner (1953) Ascetic protestantism and alcoholism. *Psychiatry* **16**, 167–176.

[11] R. D. Hawks (1987) *An Analysis of Alcohol Use Patterns Among Adolescent Members of the LDS Church.* Unpub. doctoral dissertation, Brigham Young University, UT.

[12] J. H. Skolnick (1958) Religious affiliation and drinking behavior. *J. of Studies on Alcohol* **19**, 452–470.

[13] D. Cahalan, I. H. Cisin, and H. M. Crossley (1969) American drinking practices: A national study of drinking behavior and attitude. *Monogr. Rutgers Center of Alcoholism Studies,* #6.

[14] E. H. Mizruchi and R. Perrucci (1962) Norm qualities and differential effects of deviant behavior: An exploratory analysis. *Am. Sociol. Review* **27**, 391–399.

[15] E. H. Mizruchi and R. Perrucci (1962) Norm qualities and differential effects of deviant behavior: An exploratory analysis. *Am. Sociol. Review* **27**, 398.

[16] R. F. Bales (1946) Cultural differences in rates of alcoholism. *Q. J. of Stud. on Alcohol* **6**, 480–499.

[17] E. Blacker (1966) Sociocultural factors in alcoholism. *International Psychiatry Clinics* **3** (2), 51–80.

[18] R. C. Conley and A. A. Sorensen (1971) *The Staggering Steeple* (Pilgrim, Philadelphia, PA), p. 15.

[19] J. D. Preston (1969) Religiosity and adolescent drinking behavior. *The Soc. Quart.* **10**, 372–383.

[20] J. D. Preston (1969) Religiosity and adolescent drinking behavior. *The Soc. Q.* **10**, 382.

[21] R. Straus and S. D. Bacon (1953) *Drinking in College* (Yale University, New Haven, CT).

[22] C. R. Snyder (1958) *Alcohol and the Jews* (Yale University, New Haven, CT).

[23] C. R. Snyder (1958) *Alcohol and the Jews* (Yale University, New Haven, CT), p. 191.

[24]F. E. Moss and F. V. Janzen (1980) *Types of Drinkers in Indian Communities*, Western Region Alcoholism Training Center, University of Utah, Salt Lake City, UT.

[25]W. E. Smith (1969) *The Word of Wisdom: A Test of the Predictability of Human Behavior* (Brigham Young University, Provo, UT).

[26]W. E. Smith (1969) *The Word of Wisdom: A Test of the Predictability of Human Behavior* (Brigham Young University, Provo, UT) pp. 6–1.

[27]S. L. Albrecht Alcohol Consumption and Abuse. Paper presented at Utah Academy of Arts and Sciences at Brigham Young University, UT, May, 1985.

[28]S. D. Bacon (1957) Social setting conducive to alcoholism. *JAMA* **164**, 177–181.

[29]Utah Department of Social Services. Alcohol and drug use and abuse in Utah. State Division of Alcoholism and Drugs, Salt Lake City, UT, 1985.

[30]C. R. Snyder (1962) Culture and Jewish sobriety: The ingroup-outgroup factor, in *Society, culture and drinking patterns* (D. H. Pittman and C. R. Snyder, eds.), Wiley, NY.

[31]M. M. Glatt (1970) Alcoholism and drug dependence among Jews. *Br. J. Addict.* **64**, 297–304.

[32]D. B. Kandel and M. Sudit (1982) Drinking practices among urban adults in Israel. *J. Stud. and Alcohol* **43**, 1–16.

[33]M. K. Bacon, H. J. Barry and I. L. Child (1965) A cross-cultural study of drinking II: Relations to other features of cultures. *Q. J. of Stud. Alcohol* **3**, 29–48

[34]J. V. Rachal, S. Maisto, L. L. Guess and R. L. Hubbard (1980) Alcohol use among youth, in Alcohol and Health Monograph #1 DHHS (ADM) 82-1190. US Government Printing Office, Washington DC, 55–95.

[35]D. B. Kandel (1982) Epidemiological and psychosocial perspectives on adolescent drug use. *J. Am. Academic Clinical Psychiatry* **21**, 328–347.

[36]R. Jessor, J. A. Chase and J. E. Donovan (1980) Psychosocial correlates of marijuana use and problem drinking in a national sample of adolescents. *Am. J. of Public Health* **70**, 604–613.

[37]D. E. Gersick, K. Grady, E. Sexton, and M. Lyons (1981) Personality and sociodemographic factors in adolescent drug use, in *Drug Abuse and the American Adolescent* (D.J. Lettieri and J. P. Ludford, eds.) National Institute on Drug Abuse Research Mono 38, DHEW (ADM) 81-1166. US Government Printing Office, Washington, DC.

[38]R. Briscoe (1966) *The Extent of Drug Use Among Students in Davis School District* Unpub doctoral dissertation, University of UT, Salt Lake City, UT.

[39]Utah State Office of Education. Utah 1972 statewide drug assessment. Division of Curriculum Development, Salt Lake City, UT, 1974.

[40]S. J. Bahr and A. C. Marcos (1984) Drug use among Utah secondary students, 1984. Utah Division of Alcoholism & Drugs, Salt Lake City, UT.

[41]A. Y. Amoateng and S. J. Bahr (1984) Family, religion, and adolescent drug

use (Class project). Brigham Young University, Provo, UT, Family and Demographic Research Institute .

[42] W. E. Smith (1958) An ecological study of L. D. S. orthodoxy. Brigham Young University, Provo, UT, 1958.

[43] C. W. Telford (1950) A study of religious attitudes. *J. Soc. Psych.* **31,** 217–230.

[44] J. L. Lyon (1982) Cancer in Utah Mormon men by lay priesthood level. *Amer. J. Epidemiol.* **116**(2), 243–257.

[45] J. L. Lyon (1982) Cancer in Utah Mormon women by church activity level. *Amer. J. of Epidemiol.* **116**(2), 258–265.

[46] A. M. Greeley, W. C. McCready, and G. Theisen (1980) *Ethnic Drinking Subcultures* (Praeger, New York).

[47] M. A. Flasher and S. A. Maisto (1984) A review of theory and research on drinking patterns among Jews. *J. of Nervous and Mental Disease* **172,** 596–603.

[48] R. J. Glynn, J. S. LoCastro, J. A. Hermos, and R. Bosse (1983) Social contexts and motives for drinking in men. *J. Stud. Alcohol* **44,** 1011–1024.

[49] W. M. Mathews (1975) A critique of traditional drug education programs. *J. Drug Ed.* **5,** 57–64.

[50] S. R. Burkett (1977) Religion, parental influence, and adolescent alcohol and marijuana use. *J. of Drug Issues* **7,** 263–273.

[51] T. E. Smith. (1984) Reviewing adolescent marijuana abuse. *Social Work* **29,** 17–21.

[52] T. F. Plaut (1967) *Alcohol Problems: A Report to the Nation* (Oxford University, NY).

[53] R. C. Conley and A. A. Sorensen (1971) *The Staggering Steeple* (Pilgrim, Philadelphia, PA).

[54] J. Royce (1985) Sin or solace? Religious views on alcohol and alcoholism. *J. Drug Issues* **15,** 51–61.

[55] G. N. Pearson (1970) *There Is a Way Back* (Trilogy Art, Provo, UT)

[56] R. Wootton (1976) Who Killed the Group? Unpub. manuscript, Brigham Young University, Educational Psychology Depart, Provo, UT.

[57] J. Livingstone (1981) *A Case Study of Indian Families Participating in a Church—Sponsored Alcohol Intervention Pilot Program.* Unpub master's thesis, University of Regina, Saskatchewan, Canada.

[58] R. D. Hawks and E. Buckner (1985) S.A.V.E.... more than just a four-letter word. *J. Assoc. Mormon Counselors and Psychotherapists (AMCAP)* Brigham Young University, UT, **11.**

[59] R. A. Little (1985) Mormons face alcoholism. *Alcoholism* **5,** 24,25.

Hispanic Drug Abuse

Culturally Appropriate Prevention and Treatment

Barbara V. Marin

Hispanics are a special cultural group requiring a culturally appropriate approach to drug abuse prevention and treatment. This chapter will provide background on the current drug abuse situation among Hispanics, and will show how a better understanding of Hispanic culture could aid in treatment and prevention efforts.

Drug Abuse Problem Among Hispanics

Recent reviews suggest that Hispanics are more likely than nonHispanic whites to become involved in substance abuse,[1,2] and that use of "hard drugs" remains essentially an ethnic minority phenomenon. The consequences of this drug use, including crime, health problems, prison terms, family disruption, violence, prostitution, and recently, spread of HIV and large numbers of AIDS cases in these communities, are clearly devastating to minority communities.[3,4]

Based on a thoughtful and comprehensive review of the drug abuse and drug treatment literature, Tucker[2] makes a cogent case for the need for:

1. Research on drug abuse treatment and prevention needs of minority communities;
2. Drug abuse theories that account for the special circumstances of these populations; and

3. Alternative treatment models that are culturally appropriate.

Current substance abuse treatment efforts have failed to show an impact on the drug abuse problem in minority communities, which has recently grown worse in many communities with the advent of crack cocaine.

The purpose of this chapter is to provide an understanding of cultural factors that must be considered in developing culturally appropriate drug abuse treatment and prevention programs. The next section will outline important elements of Hispanic culture and how cultural factors may influence the course of drug abuse and treatment. Based on these cultural factors, a series of ideas will be presented for developing culturally appropriate community-level prevention interventions, and data on the feasibility of these interventions will be presented. Finally, ideas for increasing the cultural relevance of current drug abuse treatment approaches are suggested.

Hispanic Culture

Allocentrism

Hispanic culture differs in important ways from the individualistic, competitive, achievement-oriented culture of mainstream US society. Hispanic culture is allocentric,[5] that is, other-oriented or collectivistic. Members of allocentric cultures are typically more concerned with the group than the individual.[6] This concern for others is expressed in Hispanic culture both in a strong family orientation and in an emphasis on smooth social relations.

Familialism

Familialism, or a strong family orientation, is a very strong cultural value that manifests itself in feelings of economic and emotional obligation among family members, as well as the tendency for family members to seek help from each other, rather than outside the family.[7] In familialistic cultures, family members are important normative referents, that is, their attitudes and values are important guides to other family members.

This family orientation manifests itself in close relationships and involvement with the extended family, including uncles and cousins. Indeed, a special category of kinship exists for Hispanics. "Compadres" and "comadres" are close family friends who are given the status of relatives (co-parents literally). These fictive kin are treated like family members in most respects. Thus, a family member who becomes motivated to reach out or talk to other family members about drug use, as suggested later in this chapter, will often feel obligated to talk to a larger number of people who are considered his or her "family."

The motivating power of this family orientation should be used in developing prevention and treatment messages. Strong family ties of Hispanics can be used as a motivator to get off drugs. Messages to Hispanics about drugs might portray the bad example that drug abuse gives to one's children or siblings or the failure of the drug-using father to protect and provide for his family. Motivation for the Hispanic drug user to seek treatment may also be increased if reconciliation with the family will be an outcome.

Hispanic family involvement in drug prevention efforts could also be very practical. Until now, prevention efforts have focused primarily on school-based activities, meaning that children from a variety of ethnic backgrounds are reached by the same message. By involving the Hispanic family as the source of anti-drug messages, intervenors are free to design messages that are specific to and supportive of Hispanic culture, thus increasing the power of the message and, hopefully, the self-esteem of the children who hear it.

Simpatia

In addition to this strong family orientation, Hispanics place great value on smooth, pleasant social relationships. "Simpatia" is a Hispanic social "script" or behavioral scheme, that describes a set of expected behaviors that maintain these smooth relationships. The "simpatico," a person who is skilled in maintaining such relationships and making others feel comfortable and happy in social settings, is a highly valued individual.[8] "Simpatia" has important implications for those designing drug treatment for Hispanics, since confrontation and assertiveness are incompatible with being "simpatico."

Respeto

Another important factor in Hispanic social relationships is "respeto," that is, a perceived need for all individuals to be treated with deference and respect. This emphasis on respect may be seen in the two forms that Spanish provides for saying "you" when addressing someone: "usted" (the more formal) and "tu." The proper use of these forms of address is very important when counseling Hispanics.[9]

Hispanic addicts may have special needs to feel respected. Wurzman, et al.[10] suggest that the addict in withdrawal is "pathetic, dangerous, and untrustworthy—the antithesis of machismo and respectability," two crucial Hispanic values. Hispanic clients must be taught that seeking treatment is not an admission of failure, but a means of achieving the respect they seek.

Gender Roles

Hispanic culture has defined certain gender role-related behaviors for both men and women. Hispanic men are expected to be strong, in control, and to provide for their families ("machismo"). Hispanic women often assume traditional gender roles, although these roles are far more complex than previously recognized.[11] Gender-role behaviors in Hispanic culture probably account for a number of differences between male and female Hispanic addicts.

The female Hispanic addict tends to differ both from male Hispanic addicts and nonHispanic female addicts. Several authors observe that Hispanic female addicts are less likely to engage in prostitution.[12,13] Hispanic females are less likely than males to be found in treatment programs, probably because of lower drug abuse in this group. Those Hispanic women who do use drugs may be more marginal to both mainstream and Hispanic society.[13-16] Traditional Hispanic culture prohibits any type of drug use among women, which has resulted in low reported use of drugs, including alcohol and tobacco, among less acculturated Hispanic women.[17,18]

Other research finds that Chicano men in drug treatment are less psychologically impaired than nonHispanic whites,[19] suggesting that drug use may be less counternormative in this group than among either Hispanic women or nonHispanic whites. This finding indicates that community projects to change norms regarding drug use could be especially effective in this group.

Acculturation

Acculturation is the process of adaptation to and adoption of mainstream cultural values by those of another culture, in this case, Hispanics. This process has been associated with a number of risk behaviors. The more highly acculturated Hispanics, that is, those who have adopted mainstream values and lifestyles, more commonly use alcohol and drugs.[20] Santisteban found children of immigrants are more involved with drug use than immigrants.[21] This increased drug use may in part be a way of coping with acculturation stress, since the assimilation process implies devaluation of who one is. In one study, Hispanic youths who were bicultural, that is, adapted to both their Hispanic heritage and mainstream culture, were rated as better adjusted than those who were oriented to only one of these two cultures.[22]

The cultural factors mentioned in the preceding paragraphs are merely hypotheses, and empirical data are needed to clarify them and identify the nuances. Other research has been conducted to identify cultural aspects of smoking cessation among Hispanics, and the results suggest the importance of this type of research. Prior to the development of a community intervention to promote smoking cessation among San Francisco Hispanics, a study of 263 Hispanic smokers and 150 nonHispanic white smokers was conducted to identify the smoking behaviors and culture-specific consequences of smoking among Hispanic smokers. It was found that Hispanics view certain consequences of smoking or quitting as much more important than nonHispanic whites. These include the effects of smoking on the health of other family members, smoking as a bad example to the children, and the bad smell of cigarets. NonHispanic smokers were more concerned about individualistic issues, such as withdrawal symptoms, as important consequences of smoking cessation.[23] This research allowed the identification of powerful cultural consequences of smoking, which were then used to promote nonsmoking effectively.

Careful research that identifies these cultural issues regarding drug use and abuse should be the basis for any intervention in the Hispanic community. The ideas proposed below to develop culturally appropriate community-level prevention interventions and drug abuse treatment programs must necessarily be based on this detailed knowledge of Hispanic culture and its relationship to drug use.

Drug Abuse Intervention Ideas

Two levels of intervention ideas will be suggested here: (1) a community-level intervention that informs the entire community about drug abuse, motivates those using drugs to stop or seek treatment, and prevents youths from becoming involved, and (2) culturally appropriate drug abuse treatment. These dual aspects are necessary because drug abuse is such a complex, multiply determined behavior. Orford[24] has recently been proposed that addiction be viewed not so much as a disease, but as a complex behavior involving some personality and biological components and also strong environmental influences. Other authors have indicated that drug addiction is strongly influenced by environmental conditions. As an illustration, several authors[25,26] found drug availability from friends and ease of acquisition to explain much adolescent drug use.

A community-level intervention can build competence, provide social support for behavior change, empower the local community, and change the social norms regarding drug abuse.[27] Community-level interventions have been effective in changing a variety of behaviors, including sexual behavior,[28,29] adolescent drug use,[30] and smoking.[31] These interventions work because they effectively change community norms and other environmental variables that influence individual behavior.

Feasibility of a Community Intervention for Hispanics

In order for a community intervention to be effective, community members must be able to contact those who are at risk and those actively abusing drugs. In a recent random-digit-dialing survey of 460 San Francisco Hispanics, 9% of those interviewed said they had a relative who injects drugs (Barbara Marin and Gerardo Marin, unpublished data). If asked about friends and acquaintances who inject drugs, the percentage would probably be much higher. This suggests that some, although not all, Hispanics currently have contact with a drug user. If we consider those who know someone at risk for drug use (including all adolescents), an intervention that encourages community members to talk to those at risk about drug use becomes very reasonable. Considering the drug user's viewpoint, Cervantes et al.[32] found that of 98 consecutive admissions to methadone maintenance, 67% lived with a family member and 75% claimed close relationships with their mothers, supporting the idea that drug users are not isolated and unreachable. Scott et al.[12] found that only 3% of their Chicano clients did not live with their families.

However, although Hispanics may have contact with or live with active drug users and those at risk, they must be willing to talk to them about drug use in order for this type of community intervention to be effective. Research by the author and others suggests that Hispanics are willing to intervene with those at risk. The same 460 Hispanic community members were asked whether they would be willing to talk to a relative who uses drugs about not using drugs, not sharing needles, and cleaning needles with bleach, and over 90% responded that they definitely would be willing to do so. These percentages did not differ by gender, although the English-speaking Hispanics were more willing to talk about cleaning needles with bleach than the Spanish-speaking. Jimenez[33] found that Puerto Rican parents who were aware of their children's drug use became angry and concerned, and approximately half of them sought some type of outside help, often from extended family members. Several authors[12,33] have also observed that Hispanic drug users have abundant family resources available to them.

Another study by the author again suggests that Hispanics would intervene with those using drugs. In a separate study, 217 Hispanic and 202 nonHispanic white community members were interviewed, as well as 28 Hispanic and 39 nonHispanic white clients of drug treatment programs. Respondents were asked to rate various reasons for intervening with a hypothetical drug using family member. The Hispanic respondents were more convinced than the nonHispanic white respondents that a family member who uses drugs would follow their advice to stop using drugs and that their advice would help to protect the drug user's wife from HIV infection.[34] Although overall Hispanic and nonHispanic white respondents were equally willing to intervene with this hypothetical drug using relative, community members of both ethnicities were significantly more willing than drug treatment clients to talk to this relative about not injecting drugs and not sharing needles. Curiously, community members were more fearful than the drug treatment clients that the drug user would be offended if these issues were raised.[35]

This study also asked respondents who they felt should intervene with the hypothetical relative who uses intravenous drugs, since Hispanics place greater value on the advice of family members and those who are older.[34] As expected, striking differences were found in responses between the two cultural groups, and these differences were consistent for both drug treatment clients and community members. When asked whether a family member, a friend, or someone else should talk to a drug user about AIDS prevention techniques, including stopping drug use, almost half of the Hispanic respondents felt the family member should talk to the hypothetical relative, but only about one-fourth of nonHispanic whites said this. When asked whether the person to intervene should be older, the same age, or younger, about 40% of Hispanics felt the person should be older, compared to only 20% of non Hispanic whites. Both Hispanics and nonHispanic whites felt the person should be the same gender as the drug user, but Hispanic community members also frequently said that the gender of the intervenor was not important. These results are consistent with Hispanic culture, with its emphasis on solving problems within the family and respect for those older than oneself.

Community Intervention Ideas

To be maximally effective, community interventions designed to change behavior must provide credible, culturally appropriate messages through all available media channels over a prolonged period.[36] Such interventions must ultimately change community norms surrounding the behaviors to be changed, reducing the social reinforcements for drug use while increasing reinforcements for alternative behavior. Community interventions should have the following elements, described in more detail below: family and community involvement, messages reaching the community through multiple channels, including radio and television, print, direct personal contact, and incentives or reinforcement for behavior change, with previously identified, culturally appropriate messages used throughout.

Family Involvement

A community-level intervention designed to prevent initiation and lower current drug abuse in Hispanic communities would seek to change the environment of the drug user by encouraging family members to become concerned and talk to the user about drug use and its dangers. Family members would use reasons for avoiding drug use that emphasize the positive values of Hispanic culture. A detailed guide for family members who wish to help drug abusing relatives, as well as understand why they abuse drugs, has already been developed by Sorensen and Bernal.[37]

Community Involvement

A community-level intervention must rely heavily on collaboration from local community members, as advisors to an intervention team, community leaders and workers in community organizations who reach out to others, and individuals talking to family and friends about drug use. Community involvement and "ownership" of this intervention will ensure that the most appropriate and effective methods are used, and community members will feel empowered to solve their own problems in creative ways.

Multiple Media

Such an intervention must utilize multiple communication channels, literally to "blanket" the community with the message.[36] Hispanics rely heavily on Spanish-language radio for information, so this medium is key, and talk shows as well as public service announcements should be used. Spanish-language television should also be utilized, including segments as part of news broadcasts. Community outreach workers should contact local groups, and present information and motivational messages directly to the community at meetings of fraternal organizations, community groups, and churches.

Printed Materials

Printed materials that present culturally appropriate messages should be developed and made available widely. The Spanish-language *Guia para dejar de fumar/Guide to quit smoking* [38] was developed based on the data about Hispanic cultural values related to smoking, and then carefully pre-tested to increase comprehension and motivating power. This guide uses testimonials from the community, graphic pictures of the effects of smoking, and culturally appropriate reasons for quitting. Full-color photographs and professional production make the booklet more costly, but also less likely to be discarded. A recent unpublished survey indicates that 25% of the Hispanic community in San Francisco have a copy of the Guide in their home after a 19 mo antismoking campaign.

Incentives

Another effective way to promote behavior change is through incentives. In work with smoking cessation, harder-to-reach men have been most effectively contacted through a quit-smoking contest. A chance for a $500 prize is offered to those who sign up to quit smoking and can prove through chemical analysis that they are not current smokers at the time the prize is given. Some monetary reward might be considered for entering drug treatment and remaining drug free, as an incentive for those who might otherwise not consider treatment. Certainly, the current situation of waiting lists for drug treatment is discouraging to many who might seek it.

Role Models

Community campaigns can use role models to teach about the behavior change in ways that are appropriate and interesting to the community. Individuals who have had drug-related experiences can explain the negative effects of drugs, how they were able to change their habit, and what benefits they have experienced. These testimonials can be used for public service announcements, documentaries, newspaper stories in local Spanish-language papers, and antidrug printed materials for drug users and adolescents. These testimonials must be carefully developed and pretested, so that they are clear, motivating, and do not conflict with other messages in the campaign.

Community-level campaigns, when developed in a culturally appropriate manner, can be effective in changing the behaviors of Hispanics. The author has been involved in a community-level intervention that employs culturally appropriate reasons to quit smoking transmitted through multiple media and other channels, and utilizing community role models. Preliminary results of this campaign indicate a major drop in smoking prevalence over preintervention levels, after 18 mo of intervention.

Improving Current Treatment Approaches

Although a community intervention may be effective in ending and preventing some drug abuse, culturally appropriate treatment programs are an important adjunct to any such intervention. This section will describe reasons for the current underutilization of treatment programs by Hispanics, as well as suggest improvements in current programs to attract and retain Hispanic clients.

Hispanics have tended to underutilize the treatment facilities currently available, but much of this underutilization may be explained by treatments that are inappropriate to Hispanic culture. In some ways, Hispanic culture can be incompatible with seeking help for a drug problem. In Hispanic culture, difficult and embarrassing problems, such as drug abuse, are solved within the family whenever possible. The loyalty of Hispanic family members to one another and the need for the family to present a good image to the outside world dictate that a problem such as drug abuse will often be hidden.[20]

Even if the Hispanic drug abuser overcomes this inherent cultural tendency to solve the problem within the family, traditional approaches to drug treatment (detoxification, methadone maintenance, and therapeutic communities) may be very unattractive. Methadone maintenance has been criticized as an "easy way out," since the client remains addicted, which contradicts a "macho" image. In therapeutic communities, the recovering-addict community becomes the addict's "family," which is culturally very inappropriate for Hispanics, who place special emphasis on their families and cannot substitute them easily.[33] In fact, the families of Puerto Rican addicts were found to be significantly more supportive and less pathological and drug-involved than the families of white nonHispanic addicts.[33]

All treatment approaches require the addicts to admit they need help and are not in control, an admission that Hispanic men find very difficult to make because of the cultural value of "machismo."[39] Any treatment approach that humiliates or degrades the individual in front of others is also problematic, since it would conflict with Hispanic cultural values of respect.[33]

Besides avoiding approaches to drug treatment that conflict with cultural values, a few changes might increase the success of current treatment programs. Hispanic family members should be more actively involved in the treatment process.[40] Family members can be encouraged to motivate the client to enter treatment, to support behavior change properly, and to provide reinforcement to prevent relapse.

Certain changes could make Hispanic drug treatment clients feel more welcome. Treatment staff should include significant numbers of Hispanics to maximize effectiveness.[14] Although it seems obvious, staff who speak Spanish and treatment materials available in Spanish are essential elements, but there is often a lack of these.[20] Written materials must be more than translations of materials currently available in English, and should incorporate cultural values and culturally appropriate reasons for behavior change.

There is an urgent need for research that identifies the culturally relevant consequences of drug abuse, so staff members can be trained to intervene more appropriately, using this information when talking to clients about reasons for change. A number of services could be routinely offered and emphasized for Hispanic addicts. Jimenez[33] suggests that treatment programs provide vocational and educational services, including English as a second language, since low levels of education, lack of work skills, language problems, and poor health are often problems of the Hispanic addict. Programs should also provide legal services and referrals, both for clients with criminal involvement and for those who are undocumented. One study has indicated that, although only a small number of Hispanic addicts entered religious programs (Pentecostal type), those who entered were highly successful at avoiding relapse,[41] suggesting that such programs may have elements that deserve further study. Certainly, such programs should routinely be made available to Hispanic addicts entering treatment.

In summary, drug abuse treatment and prevention programs targeting Hispanics must respect Hispanic cultural values of familialism, "simpatia," "respeto," and "machismo." Research to identify how these values might be used to create culturally appropriate, antidrug messages is urgently needed. Some research suggests the feasibility of motivating families to intervene with Hispanic drug users. Family focused, community-level interventions should utilize multiple media, culturally appropriate messages, and role models to reach drug users, their families, and those at risk. Drug treatment approaches for Hispanics could also benefit from a clearer understanding of and respect for Hispanic cultural values, including greater involvement of family members in treatment, more emphasis on changing the marginal conditions that lead to drug abuse, such as unemployment, and avoidance of culturally inappropriate approaches, such as confrontation.

A culturally sensitive approach to drug abuse and treatment for Hispanics has a number of advantages over current approaches. First, the interventions should be highly motivating to Hispanic drug users and community members. Second, because many of the interventions involve the entire community, the messages will affect not only those in need of drug treatment, but also those at risk. Changes in the community norms regarding drug use will have important effects on adolescents and preadolescents who tend to try drugs initially because their friends try them.

Reaching the Hispanic drug user through his or her family has the advantage of being highly culturally appropriate in a group with strong family orientation. Given Hispanics' feelings of closeness and involvement with family members as well as extended family and fictive kin, an intervention that motivates Hispanics to talk to their "family" about drug use will have far-reaching effects. Finally, this approach should enhance Hispanics' pride in their own culture and cultural values. Capitalizing on the strengths of Hispanic culture can be a key to effective drug abuse treatment and prevention in this community.

Acknowledgments

The author gratefully acknowledges the comments of Gerardo Marin and James L. Sorensen on an earlier draft of this chapter. Barbara Marin, Gerardo Marin, and James L. Sorensen, and Rolando Juarez collaborated on the previously unpub-lished study described here.

References

[1] J. Mandel and O. Bordatto (1980) DAWN: A second look—its impact on minorities and public policy. *Am. J. Drug Alcohol Abuse* **7(3,4)** 361–377.

[2] M. Tucker (1985) U. S. ethnic minorities and drug abuse: An assessment of the science and practice. *Int. J. Addict.* **20(6,7)**, 1021–1047.

[3] R. Bakeman, E. McCray, J. R. Lumb, R. E. Jackson, and P. N. Whitley (1987) The incidence of AIDS among Blacks and Hispanics. *J. Nat. Med. Assoc.* **79**, 921–928.

[4] R. M. Selik, K. G. Castro, and M. Pappaioanou (1988) Racial/ethnic differences in risk of AIDS. *Am. J. Public Health* **78**, 1539–1545.

[5] G. Marin, and H. C. Triandis (1985) Allocentrism as an important characteristic of the behavior of Latin Americans and Hispanics, in *Cross-Cultural and National Studies* (R. Diaz-Guerrero, ed.), Elsevier Amsterdam, pp. 85–104.

[6] G. Hofstede (1980) *Culture's Consequences* (Sage, Beverly Hills, CA).

[7] F. Sabogal, B. Marin, G. Marin, R. Otero-Sabogal, and E. Perez-Stable (1988) *Guia para dejar de fumar. Quit Smoking Guide.* Government Printing Office. National Cancer Institute, Washington, DC, NIH Publication No. 88-3001.

[8] H. C. Triandis, G. Marin, J. Lisansky and H. Betacourt (1984) Simpatía as a Cultural Script of Hispanics. *J. Pers. Soc. Psychol.* **47**, 1365–1375.

[9] A. Carballo-Diéguez, A. (1988) Hispanic culture, gay male culture, and AIDS: Counseling implications. *J. Counseling and Development,* **68 (Sept/Oct)** 26–30.

[10] I. Wurzman, B. Rounsaville, and H. Kleber (1983) Cultural values of Puerto Rican opiate addicts: An exploratory study. *Am. J. Drug Alcohol Abuse* **9(2)**, 141–153.

[11] H. Amaro (1988) Women in the Mexican-American community. *J. Community Psychol.* **16(1)**, 6–20.

[12] N. Scott, W. Orzen, C. Musillo, and P. Cole (1973) Methadone in the southwest: A three year follow-up of Chicano heroin addicts. *Am. J. Orthopsychiatry,* **43(3)**, 355–361.

[13] M. Anglin, M. Booth, T. Ryan, and Y.-I. Hser (1988) Ethnic differences in narcotics addition. II. Chicano and Anglo addiction career patterns. *Int. J. Addict.* **23(12)** 1011–1027.

[14] J. Langrod, L. Alksne, J. Lowinson, and P. Ruiz (1981) Rehabilitation of the Puerto Rican addict: A cultural perspective. *Int. J. Addict.* **16(5)**, 841–847.

[15] A. F. Sanchez (1978) Drug abuse and treatment of the "tecato" or Mexican-American junkie, in *A Multicultural View of Drug Abuse. Proceedings of the National Drug Abuse Conference, 1977* (S. M. D. E. Smith Anderson, M. Buxton, N. Gottlieb, W. Harvey, and T. Chung, eds.), Schenckman, Cambridge, MA pp. 574–579.

[16] A. G. Gomez and D. M. Vega (1981) The Hispanic addict, in *Substance Abuse,*

Clinical Problems and Perspectives (J. H. Lowinson and P. Ruiz, eds.), Williams and Wilkins, Baltimore, MD, pp.717-728.

[17]R. Caetano (1986) Patterns and problems of drinking among U. S. Hispanics. *Reports of the Secretary's Task Force on Black and Minority Health*. U. S. Department of Health and Human Services, Washington, DC, pp. 142-186.

[18]G. Marin, B. Marin, and E. J. Perez-Stable (1989) Cigarette smoking among San Francisco Hispanics: The role of acculturation and gender. *Am. J. Public Health* **79**, 196-198.

[19]W. E. Penk, R. Robinowitz, W. R. Roberts, M. P. Dolan, and H. G. Atkins, (1981) MMPI differences of male Hispanic-American, Black, and White heroin addicts. *J. Consult. Clin. Psychol.* **49**, 488-490.

[20]C. Smith-Peterson (1983) Substance abuse treatment and cultural diversity, in *Substance Abuse Pharmacologic, Developmental and Clinical Perspectives* (G. Bennet, C. Vourakis, and D. Woolf, eds.), Wiley, NY, pp. 370-382.

[21]D. Santisteban and J. Szapocznik (1982) *The Hispanic Substance Abuser: The Search for Prevention Strategies* (Grune & Stratton, NY).

[22]J. Szapocznik, A. Perez-Vidal, A. Brickman, F. Foote, D. Santisteban, O. Hervis, and W. Kurtines (1988) Engaging adolescent drug abusers and their families in treatment: A strategic structural systems approach. *Consult. and Clin. Psychol.* **56** (4), 552-557.

[23]B. V. Marin, G. Marin, R. Otero-Sabogal, F. Sabogal, and E. J. Perez-Stable (1990) Cultural differences in attitudes toward smoking: Developing messages using the Theory of Reasoned Action. *J. App. Social Psychol.* **20**, 478-493.

[24]J. Orford (1985) *Excessive Appetites: A Psychological View of Addictions* (John Wiley & Sons, Chichester).

[25]R. J. Akers, R. L. Burgess, and W. T. Johnson (1968) Opiate use, addiction, and relapse. *Social Problems*, **15**(4) 459-469.

[26]E. Maddahian, M. D. Newcomb, and P. M. Bentler (1986) Adolescents' substance use: Impact of ethnicity, income, and availability. *Advances in Alcohol & Substance Abuse* **5**(3), 63-78.

[27]E. L. Gesten and L. A. Jason (1987) Social and community interventions. *Ann. Rev. Psychol.* **38**, 427-460.

[28]M. L. Vincent, A. F. Clearie, and M. D. Schluchter (1987) Reducing adolescent pregnancy through school and community-based education. *JAMA* **257**(24), 3382-3386.

[29]C. Amezcua, A. Ramirez, A. McAllister, R. McCuan, C. Galavotti, and C. Reed (1989) *Effects of a Spanish-Language Community Intervention in Southwest Texas on Reported HIV Infection Knowledge. Attitudes and Behavior* (V International Conference on AIDS, Montreal, Canada).

[30]M. Pentz, J. Dwyer, D. MacKinnon, B. Flay, W. Hansen, E. Wang, and C.

Johnson (1989) A multicommunity trial for primary prevention of adolescent drug abuse: Effects on drug use prevalence. *JAMA* **261**(22), 3259–3266.

[31]P. Puska (1984) Community-based prevention of cardiovascular disease: the North Karelia Project, in *Behavioral Health: A Handbook of Health Enhancement and Disease Prevention* (J. Matarazzo, S. Weiss, J. Herd, N. Miller, and S. Weiss, eds.), Wiley, NY.

[32]O. F. Cervantes, J. L. Sorensen, L. Wermuth, L. Fernandez, and L. Menicucci (1988) Family ties of drug abusers. *Psychology of Addictive Behaviors* **2**(1), 34–39.

[33]D. R. Jimenez (1980) *A comparative analysis of the support systems of White and Puerto Rican clients in drug treatment program* (Century Twenty-One Publishing, Saratoga, CA).

[34]B. V. Marin, G. Marin, and R. Juarez (1990) Differences between Hispanics and non-Hispanics in willingness to provide AIDS prevention advice. *Hispanic J. Behavioral Sciences* **12**(2), 153–164.

[35]B. Marin, G. Marin, R. Juarez, and J. Sorensen (under review) *Prevention from Family Members and a Strategy for Preventing HIV Transmission Among Intravenous Drug Users.*

[36]B. R. Flay (1987) Mass media and smoking cessation: A critical review. *Am. J. Public Health* **77**(2), 153–161.

[37]J. L. Sorensen and G. Bernal (1987) *A Family Like Yours: Breaking the Patterns of Drug Abuse* (Harper & Row, San Francisco, CA).

[38]F. Sabogal, G. Marin, R. Otero-Sabogal, B. Marin, and E. Perez-Stable (1987) Hispanic familism and acculturation: What changes and what doesn't. *Hispanic J. Behavioral Sciences* **9**(4), 397–412.

[39]A. Alcocer (1980) Perspective: An alcohol health and research world interview feature. *Alcohol Health and Research World* **4**, 29–30.

[40]M. A. Scopetta, J. Szapocznik, O. E. King, R. Ladner, C. Alegre, and W. S. Tillman (1977) *Final report: The Spanish Drug Rehabilitation Research Project* (Spanish Family Guidance Clinic-Encuentro, University of Miami School of Medicine, Miami, FL).

[41]D. P. Desmond and J. F. Maddux (1981) Religious programs and careers of chronic heroin users. *Am. J. Drug Alcohol Abuse* **8**(1), 71–83.

Prevention of Substance Abuse Problems in Women

Barbara W. Lex

Introduction

Over the past 20 years, perceptions of women and their problems have been altered by the changing sociopolitical climate in the US. Shifts in attitudes have prompted questioning of traditional assumptions. The women's liberation movement exposed a wide range of social issues pertinent to women, and focused both public and professional attention on the legitimacy of research and treatment for women as a "special population."

Scant attention in earlier *alcohol* research appears to have been associated with various popular notions that sociocultural factors protected women from alcohol abuse, that alcohol dependence was similar in men and women, or that alcoholic women were more deviant, psychologically disturbed, and difficult to study and treat.[1-5] It is true that studies of male alcoholics present fewer logistical problems, such as retaining their surnames at marriage,[6] but it is also true that certain lines of investigation have had to await development of research techniques capable of measuring neuroendocrine hormones in females[7] and careful studies of substance use on reproductive functions in women.[8-10]

Recent events, however, have by no means closed the gap in knowledge about factors promoting or perpetuating alcohol and substance use problems in women.[3] Instead, this review discusses past knowledge and current findings, points to a number of unanswered questions, and concludes with a series of prevention recommendations that emerge from consideration of empirical data. Materials presented herein have been selected to provide a broad spectrum of information about biological, psychological, and sociocultural aspects of substance abuse as it affects women.

Gender Differences in Alcohol Use

It is now apparent that age of onset, drinking patterns, and symptoms of alcohol dependence are different for alcoholic women and men.[3-5,11-15] As noted in an earlier review,[4] onset of drinking problems in women occurs 4–8 yr later than in men, but alcohol-dependent women also drink less frequently and consume less alcohol, report having fewer binges and less continuous drinking, recall fewer blackouts, morning drinking, and delirium tremens episodes, and report that before coming to treatment they had shorter drinking histories.

However, there are still questions about significant differences between men and women in the development, expression, and consequences of alcoholism. Differential distribution of other variables, such as age, socioeconomic status, ethnicity, or psychopathology may account for several reported differences. Furthermore, once data for alcoholics of each sex have been controlled for confounding factors, such as underlying psychiatric disorder, socioeconomic status, and occupational status, the most appropriate comparisons are made with males and females in the *general population*. Writing more than a decade ago, Schuckit and Morrissey[16,17] suggested that the association between drinking practices and socioeconomic status was much more important for expression of alcohol problems in women and men than perceived gender differences. Women with lower socioeconomic status, they asserted, had drinking histories similar to those generally reported for male alcoholics, whereas those reported for women of higher socioeconomic status more closely resembled the stereotypic alcoholic female.

Frequently Cited Differences Between Male and Female Alcoholics[4]

1. **Familial/genetic factors:** Alcoholic women are more likely to have an alcoholic role model in their nuclear families and to have alcoholic spouses (assortative mating).
2. **Onset:** Women usually have drinking problems at later ages.
3. **Consumption patterns:** Women typically consume less alcohol than men, and are less likely to drink daily, to drink continuously, or to engage in binges.
4. **Course of illness:** Women progress rapidly from onset of drinking through the later stages of alcoholism—i.e., "telescoping."
5. **Attribution of etiology:** Women frequently attribute their drinking to a stress or traumatic event. Events are often related to reproductive dysfunction or crises peculiar to women.
6. **Concurrent psychological disorder:** Some alcoholic men have primary antisocial personality disorders; more women have primary affective disorders.
7. **Societal response:** Alcoholic women are more stigmatized, and women may experience more social disapproval of alcohol use.
8. **Social sequelae:** Consequences for men affect jobs or career paths. Disruptions for women more likely occur in family life. More alcoholic women are separated or divorced.
9. **Medical sequelae:** Women have more liver cirrhosis, but alcohol is a direct gonadotoxin in men.
10. **Personal response to illness:** Alcoholic women are more frequently characterized as feeling guilty, anxious, or depressed.

Thus, some alcohol problems can seem less severe for women. However, numerous reports associate alcohol abuse in women with serious reproductive (gynecological and obstetric) dysfunctions[5,8–10,18] as well as with more rapid development of dependence and cardiovascular, gastrointestinal, and liver diseases,[4,19–21] that is, with a process called "telescoping." Also, alcohol can seriously affect the developing fetus.[8,22]

Specific processes leading to these consequences are incompletely known, and the relative contributions of psychosocial and biological factors to these disease outcomes will not be identified without further systematic investigation.[4,5,8] In addition, it is also important to acknowledge that women who have alcohol problems are at risk for polysubstance use, including use of such dependency-producing substances as psychotropic prescription medications, marijuana, and cocaine.[3,4,23] A combination of environmental, familial, and genetic factors contribute to women's intercurrent polysubstance use.[3]

Gender Differences in Polysubstance Use

Many differences between male and female substance use identified over 10 yr ago still persist:[24,25]

1. **Women are socialized differently:** they have fewer assertive skills and need more supportive networks.
2. **Women's social statuses generally derive from those of men** (e.g., fathers, husbands), and their supplies of drugs also are likely to be obtained from men, whether boyfriends, conjugal partners, or physicians.
3. **Women are expected to play more key family roles.**
4. **Women are typically given most responsibility for birth control and parenthood.**
5. **Women have more medical problems,** and are perceived differently when they complain about these problems.
6. **Women have fewer and less lucrative vocational options than men.**
7. **Women are differentially perceived and responded to by the criminal justice system.**
8. **Women who commit deviant behaviors are more socially stigmatized than men.**
9. **Women addicts have often been sexually abused.**
10. **Most treatment programs have traditionally focused on men and their needs.**

More women are employed today, and some other items on the list are slowly changing, but overall there is not a great deal of difference. Investigations of women's substance abuse problems are still in their infancy,[3] so that even many basic epidemiological questions remain to be answered.

One series of studies examined sex differences in addict careers.[26-29] A total of 546 male ($n = 282$) and female ($n = 264$) clients in methadone maintenance programs in Southern California were studied. On average, women were approx 26 yr of age at admission vs 29 yr of age for men. Women and men averaged about 10.5 yr of education. Approximately 90% of men and women had been arrested, but men had their first arrest at approx 16.5 yr, and women had their first arrest at 18.5 yr. Female addicts were more likely to report poor relationships with their mothers. About 80% of men and women were married, and about 85% had lived with a partner in consensual union with an average of 2.5 children.

It is noteworthy that about 15% of women reported that they had been initiated into drug use by a spouse or common-law partner, whereas *no* men reported that their spouse or mate had initiated them into narcotics use. Instead, men were more likely to initiate use within a group context. More women than men lived with a husband or common-law partner and for a longer duration of time, and these partners were more likely to be daily users who had initiated women into drug use. None of the men reported living with a woman who was previously addicted.

Significantly more men than women used alcohol and/or marijuana daily, and for longer intervals, with approx 60% of men using marijuana and 40% using alcohol daily. White men were more likely to deal drugs than white women, but Hispanic women were more likely to be involved in drug dealing than Hispanic men. More men than women reported having been a member of a gang and reported problems in school. Men were arrested at younger ages, and men were more frequently incarcerated for longer than 30 d, and on probation.

About 25% of the addicts studied developed dependence within 1 mo of their first use of heroin. More women than men became dependent within 1 mo, and women in general took less time to become dependent. The mean number of total months from initiation into heroin use to heroin dependence was shorter for women than for men (14 vs 21 mo), and over 25% of women began daily heroin use within the first 3 wk of initial use. Women were more likely to be supplied with heroin than to supply others, and for longer time intervals.

Women were likely to sharply reduce nonnarcotic drug use and slightly decrease alcohol use during the interval from initiation of use to addiction. It was conjectured that, once a woman began to use heroin, it replaced her use of other drugs, whereas men appeared to continue to experiment with many drugs simultaneously. It was observed that women and men seemed to follow similar narcotics use patterns, but that the addiction careers of women seemed to be "compressed" into a shorter cycle. The pattern of differential time to addiction ("telescoping") is consistent with findings from other drug use studies, including alcohol.

Reasons for sustaining heroin use were more likely to be related to "hedonistic reasons," including liking the high and development of tolerance, with about 50% of men vs roughly 30% of women having reported primacy of this factor. The next most important reasons for men were economic reasons, such as ready availability or cheap price. Women were most likely to attribute social reasons, especially use by a partner (approx 36%), but 10% of men and women reported social use by friends as a reason for using narcotics. It was more likely that a woman's partner would be an addict, and influence of a narcotics-using partner was a strong factor for continued use by women.

Women took significantly less time to enter treatment, averaging about 5 yr from first drug use to admission to a methadone-maintenance program, in contrast to about 8 yr for men, and women reported shorter durations of uninterrupted daily use (23 vs 32 mo). Similar proportions (about one-third) of men and women reported having had a period of abstinence. Men were more likely to remain abstinent for longer intervals (approx 8 vs 3.5 mo), but longer durations of abstinence in men may have stemmed from their greater frequency of incarceration.

Kosten and colleagues[30] studied 522 opiate addicts, of whom 126 (24%) were female. All subjects were seen at the Yale University Drug Dependence Unit in New Haven. Addiction was defined according to RDC criteria.[31] The majority of males and females (55–63%) were ages 26–35, followed by the 18–25 yr age range (25–28%). Most had completed high school, and about 20% had additional education. Roughly 15% of women had had school failure, in contrast to 30% in males. Rates for school behavior problems were approx 50% for both men and women. Men were more likely to have full-time employment, but men also were more likely to be single.

Age at first use of opiates were similar for both men and women (approx 18 yr), and duration of opiate use also was similar (roughly 9% across groups). Men had approximately double the number (11%) of arrests than women (6%), but the rating for legal problems was similar for men and for women (3.3) on the Addiction Severity Index (ASI). ASI family and social problem (3.4) and substance abuse problem (5.4) ratings also were comparable across all groups. Employment problems also were comparable, averaging 3.3. However, women had a rating of 4.0 for psychological problems (vs 3.3 for men), and women also had higher scores for medical problems (2.5 vs 1.5). Women were twice as likely to have received their first psychiatric treatment by age 15 (10%) than men (5%).

With regard to family history of psychological disorders, women were slightly more likely (40 vs 32%) to have experienced severe family disruption. Family history of depression in fathers was approx double (10%) for women (4%) than for men, whereas family history of depression in mothers was around 10% for both men and women. Approximately 16% of men reported that their fathers had histories of alcoholism, in contrast to about 20% of women. Women were less likely (about 3 vs 7%) to report alcoholism in a sibling, but rates for drug addiction in siblings were about 25% for males and females.

Study of parental alcoholism in opioid addicts[32] examined the question of whether parental alcoholism is specifically associated with addict alcoholism. Using the same sample of 522 addicts from New Haven, the rate of addict alcoholism was 35%. The rate for alcoholism in fathers of addicts in the study was 17.6%, and the rate for mothers was 5.8%. The rate of maternal alcoholism was higher (9.7%) in alcoholic addicts than among nonalcoholic addicts (3.8%). The authors concluded that some vulnerability for substance abuse in general may be transmitted from alcoholic parents to their offspring. Rates of intercurrent psychological disorders differed significantly between male and female addicts, with females having had higher rates of affective disorder (69 vs 49%) and men having had higher rates of antisocial personality disorder (17% vs 30%). Parental alcoholism was more strongly associated with probands' alcoholism in cases of antisocial personality in female addicts and with affective disorders in alcoholic male addicts.

Dual Diagnosis Patients: Depression and Antisocial Personality Disorders

Both depression and antisocial personality disorders frequently co-occur in patients treated for alcohol dependence, as well as cocaine dependence or dependence on other psychoactive drugs.[3] Most authorities in the field of alcohol studies believe that the development of alcohol problems is a complex process for which no single factor has been shown to explain or predict why some people develop alcohol problems and others do not.[33] It is generally believed that alcoholism in women, or in men, is the result of a combination of behavioral, biological, and sociocultural variables.[5]

Several efforts have been made to distinguish subgroups of female alcoholics on the basis of psychopathology.[34-36] Schuckit and Morrissey[16] suggested that all alcoholics could be subtyped on the basis of prior diagnosis of psychological disorders: Primary alcoholics (individuals having no major preexisting psychiatric disorder) and secondary alcoholics (those who evidence alcoholism intercurrent with other psychiatric problems). Within the category of female "secondary alcoholics," Schuckit and Morrissey[16] further identified "affective disorder alcoholics" (women with primary affective disorders and secondary alcoholism) and "sociopathic alcoholics" (women with histories of serious antisocial lifestyles antedating their alcohol abuse). Other investigators have also distinguished between female alcoholics with discernible disorders preceding the onset of problem drinking or disorders developed during long periods of abstinence, and those "primary" female alcoholics who do not evidence disorders.[35,37]

A recent study of men and women hospitalized for treatment of cocaine dependence[38] compared sociodemographic characteristics, reasons for cocaine use, drug effects, psychiatric diagnoses, and depressive symptoms in 95 men and 34 women hospitalized for cocaine abuse. The ratio of male to female cocaine users was 2.8:1, so that women comprised approx 36% of the sample.

Women were significantly younger than men at the time of first drug use (mean 15.6 ± 3.5 vs 18.5 ± 7.3 yr). Women also were significantly younger at the age of their first substance abuse treatment (mean 24.6 ± 4.7 vs 29.1 ± 7.7 yr). Women had used cocaine for a significantly shorter period of time (mean 3.7 ± 2.2 yr vs mean 5.4 ± 3.2 yr). Men and women were similar in their total years of drug use (10.2 ± 5.4 vs 9.0 ± 4.7 yr), their years of heavy drug use (5.2 ± 4.2 vs 4.3 ± 3.2), the number of different drugs that had been used during the previous 30 d (3.5 ± 2.8 vs 4.4 ± 2.7), and the amount of cocaine used during the past 6 mo in grams (106.3 ± 177.5 vs 107.5 ± 148.2), but differed in the amount of money that they had spent on cocaine during the past 6 mo ($\$9,375 \pm \$10,778$ vs $\$3,050 \pm \$3,382$). More men were married (40 vs 21%), and more women than men lived with a drug-dependent partner (36 vs 21%). Men were more likely than women to be employed (78 vs 50%), and were more likely to have professional, executive, or sales jobs (61 vs 20%).

Women cited four reasons for cocaine use, including depression, feeling unsociable, family and job pressures, and health problems, but men were more likely to report that cocaine decreased libido (67 vs 38%), and overall, men cited more intoxication effects from cocaine. Men and women did not differ in their reports of cocaine effects on sexual interest, aggression, appetite, anxiety, or mood. Nonetheless, women reported significantly less guilt as a cocaine effect (47 vs 23%), but most men and women (57%) reported they used cocaine to be more sociable and recalled increased sociability.

Women were more likely to have an Axis I DSM-III-R[39] diagnosis in addition to substance abuse. Depression was the most common reported psychological disorder, and most frequently reported by women. Antisocial personality on DSM-III-R Axis II was reported only by men. In patients with depression, women reported more depression than men on the Hamilton Depression Rating Scale (HDRS) at admission, at 2 wk after admission, and at 4 wk after admission. For patients who had no diagnosis of major depression at admission, HDRS scores were similar for men and women at admission, with women having slightly elevated scores at 2 and at 4 wk postadmission. Griffin and colleagues noted that the difference in depressive symptomatology between male and female cocaine has persisted over time, despite changes in the sociodemographic characteristics of patients, with the pattern of slower recovery from depression among women remaining remarkably constant.[38]

Kandel and coworkers conducted longitudinal studies of substance abuse in young adults.[40,41] These followup studies tracked a cohort of representative adolescents first identified when they were in grades 10 and 11 in New York State in 1971. Over 1000 young men and women were reinterviewed at approx age 25. Use of alcohol, marijuana, and other illicit drugs was examined, as were effects of continued use on work and family roles, educational level, health and psychological problems, and deviant activities.

For both women and men, marijuana use in adolescence was correlated with histories of job instability at followup. Illicit drug use in both adolescence and young adulthood was the strongest predictor of intervals of unemployment among young women. Illicit drug use in young women also predicted divorce, separations, and abortions. Continued use of illicit drugs was the strongest predictor of abortion among women, and of separation or divorce among men. Use of illicit drugs in adolescence also had a deleterious effect on educational level, and also predicted antisocial behavior in the year before the followup survey, namely, theft.

Daily marijuana use strongly affected job histories (such as having four or more job changes), and daily marijuana use by women increased the likelihood of abortion fivefold. There were also differences between men and women who used marijuana daily insofar as their psychological health was affected at followup. Those who used marijuana four times per week or more consulted mental health professionals more frequently, and were more likely to have been hospitalized for psychiatric disorder. For men and women, roughly one-fifth of daily users (vs 8% of nonusers) consulted mental health professionals, and less than 1% of those who had never used marijuana but about 7% of those who currently used marijuana at least four times per week had experienced psychiatric hospitalization.

At followup, marijuana users were heavily involved in social networks where marijuana was tolerated and used frequently by others. Among women, 96% of those who currently used marijuana four times per week or more during the year prior to followup reported that most or all of their friends also used marijuana, and a similar pattern was observed for men.

For men not residing with a partner, use of other illicit drugs was a stronger predictor of continued marijuana use than friends' use of drugs. For men who were living with a partner, the effect of use by that partner was as strong a factor in continued marijuana use as the use of other illicit drugs, with use by friends next in importance. For women not residing with a partner, marijuana use by their friends was the strongest predictor of continued marijuana use, with other illicit drug use ranking second. The "husband effect" was observed for women residing with a spouse or conjugal partner insofar as marijuana use by a conjugal partner or spouse had a stronger effect on women's marijuana use than use by their friends.

Interpersonal factors were more significant for women than for men in predicting marijuana use. Male and female differences suggested that men were likely to be involved in several social networks, whereas women participated in more restricted friendships. This latter factor may have reinforced the strong effect of partners' use on women's continued drug use.

Kandel and coworkers[41] observed that drug use had a comprehensive effect on drug users' lives. In their estimation, use of a particular drug is self-reinforcing. Moreover, drug use promotes a series of consequences that, in turn, begets other consequences. In contrast, however, use of alcohol appeared to be more benign. However, use of illicit drugs by age 15 or 16 in women, or later in men, also predicted subsequent use of prescription medication, suggesting that adolescent marijuana use may ameliorate dysphoric affect. Kandel[40] also suggested that, for marijuana use to continue into young adulthood, there needed to be a facilitating social context. Apparently, after approx age 25, a shift to prescription medications would be anticipated.

In the 1970s, it was believed that marijuana smokers' social networks and peers were the best predictors for marijuana use. Since specific effects of male partner's influence is seen in women's continued use of marijuana, cocaine, and alcohol, this topic deserves further attention.

Clinically Identifiable Subgroups with Alcohol Dependence

Perhaps 40% of alcohol-dependent patients (including men and women) have a family history of alcoholism.[42] Indeed, on the basis of clinical observation, it is often asserted that all alcoholics have at least one alcoholic relative in their backgrounds. In any event, on the basis of careful study of adoption records from Scandinavian countries, it has been argued that familial and genetic factors in inheritance of alcoholism cluster into at least two clinically identifiable alcohol dependence syndromes. Recent reports have differentiated Type 1 (late onset, lower risk) from Type 2 (early onset, higher risk, less control over drinking, and more violence while drinking) forms of familial alcoholism in men.[43,44]

By using information from hospital, clinic, and registry records, a large-scale adoption study in Sweden identified two types of alcoholism in men. One subtype (Type I) was identified as "milieu-limited," because expression of alcoholism was related to interplay with environmental factors and occurred later, whereas the second type, designated as "male-limited" (Type II), was generally associated with early onset of alcohol-related problems accompanied by impulsivity, risk-taking, and criminality.

From these studies, it also has been alleged that the genetic factors in women with family histories of alcoholism are differentially expressed.[11] In the Swedish adoption studies, alcoholism in women with "milieu-limited" alcoholic fathers was found to be shaped by environmental conditions (i.e., exposure to alcohol, social status of adoptive father) superimposed on a biological substrate. In contrast, the female counterpart of "male-limited" alcoholism was found to be expressed primarily as somatization.[12,45,46] Somatic concerns were typically complaints of abdominal, back, or neck pains, but alcohol abuse or dependence occurred less frequently. Further, in the Swedish adoption studies, the highest prevalence of alcoholic relatives in the backgrounds of alcohol-dependent women was found among women with alcoholic mothers.[11]

It should be noted, however, that the typologies that have emerged from the Swedish adoption studies were drawn from records of work absences, illness treatments, and alcohol problems, but did *not* include studies of information collected directly from either alcohol-dependent men and women involved in treatment or known to the criminal justice system. Further, familial or genetic relationships between polydrug abuse and alcohol dependence do not appear to have been addressed in the Swedish studies. In the US, however, intercurrent alcohol dependence with other drug abuse or dependence is an established clinical reality in women as well as in men, and is of increasing concern.

Evidence for contributions of genetic, familial, and nonfamilial risk factors in transmission of alcoholism have drawn upon cross-sectional surveys and studies of the families of alcoholic probands. Epidemiologic Catchment Area data for two sites showed increased prevalence of alcoholism, and decreased age of onset in males and females.[12,47] In response to these findings, data from an ongoing family study of alcoholic probands and their first degree relatives in St. Louis were analyzed to identify the impact of secular trends on alcoholism prevalence, age of onset, and transmissibility.[48] Using Feighner criteria,[49] Reich and Cloninger studied 60 female and 240 male alcoholics, their fathers, mothers, brothers, sisters, offspring ($n = 831$), and spouses ($n = 125$) between 1978–1983. Alcoholism rates for sons and daughters of pro-bands were higher than rates for their fathers and mothers. It is noteworthy that male and female probands had similar numbers of first degree alcoholic relatives.[48]

When relatives of probands were grouped by age (under 25, 26–44, and over 45), 52% of male relatives ages under 25, 20% of male relatives ages 26–44, and less than 10% of male relatives ages over 45 were alcoholics. In addition, 18% of female relatives ages under 25, less than 5% of female relatives ages 26–44, and less than 5% of female relatives ages over 45 were alcoholics.[48] Ages at onset of alcohol dependence were estimated by sex and birth cohort. Lifetime prevalence for persons born since 1955 was calculated at about 22% for males and 10% for females. In contrast, prevalence for persons born before 1940 was calculated at about 12.3% for males and 4% for females.[48] Thus, the rates for females have more than doubled, while the rates for males have almost doubled.

Other findings from Reich and coworkers[48] indicate that younger cohorts are at greater risk for alcohol dependence. Younger cohorts show greater effects of transmissibility (τ^2). Heritability estimates for males varied between 0.65–0.98, and between 0.27–0.59 for females. Nongenetic transmission was detected ($\tau^2 = 0.63$), with estimates of correlations between nonenvironmental factors common to brothers and sisters varying between $\tau^2 = 0.22$–0.41. Maternal vs paternal transmission rates also were similar, and same-sex transmission rates were similar.[48] Thus, age of onset and lifetime prevalence of alcohol dependence in women appear to be approaching characteristics of men.

The increase in prevalence is strongest in children of alcoholic probands. If age of onset has shifted downward (under 25 yr), it appears that there is an overall increase in prevalence of Type II alcoholism.[48] Since Type II alcoholism in the Swedish cross-fostering studies was manifested in women as somatization, and not alcoholism, then appropriate studies could compare characteristics of women in specific populations in order to determine whether the putative Type II subtype of male alcoholism (which specifically involves legal infractions) can be identified in women.

Although putative Type II alcoholism has yet to be investigated in women with alcohol or polysubstance dependence, exploratory work can be conducted in potentially high-risk populations, such as those with involvement in the criminal justice system. For example, a national survey of women's drinking problems conducted in 1981 reported that 17% reported driving while intoxicated.[21] An increasing number of women have come to the attention of the criminal justice system in response to more stringent enforcement and penalties for drinking and driving[50] to the extent that one-third of all persons convicted for drinking and driving in Massachusetts in 1985 were female.[51] It also would be necessary to determine the extent and type of intercurrent medical disorders, concurrent substance abuse and dependence, and life circumstances that are associated with the natural history of alcohol dependence in samples of women with Type II traits.

The first 20 women civilly committed to receive alcohol treatment at a new program at the Massachusetts Osteopathic Hospital were evaluated.[23] Each patient provided information about her overall health, alcohol and drug use histories, reproductive histories, living situations, social and economic circumstances, legal problems, and background characteristics. Patients typically had completed high school, and all but one had worked at semi-skilled jobs or as homemakers. Convictions for driving while intoxicated were reported by 11 women, and three women had committed crimes against property. Patients began drinking alcohol regularly during their teens or early 20s, and age of initial sexual intercourse closely paralleled their age at initiation of alcohol use. Of importance to genetic factors, 75% of the women had a family history of alcoholism.

Since these prospective studies of women's drug and alcohol use[52,53] had found that heavy frequent use of one substance is highly correlated with use of another, patients were evaluated for polysubstance dependence and diagnosed as either alcohol dependent ($n = 12$) or polysubstance dependent ($n = 8$). The alcohol-dependent women were significantly older at admission, older at reported age of initial alcohol use, and older at age of onset of regular alcoholic use. More alcohol-dependent women lived alone or were homeless. The eight women who were polysubstance dependent did not show a uniform pattern of substance use. The range of drugs used reflected the range of ages of women in the category. Cocaine was most frequently mentioned, followed by opiates, tranquilizers/sedatives, marijuana, amphetamines, and hallucinogens.

Family history of alcoholism also was a key variable that differentiated subgroups within the sample. In this cohort, three-fourths of all patients ($n = 15$) had a positive family history of alcoholism, and of the remaining five, one woman had been adopted and had no information about her biological parents. Alcohol ($n = 8$) and polysubstance ($n = 7$) dependent patients with a positive family history of alcoholism were compared. Although alcohol dependent women were significantly older (40.6 ± 11.4 yr) than polysubstance-dependent women (27.4 ± 5.8 yr) ($t = 2.767; p = 0.016$), age did not appear to be a confounding factor that affected the number of reported relatives. There were no significant differences between the two groups for total number of reported relatives, total number of reported alcoholic relatives, or the combined total number of alcoholic relatives and mates. Numbers of male and female relatives reported by patients in each diagnostic group were then compared separately. Polysubstance-dependent women had significantly more alcoholic male relatives (mean 2.9 vs 1.8), and a trend toward a greater combined total number of alcoholic male relatives and mates (mean 3.3 vs 2.3), but there was no significant difference between the two groups for mean number of female alcoholic relatives.

Findings are similar to those reported by Hill et al.[54] for adolescent sons and daughters in high density (alcoholic fathers and at least two alcoholic brothers) families with alcoholism, and by Kosten and coworkers at Yale[55] for female opiate users. In the most extreme case, one polysubstance-dependent woman had a mother's father, mother's brother, brother, two sisters, son, and one daughter who were alcohol-dependent, and this patient also had been married to two different men who were themselves brothers and alcohol-dependent.[23]

Stress, Life Events, and Substance Use

Are life crises precipitants of substance abuse? It has been asserted that certain life stages, such as young adulthood, are associated with increased alcohol intake, and that women in particular may react to unusual events or stressful experiences by increasing alcohol intake. Accordingly, Morrissey and Schuckit[14] studied the temporal relationship of life stresses to the onset of alcohol abuse in 293 women of all social classes treated at a detoxification facility. Although 262 (89.4%) experienced a stressful gynecological event, only 8% reported temporal concordance with alcohol abuse. Fewer than one-fourth of the sample reported temporal concordance for any type of life stress, including death of a family member, separation or divorce, depression, or suicide attempt, in addition to stressful gynecological events. The closest association between stressful life events and the onset of alcohol abuse was found in the lowest social class, with the smallest association found for women in the higher social classes.

Thom[56] examined help seeking in 25 men and 25 women who were new admissions referred to an alcohol clinic serving a working-class population in England. Men tended to attribute their drinking patterns to involvement in a social network of coworkers, so that drinking problems emerged from everyday social situations where heavy drinking was part of a lifestyle. In some instances, men's consumption increased in response to stressful situations, but men's drinking was neither marked by a specific precipitating event, nor recognized until physical damage or a change in social circumstances had occurred. In contrast, women were more likely to attribute alcohol use to the aftermath of a specific distressing event or as a generalized coping method used to contend with problematic social situations. Life events cited included death of spouse or close relative, death of a baby, divorce or separation, infertility, terminal illness of a parent, and the birth of a child, which exacerbated existing marital problems. However, it should be noted that these women also were involved in social networks where heavy alcohol consumption was normative.

A number of women felt that their heavy alcohol consumption was a legitimate response to personal problems and did not perceive that it might have further complicated those problems. They seemed to share a belief that drinking for the sake of drinking was the major reason that someone should be engaged in alcohol treatment and, thus, denied that the clinic was an appropriate place for them to address their current situation. A major obstacle for men was their belief that they should be able to control their drinking on their own and, thus, found it difficult to ask for help with drinking problems. Overall, women were distressed to be formally labeled as in need of treatment from an alcohol clinic and were worried about public opinion about clinic attendance, whereas men were more concerned that they would be labeled in need of psychiatric care, and some men acknowledged that their coworkers would believe them to be lacking in masculinity if their involvement in treatment became generally known.

As reported in a related paper,[57] only three men and six women failed to recall a significant life event in the year prior to intake. No men, but eight women reported physical violence. Ten men vs two women reported job loss, and 10 men vs six women reported serious health problems. An equal number of men and women ($n = 5$) had problems with the law, and numbers experiencing death of a significant other were similar (five men and four women). Smaller numbers reported loss of a child (three men and three women), marital dissolution (three men and two women), and suicide attempts (one man and four women). Two men vs five women reported becoming homeless. However, patients did not necessarily perceive the occurrence of these events as precipitants to treatment. Serious health problems, marital breakup, loss of a child, and violence by respondents influenced help seeking, whereas job loss, deaths, legal problems, loss of adult significant others, experiencing violence, becoming homeless, and having an accident or attempting suicide did not prompt patients to seek help with alcohol problems. For men, marital disruption or threat of separation was a more frequent precipitant ($n = 9$) than for women ($n = 2$).

Intriguingly, two men and three women reported that an *encouraging* event prompted them to feel worthy and to have hope for the future, thus reinforcing the need for treatment. Influence from significant others also provided encouragement to seek help. More men ($n = 13$) than women ($n = 4$) attributed this influence to a spouse, whereas more women ($n = 6$) than men ($n = 3$) reported positive influence from their children. Four men and five women reported that friends encouraged treatment, whereas eight men vs five women reported that a general practitioner encouraged treatment. Only women reported that other relatives or coworkers encouraged treatment.

Wilsnack and colleagues provided information about women's alcohol use from retrospective data obtained in a cross-sectional survey.[21] Data were collected from a stratified sample of 917 noninstitutionalized women over age 21 studied in 1981. The sample included 500 moderate to heavy drinking women who consumed four or more drinks per week, 378 lighter drinking or abstinent women, and 39 self-reported former problem drinkers. Demographic characteristics corresponded to those of the general female population of the US in 1980, including occupational categories, racial distributions, and educational levels. Respondents answered questions about alcohol consumption, drinking context, problems associated with drinking, symptoms of alcohol dependence, attitudes and beliefs about drinking, family history, self-concept and role performance, stressful life experiences, social support, anxiety and depressive symptoms, reproductive problems, sexual experience, use of drugs in addition to alcohol, and participation in antisocial behaviors. Respondents provided data on lifetime changes in drinking, including age at onset of alcohol use, frequency of alcohol use, and quantity of consumption. Respondents were asked at what ages their drinking patterns changed, and how quantity and frequency changed. The questionnaire provided opportunity to describe six different drinking history stages, but only 2% of the sample reported as many as five stages.[21]

Since it is commonly believed that depressive symptoms and the stress regarding reproductive problems are related to drinking levels, the effects of these variables were compared. Episodes of depression were related to current drinking, but more powerfully related to maximum lifetime drinking levels. A threshold of 24 drinks/wk divided women into two groups. Those below this threshold reported few suicide attempts (3%), whereas 25% of women consuming greater amounts had attempted suicide at some time in their lives. Further, although only 10% of women below the threshold had experienced three or more depressive episodes, more than half (53%) of women drinking above the threshold reported three or more depressive episodes in their lives. Reproductive problems were less strongly related to consumption in excess of the 24 drink/wk threshold.[21]

The majority of women who reported drinking in association with stressful life events stated that drinking increased *after* the occurrence of the event, and this relationship held across different age cohorts. Health-related experiences were readily recalled, and 98% of the women answered pertinent questions, with 93% able to recall age of first occurrence. The median ages for first experiences of four reproductive problems occurred during the mid-20s. Miscarriage or stillbirth was reported by 28% of women who had ever been pregnant. Premature delivery also occurred in mid-20s, as did birth of a baby with birth defects and infertility lasting for at least one year's duration. Depressive episodes preceded heavy drinking, at a median time lag of 5 yr. In instances of reproductive problems, onset of increased drinking usually occurred after one decade or more.[21]

Thus, excessive alcohol consumption may function as both cause and result of stressful life experiences, marital problems, employment problems, physical illness, or depression. Consumption rates may fluctuate through time, and also may be inadequate to predict future alcohol use. Further, the effects of excessive drinking may be age-specific, or may be circumscribed, delayed, or accumulate over time. Cooke and Allan[58] also examined the relationship between life events and alcohol consumption in a cross-sectional survey of 230 women in Scotland. Findings showed that women's consumption generally was moderate. Speculation that increased alcohol consumption occurs in the aftermath of stressors (e.g., bereavement, divorce) was unfounded. The belief attributing women's alcohol abuse to stressors may have arisen as a way to explain or excuse excessive drinking by some women.

Differences in Alcohol Consumption, Absorption, Metabolism, and Health Consequences

Generally speaking, patterns of alcohol intake differ for women and men,[10] with women's consumption patterns being more variable than men's. Similarly, rates of alcohol absorption differ for women and men. Women's absorption rates also are more variable, and affected by progesterone levels that fluctuate across the menstrual cycle (rising after ovulation and before onset of menses) or during pregnancy. It is estimated that women have lower mean body water volume (Vd) (51%) than men (65%). Since alcohol is water soluble, at the same dose of alcohol, women will attain higher peak blood alcohol levels. In addition, there is evidence that shows that higher blood alcohol levels are attained by women during the luteal phase of the menstrual cycle, after ovulation and before the onset of menses.[10]

It has long been known that alcoholism is associated with severe disruption of reproductive function in men. Impotence, low testosterone levels, testicular atrophy, gynecomastia, and diminished sexual interest are consistently reported,[7] but until very recently, there has been relatively little research on alcohol's effects on the reproductive function in women.[8,9] Pathophysiologic effects of chronic alcohol intake on reproductive function may be the result of direct toxic effects of alcohol on the hypothalamus, pituitary, or ovaries, or of interaction effects. Some of the major alcohol-related disorders of the female reproductive system include amenorrhea, anovulation, luteal-phase dysfunction, ovarian atrophy, spontaneous abortion, and early menopause. In women of reproductive age, amenorrhea is defined as complete cessation of menses for intervals of months or years. Women who continue to menstruate may experience anovulation and luteal-phase dysfunction. Anovulation is defined as the absence of ovulation, whereas luteal-phase dysfunction is defined either as a short luteal phase defect of eight days or less from ovulation to menses or an inadequate luteal phase when progesterone levels are abnormally low, wherein the interval from ovulation to menstruation is of normal length. Alcohol abuse also increases the risk of spontaneous abortion. Further, alcohol abuse also may promote early menopause, and postmortem studies of alcoholic women have found evidence of ovarian atrophy.[9]

Endocrine profiles were studied for the first 18 consecutive women (age 17–58) receiving court-ordered treatment of alcohol or polysubstance dependence under civil commitment in a Massachusetts hospital.[59] Twelve women were diagnosed as alcohol-dependent or abusers according to DSM-III-R criteria,[39] and their alcohol consumption ranged from 42–324 g/p d. Six women were diagnosed as polydrug-dependent. In addition to alcohol (84–830 g/d), cocaine was the most frequently abused drug followed by tranquilizers, sedatives, marijuana, amphetamines, and opiates. All women received a thorough physical examination and laboratory studies, including blood hemogram and chemistry. Blood samples for LH, FSH, prolactin, estradiol, progesterone, and cortisol were obtained. All patients were detoxified and showed no signs of withdrawal at sample collection.

Fifty percent of the alcoholic women had hyperprolactinemia (22.3–87.5 ng/mL) independent of amount and duration of alcohol use, and one patient had secondary amenorrhea with a normal prolactin level and low levels of LH and estradiol. Two polysubstance-dependent women had hyperprolactinemia (25.7 and 29.6 ng/mL), and one had secondary amenorrhea, with normal prolactin but low LH, FSH, and estradiol. Hormone levels were consistent with reported menstrual cycle phase or menopausal range in 16 patients. Although specific mechanisms of alcohol- and drug-induced derangements of the reproductive dysfunction have yet to be determined, hyperprolactinemia may cause amenorrhea and disruptions of the menstrual cycle.

In another study of these women,[23] two subgroups within the sample were differentiated on the basis of their reported type of drug use, and at least 40% of the women reported dependence on one or more drugs in addition to alcohol. As noted, drug-use patterns were heterogeneous, when cocaine was the most frequently reported dependency-producing drug, followed by opiates, tranquilizers and sedatives, and marijuana. Polysubstance-dependent women also reported beginning sexual activity at an earlier age (mean = 15.7 yr ± 2.6) than alcohol-dependent women (mean = 18.6 yr ± 3.3). Although 50% of alcohol-dependent women had had no live births, one polysubstance dependent woman reported 12 conceptions, resulting in six live births, one stillbirth, and five spontaneous abortions. Thus, the consequences of substance use on reproductive capacity are far from clear and, in all likelihood, are affected by other environmental factors, such as nutrition or trauma.

Hugues and colleagues[60] studied hypothalamo-pituitary function in 31 chronic alcoholic women aged 29–66 yr. All 31 patients had chronic pancreatitis or cirrhosis of the liver. The majority (67%) had a current history of amenorrhea. These subjects were compared with 12 healthy postmenopausal and 10 normal women of reproductive age. Four women had severe oligomenorrhea (scanty or infrequent menstrual flow), six had mild oligomenorrhea or cycles of normal length. *En toto,* several distinct patterns of hypothalamic-pituitary-ovarian activity were found. Normal menopause was seen in eight of the amenorrheic patients. Women in this group had low estrogen levels, high basal gonadotrophin secretion, and a distinct LHRH-induced gonadotrophin response. Five women comprised a second group with a hypothalamic amenorrhea associated with low estrogen output, low gonadotrophin levels, and adequate response to LHRH. In the third group were eight perimenopausal women, ages 43–51 yr and characterized by adequate estradiol levels with a preferential FSH increase. Some subjects could still respond to ovarian stimulation, six women had inadequate luteal phase, and five women had anovulation related to defects in cyclic control of gonadotrophin secretion.

Other studies have approached the question of reproductive compromise in women through screening for alcohol-related problems in obstetric-gynecologic treatment samples. Russell and Bigler[61] screened 499 women seen in an obstetric-gynecologic outpatient clinic of a general hospital in the inner city of Buffalo. Patients responded to a self-administered questionnaire comprised of 31 questions, eight sociodemographic characteristics, one tobacco smoking, twelve alcohol use, and ten alcohol-related problems. Criteria for alcohol-related problems were reports of heavy alcohol consumption (QFV), whereby heavy drinking was defined as consumption of three or more drinks daily regardless of quantity for patients drinking two to three times a month or having five or more drinks on more than one-half of all drinking occasions. Reports of heavy drinking ranged from between 10–14%.

A combination of factors was required to identify all heavy drinkers in the sample. Individuals who were identified as problem drinkers by counselors rather than through screening procedures were more likely to be younger (mean 26 yr ± 12) women who consumed a mean of 2.5 ± 1.8 oz alcohol/episode. These individuals were sufficiently young to have avoided consequences of heavy alcohol intake, since they had no work or steady involvement to interfere with drinking and they were associating with people who did not criticize their consumption. The most frequently endorsed questionnaire items associated with heavy alcohol intake were having a blackout (55%), feeling the need to cut down on drinking (48%), reporting that parents had a drinking problem (42%), seeking help for emotional problems (33%), experiencing family problems associated with drinking (28%), friends or relatives concerned about their drinking (25%), having siblings with a drinking problem (23%), receiving a physician's advice to cease drinking (21%), and having a husband with a drinking problem (18%). Heavy alcohol consumption also was associated with obstetric/gynecological clinic patients under age 40 who reported gastrointestinal pain and obesity. In addition, women in this category were more likely to report experiencing one or more physical complaints, or one or more psychological problems.

Work by Halliday and colleagues[20] replicated earlier work of Russell and Bigler, but studied women treated in two private practice settings in the Boston area. One setting was an obstetric/gynecology practice in a middle-class suburb, whereas the other was a solo practice drawing patients from the metropolitan area. All women between the ages of 18 and 44 were screened for alcohol consumption patterns. Heavy drinking was more frequent in gynecological patients (19%) than in obstetric patients (11%).

Systematic study of adverse effects of alcohol on the fetus and infant began only within the last 15 yr.[62,63] Research on this topic was stimulated by the independent reports of Jones and Smith[64] and Jones et al.[65,66] in the U.S., and Lemoine et al.[67] in France, which described a common pattern of abnormal growth, morphogenesis, and behavioral impairment called the fetal alcohol syndrome (FAS) that occurred in some children of alcoholic mothers who drank heavily during pregnancy.

The effects of alcohol on the fetus are complex, with multiple biochemical pathways and pathophysiological alterations potentially involved in embryonic and fetal growth and development at different stages of gestation.[63] Clinical descriptions of FAS include: growth and performance abnormalities (pre- and postnatal growth deficiency microencephaly, fine motor dysfunction); characteristic craniofacial defects (short palpebral fissures, epicanthal folds, maxillary hypoplasia, cleft palate, micrographia); and limb abnormalities (joint anomalies, altered palmar crease pattern). Various other abnormalities, such as cardiac defects, anomalies of external genitalia, small hemangiomas, and deformed ears, have also been observed.[68] Once seen and described, this syndrome was easily recognized.[69] Streissguth[69,70] reported that the most disabling aspect of FAS is mental impairment, ranging from borderline intellectual functioning to moderately severe impairment. In all cases, the severity of intellectual deficit was positively correlated with the severity of dysmorphogenesis. The prognosis for mental retardation in FAS children is poor, with only limited response to environmental intervention.[22]

Other substances are also fetotoxic, including marijuana.[71] A case-control study[72] of very low birthweight (VLBW) (≤1500 g) infants delivered to impoverished black women in a Washington, D.C., public hospital found that alcohol abuse was only one of at least ten interactive factors that profiled high-risk mothers. At highest risk of VLBW infants were mothers who were underweight, abusers of alcohol and nicotine, ineffective contraceptors, frequently pregnant, rural migrants, chronically ill, depressed and lacking social supports, victims of psychological or physical violence, with histories of poor pregnancy outcome. No evaluation was made of other psychotropic drug use, but use of nicotine, alcohol dependence, poor nutrition, and social and psychological adjustment problems were found to combine for socioeconomically disadvantaged women when added to ineffective contraception and inadequately spaced pregnancies.

Amenorrhea and anovulation, as well as spontaneous abortion can occur in association with alcohol, marijuana, cocaine, and opiate use. Luteal-phase dysfunction also can occur in association with alcohol, marijuana, and opiate use.[9] More importantly, cocaine, marijuana, and opiate use also have been shown to compromise fetal growth and development.[22,73–75]

Substance abuse has both prenatal and postnatal effects on children. In a study of family violence in the Commonwealth of Massachusetts during 1988, it was noted that the Department of Social Services received over 40,000 reports of child abuse, neglect, emotional maltreatment, or sexual abuse.[76] Of the 60,000 children involved, 65% were screened. In order to identify the extent of the relationship between substance abuse and child abuse and neglect, a period prevalence study analyzed all substantiated cases completed in the city of Boston between December 5, 1988 and December 18, 1988 for evidence of substance abuse, characteristics of abuse or neglect, medical status of children, and family composition and demographics. The city of Boston was selected as a study site because of its high reporting rate. During the study interval, 108 cases were examined, and 64% (69 cases) involved substance abuse. Categories of drugs used in those 69 cases included cocaine (65%), alcohol (48%), and other opiates (35 cases), including heroin (9%) and methadone (41%), with some cases involving abuse of more than one substance.

Ninety-two percent of cases involved a single parent (usually the mother) family. Children under the age of 1 yr for whom reports of child abuse or neglect were substantiated were from households where one or more family member was an identified substance abuser (34 out of 38 cases, or 89%). Moreover, 23 of these 34 cases involved hospital reports of infants who were born addicted to methadone or heroin (six cases), who had positive drug screens for cocaine (20 cases), or who showed symptoms of FAS (four cases).

Of the 20 mothers who had used cocaine, seven had received minimal or no prenatal care. Cases in which urinalysis of infants tested positive for cocaine indicated that the mother had used cocaine within 48 h or less prior to delivery. Of these babies, eight were premature or had low birth weight, and five others had other medical problems. In some instances, a baby showed the effect of more than one drug, especially when heroin was a primary drug of use.

Cocaine also was implicated in documentation of severe and chronic neglect of older children. Upon investigation, caseworkers found no food, milk, or diapers in the home, lack of medical attention for serious and acute injuries or illnesses, poor or nonexistent housekeeping standards, and absence of care and supervision for children under five yr. In the latter cases, children might have been left with relatives, friends, or neighbors, as well as simply left unsupervised.

Friends or neighbors made one-fourth of the reports of substance-abuse-related cases. If hospital reports are excluded, then family, friends, and neighbors constituted the largest group (44%) reporting cases of substantiated abuse or neglect. In some instances, children were placed with extended family who were concerned about the children's welfare.

Apart from reproductive problems, findings from a number of studies suggest that women are at greater risk for the development of physical morbidity related to alcohol abuse than men. Studies of Swedish public health insurance societies indicate that female alcoholics begin to experience moderate increases in morbidity 5–6 yr prior to treatment for alcoholism, but exceed men and women in the general population, as well as male alcoholics, in their amount of disability rates, sickness days, and duration of illness both before and after treatment.[77,78]

Liver disease is an important consequence of alcohol abuse. Early observers, such as Spain,[79] Summerskill et al.,[80] and Wilkinson et al.,[81,82] reported women were more susceptible to the development of alcoholic liver disease than men. Among women, increased prevalence of both alcoholic hepatitis and liver cirrhosis has been found despite shorter duration of excessive alcohol intake.[81,83,84] Menopause appears to increase the risk for cirrhosis of the liver in alcoholic women, and early menopause can be a consequence of chronic alcohol abuse.[85-87] Wilkinson and colleagues[81] found a dramatic increase in prevalence of liver cirrhosis in women aged 40–60, but only a slight increase for men in that age range. On average, women die from liver cirrhosis 10.5 yr earlier than men, despite having later onset of drinking, and reduction or cessation of alcohol intake does not appear to alter the progress of liver cirrhosis.[10]

Special Populations

Minority Women

Relationships have been established between a number of sociodemographic factors and various patterns of alcohol consumption. National drinking practices surveys have demonstrated statistical correlations between extent of drinking and age, sex, socioeconomic status, ethnic background, education, occupation, and degree of urbanization.[88-90] In general, national surveys indicate that the percentage of drinkers increases as social status increases. However, rates of heavy drinking, heavy "escape" drinking, and problem drinking are highest in lowest status groups. Lower-status women report higher rates of abstinence than upper-status women, but when they drink, they are more likely to drink heavily. This pattern is particularly characteristic of Black women, and it has also been described for some American Indian women and an increasing number of Hispanic women.[4] The disproportionate rate of alcoholism among minority women may warrant special attention, especially if different sociocultural factors contribute to the development and expression of their alcohol problems.

Until recently, the major source of information about Black drinking was the 1960s drinking practices survey, of which Blacks comprised a 9% subsample.[88] Abstinence was reported by 38% of Black men, 31% of white men, 51% of Black women, and 39% of white women. Rates for heavy drinking were similar for Black (19%) and white (21%) men, but were almost three times higher for Black women (11%) than for white women (4%). Comparable patterns for Blacks were obtained in a 1979 national household survey of adults.[91] However, findings from the recent Epidemiological Catchment Area (ECA) studies that used DSM-III[92] criteria for alcohol abuse and alcohol dependence found no significant differences in mean lifetime prevalence rates between Black (14.5%) and white (13.4%) adults in three cities.[47]

Rimmer et al.[93] compared alcoholic white and Black men and women in public and private psychiatric hospitals. More Blacks (52%) than whites (11%) had medical complications. Blacks had almost triple rates of alcoholic hallucinosis (47 vs 16%) and double rates of delirium tremens (54 vs 26%). Black women reported more prior hospitalizations and more binge drinking than white women. In a more recent study, Dawkins and Harper[94] compared the backgrounds of white and Black women treated for alcoholism. Black women were significantly younger when they began to drink, when they began to drink heavily, and when they began to seek alcoholism treatment. Black women also were more likely to drink in the street and to drink with groups of friends or with a female friend, and they drank more on holidays and in the morning. A study of 32 Black and 118 white women entering alcoholism treatment[95] found no significant differences in the age of onset of drinking (mean 21.4 vs 20.5 yr), age of onset of problem drinking (mean 37 vs 34 yr), duration of drinking before entering treatment (mean 6.3 vs 5.7 yr), number of drinks per day (mean 11.81 vs 11.03), or type of preferred beverage (distilled spirits). In contrast to alcoholic white women, however, alcoholic Black women were significantly less likely to drink alone (59 vs 75%) or to drink in bars or restaurants (28 vs 74%), but were more likely to have heavy-drinking female friends (47 vs 21%). Black women also were less likely to hide their drinking (53 vs 69%) or to conceal the amount that they drank (47 vs 70%). In addition, Black women were less likely to be concerned about their emotional health (22 vs 50%), and their husbands were less likely to criticize their drinking behavior (9 vs 30%). Although this sample was small, these findings suggest that the social context of drinking among Black alcoholic women differs from that among white alcoholic women, and that peer and family factors may be important in maintaining abusive drinking patterns.

It has been observed that, relative to Black men, Black women are at higher risk for developing alcoholism[96] than are white women in comparison to white men.[97] Several interpretations of this phenomenon have been offered. Bailey et al.[96] attributed alcoholism in Black women to a combination of stresses associated with dual social roles and permissive cultural norms. Knupfer et al.[98] suggested that the extent to which women have economic independence from men delimits other behaviors, including drinking patterns. Thus, purported greater economic independence is thought to permit Black women to drink like Black men.

Study of sex differences in the use of psychoactive drugs[25] provides further illumination. Although this analysis omitted alcohol use, for both licit and illicit psychoactive drugs, males generally control production and distribution, influence drug availability, and determine context of use. Access, however, is also affected by legal status of a drug, so that alcohol is more like tobacco, i.e., legal and widely available, than it is like cocaine or heroin, i.e., illegal and obtained only via highly restricted distribution channels. Legal drugs are also far less expensive than illegal drugs, so that the legal status of alcohol contributes to its relatively small cost and wide availability. Higher rates of heavy drinking by Black women cannot be explained by greater availability of disposable income, because Blacks earn less than whites. Exposure to heavy-drinking males, proportionately more numerous among Blacks, as well as to other heavy-drinking women, may account for some portion of influence on the heavy drinking rate among Black women, as may differences in values regarding expenditures.

Black women also have been shown to have poorer treatment outcomes than white women.[95,99] A 1-yr followup study of Black and white women treated for alcoholism[95] found that only 13% of Black women (vs 41% of the combined sample) abstained, and 9% (vs 12% of the combined sample) drank on rare occasions. No difference was found in the likelihood of remaining in treatment. However, two-thirds of the Black women were of lower socioeconomic status, whereas the white women were distributed across several socioeconomic strata. Black women scored a mean of 9.3 on a psychiatric impairment scale vs a mean of 4.9 for white women; and on a case-by-case basis, Black women also were found to have fewer social and emotional supports and greater exposure to heavy-drinking mates and friends. In a 12-yr followup study of 24 Black and 24 white female alcoholics matched for age and hospitalization,[99] 69% of Black women were found to be uncontrolled drinkers, whereas 78% of the white women had become abstinent. Mortality among Black women (10 deaths) was double the rate for white women (five deaths). No significant differences were found between Black and white women for religious affiliation, educational level, marital status, age at index admission, number of alcohol-dependence symptoms at index admission, or site of hospitalization.

Hispanic women also are reported to have higher rates of abstinence.[100] Drinking patterns among 402 Spanish-speaking men and women in three California areas showed rates of heavy drinking that ranged from 8–43% for men and from 2–10% for women and showed rates of abstinence that ranged from 11–39% of men and from 37–68% of women.[101] Hispanic youths have reported less alcohol use and may abstain more than whites.[100] Some Hispanic youths prefer inhalants, depressants, or marijuana.[102,103]

In 1977, 9% of all clients (27,000 persons) who received outpatient treatment in programs funded by the National Institute on Alcohol Abuse and Alcoholism were of Spanish origin.[104] In comparison with other clients, Spanish-origin clients entered treatment at higher rates (46 vs 41%), and higher percentages of clients were male (89–95% vs 83–88%). At admission, Spanish-origin clients were younger (aged 33–38 yr), had longer histories of heavy drinking (from 8.9–12.1yr), consumed less absolute alcohol per day (2.6–5.6 oz), and had less prior treatment. Spanish-origin clients were more likely to be married, to have 1–2 yr less education, and to earn about $1,750 less per year. Spanish-origin clients also were more likely to have been referred for treatment via the criminal justice system or to require detoxification. Caetano[105] compared rates of self-reported intoxication in California Hispanics with rates for the general population. Frequencies of drinking until intoxicated once a month or more were at least double for Hispanic men and women of all ages. In addition, frequency of intoxication in Hispanic men increased with age, but declined with age for men in the general population.

Contemporary American Indians comprise slightly less than 1% of the US population, but they are heterogeneous in tribal origin, preservation of traditions, and degree of urbanization.[106,107] About one-half live in cities, and the remainder live in remote, widely separated areas. No broad-scale drinking practices or drinking problems surveys have studied samples across tribes or communities,[107] and American Indians were not included in the national sample of 1979.[91]

With few exceptions, studies of Indian drinking have focused on public drinking by men, and data about women's drinking are scanty.[107,108] The highest alcohol use occurs among men aged 25–44 yr, but the number of women who drink may be increasing.[107,109,110] FAS is disproportionately found in offspring of Native American women,[22] but concentrated in Plains tribes. The likelihood that a woman who bears one affected child will bear others is roughly 25%.[110]

Partly in response to greater efforts to enforce drinking and driving laws and more stringent penalties for drinking and driving, an increasing number of women have come to the attention of the criminal justice system.[50] Relatively few women have entered treatment involuntarily,[111] and the quality of treatment programs for women generally has lagged behind those for men.[112,113] The recent study that compared characteristics of men and women arrested in Massachusetts for "Driving Under the Influence of Liquor" (DUIL) concluded that severity of alcohol-related problems among women generally paralleled those of men, but that women might have greater need for comprehensive treatment programs, since they had fewer economic resources and social supports.[50] Argeriou and colleagues reported data for female DUIL offenders in Massachusetts during the years 1983–1984. Second DUIL offenders were referred to 14-d residential treatment programs, and third DUIL offenders were incarcerated for 60 d. In comparison to men in that population, women had fewer economic resources and social supports. Among second and third DUIL offenders, almost twice as many women as men (40%) were separated or divorced. Their mean age was 32.0, and the majority had finished high school. Among female second offenders, about 11% were unemployed and 18% had concurrent drug problems.

Engaging in Treatment, Treatment Effects, and Treatment Outcome

Alcoholism treatment programs traditionally have been geared to the needs of males—their most numerous clients.[114] A review by Duckert[115] noted that women alcoholics are less likely than male alcoholics to seek treatment in conventional alcoholism services. Moreover, women with alcohol problems appear more likely to seek help specifically for marital problems, family problems, physical illness, or emotional problems, but do not associate these problems with alcohol abuse. Because women may receive psychotropic medications, the problem of dual addiction arises.

A number of investigators have reported differential treatment experiences of women vs men. Beckman and Amaro[116] reviewed distinctions between female and male alcoholics. In their summary, they noted that intercurrent psychiatric diagnoses, psychological problems, and intercurrent medical illness all occur with greater frequency in female alcoholics. In addition, female alcoholics are more likely to have alcoholism in their family background, to experience greater marital disruption, and are more likely to have alcoholic husbands. Female alcoholics are more likely to have experienced sexual or physical abuse, and were also reported to have lower feelings of self-worth. In addition, a number of investigators have remarked that females are more likely to attribute their onset of alcoholismic drinking to the consequences of some significant life event. Further, women are more likely to have concerns about their role as family caretakers.

Thom[57] examined barriers to help seeking in 25 men and 25 women who were new referrals to an alcohol clinic. Few, only four women and no men, reported that there were practical problems that made it difficult to attend the clinic. Child care did not seem to be a salient issue for women; instead obtaining time off from work was considered to be awkward. An equal number of men and women ($n = 5$) were afraid of the hospital context. Fears included shame and embarrassment about discussing personal problems, fear and lack of knowledge about what treatment what might entail, fear of being told never to drink again, general anxiety and fear of hospitals, and fear of the authority figure of the physician.

Reasons for referral in this sample also were examined.[57] Half of the men and women had first sought treatment within the year prior to the interview. Similar numbers of men ($n = 16$) and women ($n = 14$) were referred to the alcohol clinic by general practitioners. However, almost double the number of women ($n = 9$ vs $n = 5$) were referred to the alco-hol clinic from an emergency clinic, suggesting that women may delay treatment until health problems become urgent.

Beckman and Amaro[116] investigated the effects of three types of characteristics that might differentiate the experiences of men and women in treatment settings. Major potential obstacles to obtaining treatment were the typically lower levels of disposable income and paucity of economic resources available to women. This study[116] compared 67 white women and 54 white men who sought treatment for alcohol problems in 23 California treatment facilities. Men and women were similar in the type of treatment facility, frequency of prior treatment, and number of days in their current treatment. Measures included interview items pertinent to health perceptions, locus of control, behavioral impairment, socioeconomic status, self-esteem, and social isolation. Respondents were queried regarding whether they believed that successful treatment could occur for themselves and others, the extent to which they experienced their own drinking as a serious problem, the extent to which family background, heredity, or life circumstances promoted alcoholism, satisfaction with treatment services, problems associated with drinking, and problems associated with treatment.

Since women traditionally have been more willing to seek care for medical and psychological problems, this factor was predicted to differentiate male and female expectations of efficacy of alcoholism treatment. Next, since it had been frequently reported that alcoholic women experience far greater stigma than alcoholic men, it was predicted that women would experience greater obstacles in seeking and obtaining treatment. In addition, it was predicted that women would identify more impact of alcoholism on their roles as family caretakers and have need for child care, whereas men would be more concerned about job-related factors. Lastly, it was predicted that women would thus receive less social support for engagement in treatment.

However, women and men did not differ in ratings of seriousness of drinking problems, satisfaction with treatment, or expectations of treatment outcomes. Further, women and men did not differ in health consequences or problems with their children. Women were more likely than men to acknowledge family problems, problems with their friends, and financial problems. Roughly one-half (48%) of women reported having had one or more types of treatment-related problems, in contrast to one-fifth (20%) of men. Men and women were similar in their concerns about health and expectations of medical care, and men and women were similar in their scores on locus of control scales.

Women and men were asked to indicate whether members of their family, friends, health professionals, employers, coworkers, or police had encouraged their seeking treatment. The vast majority of men (72%) and women (59%) reported social support from more than one source. Men were more likely to receive encouragement from spouses, whereas women were more likely to receive encouragement from their parents. Children were more likely to support treatment for women than for men. Both men and women received limited encouragement from sources other than family and friends, and these sources did not differ between men and women. However, in this sample all respondents had been employed, but 64% were currently unemployed. Roughly 2% of men reported opposition from family and friends during the months prior to treatment, in contrast to over 20% of women. Opposition to women's treatment came from husbands, friends, and other family members. In contrast, only one man reported opposition to treatment, which came from a drinking companion. Finally, women were three times more likely than men to report that they needed child care, but the rates were very small (6 vs 2%). There also was a tendency for women to report that they felt a need for educational counseling.

A step-wise discriminant function analysis examined 12 independent variables, including health perceptions, health locus of control, drinking-related problems, negative effects of obtaining treatment, and negative effects of not obtaining treatment. Other variables included satisfaction with treatment, perceived success of treatment, and beliefs about family or genetic contributions to alcoholism. In contrast to predictions, negative attitudes about health providers were stronger in women. However, men reported slightly greater social support for entering treatment, women had higher depression scores, and men had higher scores for amount consumed per day.[116]

Findings generally supported the contention that women experience more difficulties in entering treatment. Family therapy and environmental intervention strategies could counterbalance these obstacles. Another important factor was co-morbidity of affective disorder in women. This finding suggested that family history evaluations include history of affective disorder as well as history of alcohol problems. Data also suggested that women may have had more difficulties than men in establishing trust in their alcohol counselor or therapist.

Patterns of Compliance in Men vs Women

Allan and Phil[117] studied 112 men and women with drinking problems enrolled in a community-based volunteer agency over a 6 mo period. Their study examined assumptions that alcoholic patients were difficult to engage in treatment, were highly ambivalent about treatment, and showed poor motivation for treatment, with attrition rates for the first month after engaging in treatment ranging from 28–80%, and that patients who dropped out of treatment had poor prognoses.

In Great Britain, local Councils on Alcohol have adopted a different approach from the typical medical model. Counselors are volunteers, services do not include either detoxication or direct access to psychiatric or medical care, and self-referrals constitute the major proportion of those who seek help. Accordingly, results from these services contrast with services that require a referral from a general practitioner, the courts, or employers. Councils on Alcoholism have reported to be more successful in attracting problem-drinking women. Female counselors are available to female clients, which may reduce stigma, appointment scheduling is flexible, and individual counseling is emphasized.

All 112 clients[117] were problem drinkers requiring treatment. About one-half (52%) were married, with about 25% separated or divorced, and the remainder (21%) were single. Ages ranged from 18–65 yr with a mean of 40 yr. Sixty-one percent were employed. Twenty-seven percent of the sample were seen only once. By 4 wk, 37 additional referrals dropped out of the program, and by 6 mo an additional 29% had dropped out. Thus, only 7% were still in treatment at the 6 mo mark. Other statistics indicated that 72% of the 112 clients did not respond to any followup attempts. Formal discharge occurred for 21% of the sample, leaving the remaining 7% still in need of services.

Gender differences were reflected in the number of individuals who chose to participate in only one interview, 35% of men vs 21% of women. Men had a mean of 4.7 sessions during 6 wk, whereas women had an average of 3.3 sessions over 4 1/2 wk. Only men (11% of original referrals) attended the clinic for 6 or more mo, while no women remained in treatment for 6 mo.

Gender of counselors did not affect treatment retention, since 78% of the women had been assigned to female counselors, but the source of referral proved to be important. About one-half (49%) were self-referrals, with the remainder referred by general practitioners, hospitals, and shelters. Individuals who had been referred by agencies remained in treatment longer, with 14% of agency-referred clients remaining in treatment 6 mo, vs only 1.8% of self-referrals. However, there were no significant differences in age, marital status, or employment status. Referrals made by shelters, employers, or courts were associated with higher rates of attendance, with individuals referred from these sources maintaining a regular attendance record and sustaining engagement in treatment for significantly longer intervals than individuals who were self-referred. Individuals referred by courts, employers, or shelters had an average of 6.1 appointments over 9.1 wk, whereas self-referrals attended 3.4 sessions over 3.7 wk. Only one-half of the clients referred from coercive sources spontaneously left treatment, in contrast to 80% of the self-referred. Only two women were referred by coercive sources, namely, employers. Since the vast majority of women were self-referrals or referred by noncoercive sources, high attrition may have been associated with low motivation. The author concluded that, since the majority of clients were only seen once, the initial interview should have been targeted for thorough evaluation, with the results incorporated into a highly specific treatment plan. Further, lack of motivation by women was considered to reflect the absence of coercive factors in referrals as opposed to greater pathology.

Treatment Outcome

Valid treatment outcome data for women have lagged behind outcome data for men. Vannicelli and Nash[112] evaluated 259 studies that were published between 1972–1980 in order to assess whether sex bias was a contributing factor to underrepresentation of women. In studies wherein males and females were analyzed separately, at most 2,459 women were studied between 1972–1980. Only 7.8% of over 64,000 subjects for whom data were pooled were female. Of these 259 studies, over 80% had male first authors. The likelihood of followup was increased when women investigators studied treatment samples. Overall, female investigators sampled three times the number of women when compared by the number studied by male investigators. (Although 13.4% of all individuals sampled by female authors were women, women comprised only 4.3% of all individuals studied by male investigators.)

Rationale for inattention to women argues that more men than women are alcoholic or heavy drinkers, that women are often excluded since their numbers are small and inclusion of their data might generate unstable statistics, or that followup studies on women are complicated should their names change following divorce or marriage. However, when Vannicelli and Nash[112] recalculated outcome data for 23 studies (out of 259) that had differentiated between male and female alcoholics, 78% (18) showed no differences in outcome between men and women, and four studies showed better outcome for women, but no studies showed better outcome for men. Thus, no scientific evidence supported the contention that women responded poorly to treatment.

Herr and Pettinati[118] presented outcome data for 48 homemakers and 24 employed women who had received inpatient alcoholism treatment in a psychiatric hospital. Average age at admission was 43 yr. Outcome was assessed at the end of 4-yr intervals following a 28-d treatment experience. As might be expected, more homemakers were married (85 vs 33%), whereas more working women were divorced or separated (42 vs 8%). Women who were homemakers reported longer intervals of drinking (mean 9.2 vs 5.8 yr).

Adjustment was categorized as good, poor, or inconsistent. Approximately one-half of the homemakers and workers maintained a good adjustment over the 4-yr interval, whereas 24% of homemakers vs 14% of employed women showed a poor adjustment. Roughly equal percentages (32% homemakers vs 36% employed women) had inconsistent adjustment ratings during the 4-yr followup interval. These differences could not be attributed to marital status.

More than half of the patients maintained the same occupation at the followup interview, with 60% still functioning as homemakers and 59% still in the labor force. Improvement in adjustment and change of occupation were examined. Of 10 women who changed occupation, nine improved at followup, in comparison with seven of 13 who had maintained the same occupation. A smaller number of women (three homemakers and three women in the labor force) did not change marital status at the time they changed occupations, suggesting that improvement in adjustment might be more related to change in occupation but independent from change in marital status. However, change in occupation cannot be considered to be a single variable, since such a change might prompt a reallocation of leisure time or might reflect a consequence rather than a reason for improvement.

A series of reports by Haver[119-121] presented data from a followup study of 44 Norwegian women who had been treated for alcohol problems in the interval 1970–1980. Followup interviews occurred approx 6.5 yr after first admission, when the mean age of the women was 32.2 yr. Exactly one-half of the women reported that violence had occurred between their parents or between a parent and themselves. In the majority of cases, fathers abused mothers, followed by fathers abusing patients, mothers abusing patients, and mothers abusing fathers. Twenty-four women reported that one or both parents were alcoholic. Alcoholism was slightly more frequently associated with intrafamilial violence. At treatment, 80% of the women had had at least one partner, 57% had lived with an alcohol abuser, and 18% had experienced violence. In this sample, four women had a history of residing with one or more partners who were alcoholic, violent, or both.

A woman's experience of physical abuse by her father, or of witnessing abuse of her mother by her father, was significantly correlated with the number of violent partners that patients had during the followup interval. Thus, the more that these female patients had experienced violence as children, the greater the likelihood that they would be involved in violent relationships in their adult lives. Women who had experienced violence from their mothers had poorer outcome and a history of residing with violent partners. In contrast, during the followup interval, women who had no family history of childhood violence were more likely to break off relationships with a violent partner.

Past and present domestic violence contributed significantly to poor outcome. A multiple regression analysis indicated that childhood violence experiences explained 11% of variance in outcome, and living with a violent partner after treatment increased the explanation of variance to 25%. Significant associations also were observed among childhood violence experiences, prevalence of antisocial and/or borderline personality disorders, and violence in a cohabiting partner. Personality disorders added an additional 9% to explained variance in outcome. It was concluded that childhood violence may have promoted symptoms reminiscent of posttraumatic stress disorder, and that these aftereffects may have contributed to a woman's inability to cope with life problems.

The same 44 women were evaluated for alcohol consumption during the year prior to the followup interview. All of the women had consumed alcohol, but at the followup, their alcohol consumption differed. Drinking patterns could be classified as abstinence, light drinking, moderate drinking, and heavy drinking. Of the eight women who reported no alcohol consumption in the previous year, six had been abstainers for several years. An additional 12 women consumed about the average amount of alcohol (2 L) reported by women in the general Norwegian population. Seven more women drank less than 7 L/yr, and the remainder (39% or 17 women) were heavy drinkers whose consumption ranged from 8–180 L in a year's span. Almost all of the women who consumed more than 20 centiliters of pure alcohol (roughly two-thirds of a bottle of spirits) on any single drinking day met one or more criteria for pathological alcohol use. In contrast, no women who reported consuming less than 14 centiliters met any criteria for pathological alcohol abuse. Four women shifted from moderate to heavy drinking, and four women shifted from heavy drinking to moderate drinking. Among the abstainers, all had relapsed one or more times following treatment.

Six women were long-term abstainers who changed their identities to nondrinkers by informing their drinking partners that they chose to abstain, by avoiding or coping with situations in which other people drank, by attending self-help groups, or through religious participation. Interestingly, however, even long-term abstainers who relapsed into heavy drinking alleged that they were prompted by a life crisis. Although it can be argued that these factors were consequences and not predictors, typical life crises were divorce or removal of children from the household. Thirty-seven percent (16) of the women were short-term abstainers who attempted to remain sober over time, but could not maintain sobriety over the entire followup interval. These women appeared to be able to respond to responsibilities, such as holding a job or caring for children, by reducing their frequency and consequences of drinking. A shift to social drinking was reported by 39% (17) women, but a check of registry records indicated that only eight of the women provided valid information. In the case of these eight individuals, abstinence occurred over months or years after treatment. Life situations changed for the better, with some women separating from heavy drinkers and living either with their children, with a new partner, or by themselves. Their problem drink-ing appeared associated with emotional crises and difficult life circumstances.

Accordingly, these women shifted to social drinking and did not seek intoxication. Their average consumption ranged from one or two glasses of an alcoholic beverage to four to six glasses. Among the heavy long-term drinkers, four women maintained heavy drinking following treatment and two retained jobs, whereas two had unstable employment.

A 1-yr followup study of 93 alcoholic women in Ontario found 56% abstinent.[122] Fewer life problems (financial, health, marital) and strong social supports were associated with favorable outcome. Silvia and coworkers[123] compared biological, psychological, and sociocultural variables in 60 alcoholic vs 60 nonalcoholic women. Alcoholic women had significantly more alcoholic relatives, more health problems, more depression symptoms, lower levels of self-esteem, believed themselves to be less "feminine," and believed that they were less able to meet the expectations of others.

Vannicelli[124] evaluated 15 treatment outcome studies. Twelve showed no significant differences in outcome for men vs women, two showed superior outcome for women, and one showed superior outcome for men. Consequently, there appears to be little evidence indicating a poorer prognosis for women than for men. However, concerns about social conditions peculiar to women as mothers have promoted development of all-female treatment programs. A number of these programs provide child care or are targeted toward pregnant women. Some treatment programs have stemmed from feminist ideology. However, it is the case that in-patient treatment may be more difficult for women, since residential treatment in most instances necessitates a woman's absence from her family. Treatment outcomes for programs specifically targeted to women were also reviewed by Duckert.[115] Results from 15 studies indicate that improvement rates ranged from 20% to close to 60%.

Vannicelli[124] found that treatment providers had beliefs that erected three barriers to efficacious treatment of alcoholism in women. These beliefs

1. Reflect negative expectancies that alcoholic women will not profit from treatment because they are perceived as more depressed, experience mood swings, and are self-centered
2. Incorporate stereotypic views of female sex role expectancies that are thought to limit alcoholic women's potential for change, and
3. Demonstrate lack of information about prognosis for alcoholic women.

These expectancies were are held by both male and *female* alcohol treatment providers,[124] and case vignettes amply illustrate the extent to which providers infantilized female alcoholics, thus undercutting the growth and strength of female clients in the course of treatment.

In recent years, advocates of the needs of alcoholic women have argued for sexually segregated facilities to provide emotionally and socially sensitive treatment. This position has been viewed as overdrawn, as well as supported by little empirical evidence.[124,125] One study of structural factors in treatment utilization of 53 alcoholism treatment facilities in two California counties[126] found women more likely to choose agencies with higher percentages of professional staff, aftercare services, and treatment programs for children. Neither provider attitudes toward female alcoholics nor the type of agency (public or private) was associated with women's utilization rates, and support services, such as transportation, vocational counseling, or legal aid, were found to be of lesser importance to women than child-related services. Thus, the alcoholic women in this study appear to have chosen treatment for themselves and their children that addressed the central impact of alcohol problems, whereas social support requirements were of less importance.

However, recent results from a comparison of women assigned to a specialized women's alcoholism treatment unit were contrasted with a matched number of control women assigned to a conventional unit treating both men and women.[127] All women were patients from the Stockholm metropolitan area. The early treatment (EWA) program sought to reach women in early stages of alcohol dependence, and give them broad assistance in a specialized inpatient ward and outpatient clinic. EWA staffing included two physicians, a nursing staff, one social worker, one psychologist, and one child psychiatrist available for consultation. Specialized treatment included medical care, individual and group therapy, social work support, occupational therapy, and physical therapy. Employment and family conditions were examined, and women received help and support in these areas as well as help with their children from a child psychiatrist. The duration of treatment was a minimum of 1 yr, and program-specific aspects included individualized treatment planning, close contact with staff, family therapy, and a focus on women's problems with group support. Controls received briefer treatment, and they did not have access to long-term supports, but did have access to disulfiram treatment. No women in either group had had prior treatment for alcoholism, and none had serious medical disorders including liver cirrhosis. Approximately one-third of each group exhibited withdrawal symptoms upon admission. The majority of women (85%) were self-referred, with the remainder having physician referrals.

One-half of the women admitted to the EWA program vs 31% of controls were inpatients. The median length of treatment was 8 mo for women in the EWA program vs 5 mo for controls, and 36% in the EWA program vs 21% of controls remained in treatment for 12 or more mo. At 2 yr postadmission, 75 patients in the EWA program and 68 controls were available for followup. Only 8% of patients in the EWA program had a reduced capacity for work vs 30% of controls.

At followup one-quarter of the women in both groups were divorced from their partners. Although 36% of controls had obtained a new partner, none of the patients in the EWA program had acquired a new partner. Indeed, women who had not been divorced reported improved relations in their marital life (40% in the EWA program vs 26% of controls). Moreover, 35% of patients in the EWA program vs 12% of controls reported improved relations with children, a result attributed to availability of help from a child psychiatrist. Only 5% of patients in the EWA program, but 25% of controls, voluntarily surrendered their children to foster homes.

Double the number of controls (31 vs 16%) relapsed and required inpatient care. However, one-third of the women in each group were hospitalized for a nonalcohol-related disorder. Although employed women in the greater Stockholm area averaged 22.5 d of illness/yr, women in both study groups had more than 30 d of illness.

In this study, abstinence was defined as absence of alcohol use for 300 or more days per year, with 67% of patients in the EWA program vs 45% of controls attaining that goal during year one, and 59% of patients in the EWA program vs 48% of controls attaining that level in year two. Interestingly, when relapse did occur, patients in the EWA program drank a median of 62.5 g of absolute alcohol/d vs 125 g/d for controls. Again, double the number of patients in the EWA program reported being able to drink socially (42%) in contrast to 20% of controls. Only 8% of patients in the EWA program, in contrast to about 30% of controls, relapsed to daily alcohol consumption. Additional gains seen for patients in the EWA program at 2-yr followup included fewer blackouts (25 vs 40%), less mood change during intoxication (16 vs 40%), and improvement of anxiety symptoms (43 vs 18%). For both groups, the longer patients remained in treatment, the better the outcome.

Since the assignment to two types of treatment had been entirely random, it is reasonable to assume that specialized attention and tailored design of the EWA program were the major factors determining outcome. Since no multiple regression analysis was performed, it is not possible to discern which aspects of the women's program were most strongly related to favorable outcome. The authors concluded that women in the early stages of alcohol dependence are unwilling to be confronted by male patients and are concerned about the effects on their children should their alcoholic status become known to social welfare agencies. The specialized women's program described in this study appeared to attract "hidden alcoholics." One interesting observation was that wine consumption was related to continuous drinking and development of alcohol dependence in women. The authors noted that, when couples adopt a pattern of daily wine drinking, women become more intoxicated and/or are more likely to experience difficulties in controlling their consumption sooner than their male partners. It also was noted that wine was used as a tranquilizer, and indeed one-quarter of patients in each group had used benzodiazepines. Since, in general, patients enrolled in the women's program had more favorable outcome, the positive aspects of the program are highlighted. However, it also is important to note that partner relationships, especially in pattern of consumption, again were found to be related to the women's alcohol problems.

Outcome studies of narcotics users by Anglin and coworkers[29] found that Hispanic women received significantly less social support for remaining in treatment than white women or white or Hispanic men. Underhill[128] observed that the history of physical and sexual abuse of women by men argued for separate services for women. This may be especially true, since it was also observed that men's problems tended to dominate group discussions, and women resorted to traditional patterns to support men, thus submerging their own problems.[128]

There are too few well-documented treatment research studies to provide a sound basis for retargeting treatment approaches to female alcoholics. For example, there is insufficient evidence to permit assessment of the impact of individual therapy vs group therapy, the value of family therapy, the need for women to be treated separately or in mixed groups, and the impact of a female vs male therapist.[112] The heterogeneity of substance use history among many women now receiving treatment also imposes a challenge to a treatment program primarily designed to focus on alcohol problems. Similarly, although child care during treatment may be an important issue for some women, others may have children in foster care and have quite different needs vis-á-vis their children, such as acquisition of parenting skills and planning for visitation.

Toward Prevention Throughout the Life Cycle

As already demonstrated by the lengthy discussion of the scope and nature of substance abuse-related problems in women, there are a number of factors that can be identified repeatedly. For heuristic purposes, these factors can be grouped into three interacting subsets: First are predisposing sociocultural factors, then predisposing biological factors, and finally, pharmacological effects of the substances themselves. All of these factors interact to exacerbate substance abuse problems.

With regard to predisposing cultural factors, there is evidence pro and con about cause-and-effect relationships between life crises and substance use. Accordingly, those who counsel women experiencing stress should be aware of potential risk for substance abuse. Preventative strategies would include bringing tendencies to alleviate psychic pain through the use of alcohol or drugs into awareness, and offer concrete suggestions for problem-solving alternatives. It is also important to examine the influence of male partners in women's social environments to consider the environmental effects of a family history of alcoholism or other substance abuse, and to assess the impact of domestic violence, whether experienced in childhood or adulthood and whether it involves physical or sexual abuse. The impact of socioeconomic factors also cannot be discounted.

Predisposing biological factors also include effects of family history of alcoholism and other substance abuse as a risk factor, the existence of comorbidity with other psychological disorders, such as depression and antisocial personality disorder, and reproductive dysfunction. Pharmacologic effects of alcohol and other substances again may be modulated by family history of alcoholism, dysphoria that accompanies heavy consumption also has a significant impact, and the disruption of reproductive function by excessive intake is additionally important. Socioeconomic status—primarily considered a sociocultural factor—

nonetheless can exert an influence on biological factors as well as pharmacologic effects (e.g., through nutritional status).

Midanik[129] indicated that more women than men surveyed in a cross-sectional sample reported having a family history of alcoholism. Cloninger and coworkers[12] have argued that the prevalence of family history of alcoholism is increasing in response to a secular trend that results from promotion of greater overall alcohol consumption in American society. Although Cloninger and coworkers[12] did not specifically indicate an increased prevalence of Type II alcoholism in young women, our own work with women civilly committed to receive treatment[23,59] indicates that this population may include a substantial number of women with both family history of alcoholism, polysubstance dependence, hormonal disruption, and reproductive dysfunction. Further, these women were of lower socioeconomic status and had had encounters with the criminal justice system. Some of them had been victims of violence, including rape and incest, and all had experienced heavy consumption and accompanying dysphoria. However, the time to intervene with women who became subjects of those studies was much earlier in their lives.

Suggestions for prevention of substance-related child abuse include strengthening the system of prenatal care and delivery that is targeted to high-risk communities. In addition, there may be positive benefits to alcohol and drug prevention programs targeted to 11th and 12th graders. However, since young women who drop out of school may be at higher risk, special attention through outreach should be addressed to their needs. Other related efforts require coordination for increased access to prenatal care, especially for minority women, as well as ongoing health care, social services, day care, and employment and financial assistance services.

With regard to more specific predisposing biological factors, family history of alcoholism may convey a differential sensitivity to the effects of alcohol,[130] and perhaps to other substances. There also have been reports that women with unspecified family histories nonetheless exhibit differential responses to alcohol effects.[131,132] However, a close reading of pertinent materials indicates that psychosocial factors also may shape women's expectancies of alcohol effects.

Certainly, comorbidity with other psychological disorders is an important factor in women's substance use, as witnessed by reports by Griffin et al.[38] for female cocaine users, as well as by other reports of dysphoria consequent to drug use emanating from studies in our laboratories.[133,134]

Moreover, reproductive dysfunctions[9,23,59] accompany use of alcohol, marijuana, cocaine, and opiates. The extent to which reproductive dysfunction may precede substance abuse problems is possibly substantiated by the work of Cloninger and colleagues[12,43,44] regarding the female offspring of Type II (early onset of alcohol-dependent men with concomitant histories of poor-impulse control, criminal behavior, and violent behavior) alcoholics who showed increased symptoms of abdominal pain. Since in the sample studied by Lex et al. the women receiving civil court-mandated treatment exhibited both problems with reproduction and encounters with the criminal justice system,[23] it is likely that Type II alcohol problems in women in the US may manifest themselves in patterns different from those observed in Scandinavia. Again, although these factors may be primarily considered biological, the effect of sociocultural factors, familial factors, and psychological factors also cannot be discounted. In addition, the socioeconomic status of women manifesting this cluster of symptoms is generally low.

Although at first glance pharmacological effects of substances may appear more clear-cut, again these factors intersect with other major categories of factors. Family history of alcoholism may affect perception of sensitivity to alcohol and other substances,[130] and also be related to mood states associated with consumption.[135] For example, Birnbaum and coworkers[136] found that even social drinkers who became abstinent for the duration of a 90-d study reported improved moods after cessation of alcohol intake. In addition, reproductive dysfunction may be preexisting, as in the case of infertility, but also exacerbated in the presence of substance abuse.

With all of these interlocking factors, it is important to choose appropriate junctures in the cycle for intervention. One dominant area pertains to family history of alcoholism. It is asserted that close to 28 million individuals in the US,[137,138] slightly more than half of whom may be female,[129] constitute a large population who have shown evidence of gaining awareness of the high risk conveyed by their familial and genetic legacy of substance abuse. Since this legacy can include domestic violence, and is believed by some to foster assortative mating with men who also have substance abuse problems, the sheer magnitude of size of this population invites an educational initiative.

Further, this initiative is most appropriately targeted to all age groups. Thus, girls as well as boys should learn that familial and genetic factors associated with parental substance abuse may have a strong impact on their adolescent and adult lives. Issues of responses to physical and emotional abuse and neglect, as well as interaction with substance-abusing significant others are topics that can and must be addressed at early ages. Moreover, as girls mature into their reproductive years, it is important to include education about substance abuse into education about female reproductive capacity. As young women (and men) begin to date during their teen years, they need to be exposed to information about the possible deleterious effects of influence from male partners who encourage women to engage in substance use. This topic intersects with emerging ideas of less traditional female roles, including development of assertiveness, limit-setting, and ability to form independent social judgments. Since comorbidity with depression in particular may be a predisposing factor, it is incumbent upon educational campaigns and health-care providers as well as educational personnel to make young women aware of the relationship between dysphoria and excessive alcohol, cocaine, marijuana, and other substance intake.

Educational campaigns that include information about pharmacological effects of drugs must underscore the potential vulnerability of individuals with family histories of substance use, indicate the psychological consequences of consumption, and warn of reproductive hazards. Evidence from studies of women seeking obstetrical and gynecological care[20] indicate that obstetrical and gynecological practices are other domains for disseminating information about substance abuse and engaging in prevention or treatment outreach. If reproductive events (miscarriage, stillbirth, infertility, hysterectomy) promote excessive drinking or other substance use in vulnerable women, then obstetrical and gynecological practices are potential resources for patient education. Since the time course and prognosis for recovery from reproductive disorders during abstinence and the extent to which the reproductive system develops tolerance to disruptive effects of chronic alcohol and drug abuse are unknown, it is important that programs treating female substance users also should evaluate neurendocrine status, such as hormone levels, especially reproductive hormones.[59] Outreach programs targeted to other vulnerable populations,[72] including pregnant teenagers, also are important vehicles for disseminating information about substance abuse and its consequences. Again, since the male to female vector is a common one, these outreach programs also are important contexts for discussion of relationships between women and men.

Further, substance abuse treatment programs reaching identified patients often include a family therapy and/or marital therapy component. It is also appropriate in this modality to include educational and intervention component specifically targeted toward women. It is not enough to discuss the overall disruption by substance abuse in families and households when the physically deleterious consequences for women and children can be so serious.[76] Women's demonstrated needs for social supports[139] also argue for "inoculating" vulnerable individuals by increasing awareness of appropriate affiliative behaviors as a prevention strategy and facilitating support groups as a treatment strategy.

In summary, creative prevention programming would examine existing facilities' programs and identify appropriate information and junctures for intervention that include detailed information for girls and women who are at high risk for substance abuse and its deleterious effects on themselves, their families, their offspring, their significant others, employers, and society at large.

Acknowledgment

Preparation of this manuscript was supported in part by Grants AAO 6252 and AA 06794 from the National Institute on Alcohol Abuse and Alcoholism and Grant DA 04870 from the National Institute on Drug Abuse. I am grateful to Carol Buchanan for her diligent and careful preparation of the manuscript.

References

[1] J. Barnes, C. Benson, and S. Wilsnack (1979) Psychosocial characteristics of women with alcoholic fathers, in *Currents in Alcoholism, Treatment and Rehabilitation and Epidemiology, vol. 6*. (M. Galanter, ed.) Grune, Stratton, NY, p. 209.

[2] P. G. Bourne and E. Light (1979) Alcohol problems in Blacks and women, in *The Diagnosis and Treatment of Alcoholism*, (1st Ed.) (J. H. Mendelson and N. K. Mello, eds.), McGraw-Hill, NY, p. 83

[3] R. L. Clayton, H. L. Voss, C. Robbins, and W. F. Skinner (1986) Gender differences in drug use: An epidemiological perspective, in *Women and Drugs: A New Era for Research* (B. A. Ray, and M. C. Braude, eds.), NIDA Research

Monograph No 65, DHHS Publ No (ADM) 86-1447, Rockville, MD, p. 80.

[4]B. W. Lex (1985) Alcohol problems in special populations, in *The Diagnosis and Treatment of Alcoholism* (2nd Ed.) (J. H. Mendelson and N. K. Mello, eds.), McGraw-Hill, NY, p. 89.

[5]N. K. Mello (1980) Some behavioral and biological aspects of alcohol problems in women, in *Alcohol and Drug Problems in Women* (O. J. Kalant, ed.) Plenum, NY, p. 263.

[6]M. M. Hyman (1976) Alcoholics 15 years later. *Ann. NY Acad. Sci.* 273, 613–623.

[7]T. J. Cicero (1980) Sex differences in the effects of alcohol and other psychoactive drugs on endocrine function: Clinical and experimental evidence, in *Alcohol and Drug Problems in Women* (O. J. Kalant, ed.), Plenum, NY, p. 545.

[8]N. K. Mello (1988) Effects of alcohol abuse on reproductive function in women, in *Recent Developments in Alcoholism, vol. 6* (M. Galanter, ed.), Plenum, NY, p. 253.

[9]N. K. Mello, J. H. Mendelson, and S. K. Teoh (1989) Neuroendocrine consequences of alcohol abuse in women. *Ann. NY Acad. Sci.* 562, 211–240.

[10]D. H. Van Thiel and J. S. Gavaler (1988) Ethanol metabolism and hepatotoxicity: Does sex make a difference? in *Recent Developments in Alcoholism, vol. 6* (M. Galanter, ed.) Plenum, NY, p. 291.

[11]M. Bohman, S. Sigvardsson, and C. R. Cloninger (1981) Maternal inheritance of alcohol abuse cross-fostering analysis of adopted women. *Arch. Gen. Psychiatry* 38, 965–969.

[12]C. R. Cloninger, S. Sigvardsson, T. Reich, and M. Bohman (1986) Inheritance of risk to develop alcoholism, in *Genetic and Biological Markers in Drug Abuse and Alcoholism* (M. C. Braude and H. M. Chao, eds.) NIDA Research Monograph No. 66, DHHS Publ No (ADM) 86-1444, Rockville, MD, pp. 86–96.

[13]M. N. Hesselbrock, R. E. Meyer, and J. J. Keener (1985) Psychopathology in hospitalized alcoholics. *Arch. Gen. Psychiatry* 42, 1050–1055.

[14]E. R. Morrisey and M. A. Schuckit (1978) Stressful life events and alcohol problems among women seen at a detoxication center. *J. Stud. Alcohol* 39, 1559–1576.

[15]M. A. Schuckit (1985) Genetics and the risk for alcoholism. *JAMA* 254(18), 2614–2617.

[16]M. A. Schuckit and E. R. Morrissey (1976) Alcoholism in women: Some clinical and social perspectives with an emphasis on possible subtypes, in *Alcoholism Problems in Women and Children* (M. Greenblatt and M. A. Schuckit, eds.), Grune, Stratton, NY, p 5.

[17]M. A. Schuckit (1978) Alcoholism in women. *Adv. Alcohol* 1, 1–3.

[18]J. S. Gavaler (1988) Effects of moderate consumption of alcoholic bever-

ages on endocrine function in post-menopausal women: Bases for hypotheses, in *Recent Developments in Alcoholism, vol. 6* (M. Galanter, ed.). Plenum, NY, p. 229.

[19]S. B. Blume (1986) Women and alcohol: A review. *JAMA* **256**(11), 1467–1470.

[20]A. Halliday, B. Booker, P. Cleary, M. Aronson, and T. Delbanco (1986) Alcohol abuse in women seeking gynecologic care. *Obstet. Gynecol.* **68**, 322–326.

[21]S. C. Wilsnack, R. W. Wilsnack, and A. D. Klassen (1984) Drinking and drinking problems among women in a U.S. national survey. *Alcohol Health Res. World* **9**(1), 3–13

[22]A. P. Streissguth, P. D. Sampson, and H. M. Barr (1989) Neurobehavioral dose–response effects of prenatal alcohol exposure in humans from infancy to adulthood. *Ann. NY Acad. Sci.* **562**, 145–158.

[23]B. W. Lex, S. K. Teoh, I. Lagomasino, N. K. Mello, and J. H. Mendelson (1990) Characteristics of women receiving mandated treatment for alcohol or polysubstance dependence in Massachusetts. *Drug Alcohol Depend.* **25**, 13–20.

[24]R. G. Ferrence (1980) Sex differences in the prevalence of problem drinking, in *Research Advances in Alcohol and Drug Problems, vol. 5 Alcohol and Drug Problems in Women* (O. J. Kalant, ed.) Plenum, NY, p. 69.

[25]R. G. Ferrence and P. C. Whitehead (1980) Sex differences in psychoactive drug use: Recent epidemiology, in *Research Advances and Drug Problems, vol. 5, Alcohol and Drug Problems in Women* (O. J. Kalant, ed.), Plenum, NY, p. 125.

[26]Y. I. Hser, M. D. Anglin, and W. McGlothlin (1987) Sex differences in addict careers. 1. Initiation of use. *Am. J. Drug Alcohol Abuse* **13**(1&2), 33–57.

[27]M. D. Anglin, Y. I. Hser, and W. H. McGlothlin (1987) Sex differences in addict careers. 2. Becoming addicted. *Am. J. Drug Alcohol Abuse* **13**(1&2), 59–71.

[28]Y. I. Hser, M. D. Anglin, and M. W. Booth (1987) Sex differences in addict careers. 3. Addiction. *Am. J. Drug Alcohol Abuse* **13**(3), 231–251.

[29]M. D. Anglin, Y. I. Hser, and M. W. Booth (1987) Sex differences in addict careers. 4. Treatment. *Am. J. Drug Alcohol Abuse* **13**(3), 253–280.

[30]T. R. Kosten, B. J. Rounsaville, and H. D. Kleber (1985) Ethnic and gender differences among opiate addicts. *Int. J. Addict.* **20**(8), 1143–1162.

[31]R. L. Spitzer, J. Endicott, E. Robins (1978) *Research Diagnostic Criteria (RDC) for a Selected Group of Functional Disorders* (New York State Psychiatric Institute, NY).

[32]T. R. Kosten, B. J. Rounsaville, and H. D. Kleber (1985) Parental alcoholism in opioid addicts. *J. Nerv. Ment. Dis.* **173**(8), 461–469.

[33]N. K. Mello, and J. H. Mendelson (1978) Alcohol and human behavior, in *Handbook of Psychopharmacology, vol. 12. Drugs of Abuse* (L. L. Iversen, S. D. Iversen, S. H. Snyder, eds.) Plenum, NY, p. 235.

[34]M. Schuckit, F. M. Pitts, Jr., T. Reich, L. J. King, and G. Winokur (1969) Alcoholism I: Two types of alcoholism in women. *Arch. Gen. Psychiatry* **20**, 301–306.

[35]J. Rimmer, T. Reich, and G. Winokur (1972) Alcoholism: V. Diagnosis and clinical variation among alcoholics. *Q. J. Stud. Alcohol* **33**, 658–666.

[36]M. A. Schuckit (1972) Sexual disturbance in the woman alcoholic. *Hum. Sexuality* **6**, 44–65.

[37]L. J. Beckman (1976) Alcoholism problems and women: An overview, in *Alcoholism Problems in Women and Children*. (M. Greenblatt and M. A. Schuckit, eds.) Grune, Stratton, NY, p. 65.

[38]M. L. Griffin, R. D. Weiss, S. M. Mirin, and U. Lange (1989) A comparison of male and female cocaine abusers. *Arch. Gen. Psychiatry* **46**, 122–126.

[39]*American Psychiatric Association: Diagnostic and Statistical Manual of Mental Disorders* (3rd Ed. revised), (1987) American Psychiatric Association, Washington, DC.

[40]D. B. Kandel (1984) Marijuana users in young adulthood. *Arch. Gen. Psychiatry* **41**, 200–209.

[41]D. B. Kandel, M. Davies, D. Karus, and K. Yamaguchi (1986) The consequences in young adulthood of adolescent drug involvement. *Arch. Gen. Psychiatry* **43**, 746–754.

[42]M. A. Schuckit (1987) Biological vulnerability to alcoholism. *J. Consult. Clin. Psychol.* **55**(3), 301–309

[43]C. R. Cloninger, B. Bohman, and S. Sigvardsson (1981) Inheritance of alcohol abuse cross-fostering analysis of adopted men. *Arch. Gen. Psychiatry* **38**, 861–868.

[44]C. R. Cloninger, M. Bohman, S. Sigvardsson, and A. L. Von Knorring (1985) Psychopathology in adopted-out children of alcoholics the Stockholm adoption study. *Recent Dev. Alcohol* **3**, 37–51.

[45]C. R. Cloninger (1983) Genetic and environmental factors in the development of alcoholism. *J. Psychiat.Treat Eval.* **3**, 487–496.

[46]C. R. Cloninger, K. O. Christiansen, T. Reich, and I. I. Gottesman (1978) Implications of sex differences in the prevalences of antisocial personality, alcoholism, and criminality for familial transmission. *Arch. Gen. Psychiatry* **35**, 941–951.

[47]L. N. Robins, J. E. Helzer, M. M. Weissman, H. Orvaschel, E. Gruenberg, J. D. Burker, Jr., and D. A. Regier (1984) Lifetime prevalence of specific psychiatric disorders in three sites. *Arch. Gen. Psychiatry* **41**, 949–958.

[48]T. Reich, C. R. Cloninger, P. Van Eerdewegh, J. P. Rice, and J. Mullaney (1988) Secular trends in the familial transmission of alcoholism. *Alcohol Clin. Exp. Res.* **12**(4), 458–464.

[49]J. Feighner, E. Robins, S. B. Guze, R. A. Woodruff, G. Winokur, and R.

Munoz (1972) Diagnostic criteria for use in psychiatric research. *Arch. Gen. Psychiatry* **26,** 57–63.

[50]M. A. Argeriou, D. McCarty, D. Potter, and L. Holt (1986) Characteristics of men and women arrested for driving under the influence of liquor. *Alcohol Treat. Quart.* **3,** 127–137.

[51]D. P. LeClair, L. Felici, and E. Klotzbier (1987) The use of prison confinement for the treatment of multiple drunken driver offenders: An evaluation of the Longwood Treatment Center. Department of Corrections, Commonwealth of Massachusetts, Boston, MA.

[52]B. W. Lex, M. L. Griffin, N. K. Mello, and J. H. Mendelson (1986) Concordant alcohol and marijuana use in women. *Alcohol* **3,** 193–200.

[53]B. W. Lex, S. L. Palmieri, N. K. Mello, and J. H. Mendelson (1987) Alcohol use, marijuana smoking, and sexual activity in women. *Alcohol* **5,** 21–25.

[54]S. Y. Hill, J. Armstrong, S. R. Steinhauer, T. Baughman, and J. Zubin (1987) Static ataxia as a psychobiological marker for alcoholism. *Alcohol Clin. Exp. Res.* **11,** 345–348.

[55]T. R. Kosten and B. J. Rounsaville (1988) Familial alcoholism in opioid addicts. (Abstract) 50th Annual Meeting: Committee on Problems of Drug Dependence, Falmouth, MA.

[56]B. Thom (1986) Sex differences in help-seeking for alcohol problems: 1. The barriers to help-seeking. *Br. J. Addict.* **81(6),** 777–786.

[57]B. Thom (1987) Sex differences in help-seeking for alcohol problems—2. Entry into treatment. *Br. J. Addict.* **82,** 989–997.

[58]D. J. Cooke, and C. A. Allan (1984) Stressful life events and alcohol abuse in women: A general population study. *Br. J. Addict.* **79,** 425–430.

[59]S. K. Teoh, B. W. Lex, J. Cochin, J. H. Mendelson and N. K. Mello (1989) Anterior pituitary gonadal and adrenal hormones in women with alcohol and polydrug abuse, in 60th Anniversary Fifty-First Annual Scientific Meeting Abstracts, Keystone, The Committee on Problems of Drug Dependence, Inc., Keystone, CO.

[60]J. N. Hugues, T. Coste, G. Perret, M. F. Jayle, J. Sebaoun, and E. Modigliani (1980) Hypothalamo-pituitary ovarian function in thirty-one women with chronic alcoholism. *Clin. Endocrinol.* **12,** 543–551.

[61]M. Russell and L. Bigler (1979) Screening for alcohol-related problems in an outpatient obstetric-gynecologic clinic. *Am. J. Obstet. Gynecol.* **134(4),** 4–12.

[62]R. H. Warner, and H. Rosett (1975) The effect of drinking on offspring: An historical survey of the American and British literature. *J. Stud. Alcohol* **36,** 1395–1420.

[63]H. L. Rosett (1980) The effects of alcohol on the fetus and offspring, in *Alcohol and Drug Problems in Women, Research Advances in Alcohol and Drug Problems, vol. 5* (O. J. Kalant, ed.), Plenum, NY, p. 595.

[64]K. L. Jones, and D. W. Smith (1973) The fetal alcohol syndrome: Recognition in early infancy and historical perspective. *Lancet* **2,** 999–1001.

[65]K. L. Jones, D. W. Smith, C. N. Ulleland, and A. P. Streissguth (1973) Pattern of malformation in offspring of chronic alcoholic mothers. *Lancet* **1,** 1269–1271.

[66]K. L. Jones, D. W. Smith, A. P. Streissguth, N. C. Myrianthopoulos (1974) Outcome in the offspring of chronic alcoholic women. *Lancet* **1,** 1076–1078.

[67]P. Lemoine, H. Harousseau, J. P. Borteyru, and J. C. Menuet (1968) Les enfants des parents alcoholiques: Anomalies observees a propos/de 124 cas. *Arch. Fr. Pediatr.* **25,** 830,831.

[68]S. K. Clarren and D. W. Smith (1978) The fetal alcohol syndrome. *NEJM* **298,** 1063–1067.

[69]A. P. Streissguth (1976a) Maternal alcoholism and the outcome of pregnancy: A review of the fetal alcohol syndrome, in *Alcohol Problems in Women and Children* (M. Greenblatt, and M. A. Schuckit (eds.) Grune, Stratton, NY, p. 251.

[70]A. P. Streissguth (1976b) Psychological handicaps in children with fetal alcohol syndrome. *Ann. NY Acad. Sci.* **273,** 140–145.

[71]J. H. Mendelson (1987) Marijuana, in *Psychopharmacology: The Third Generation of Progress* (H. Y. Meltzer, ed.), Raven, NY, p. 1565.

[72]M. S. Boone (1982) A socio-medical study of infant mortality among disadvantaged blacks. *Human Organization* **41,** 227–236.

[73]I. J. Chasnoff, and D. R. Griffith (1989) Cocaine: Clinical studies of pregnancy and the newborn. *Ann. N.Y. Acad. Sci.* **562,** 260–266.

[74]P. A. Fried, (1989) Postnatal consequences of maternal marijuana use in humans. *Ann. NY Acad. Sci* **562,** 123–132.

[75]G. S. Wilson (1989) Clinical studies of infants and children exposed prenatally to heroin. *Ann. NY Acad. Sci.* **562,** 183–194.

[76]J. Herskowitz, M. Seck, C. Fogg, S. Osgood, J. Powers, and D. Makin (1989) Substance abuse and family violence Part I. Identification of drug and alcohol usage during child abuse investigations in Boston. Commonwealth of Massachusetts Department of Social Services, Boston, MA.

[77]A. Medhus (1974) Morbidity among female alcoholics. *Scand. J. Soc. Med.* **2,** 5–11.

[78]L. Dahlgren and C. M. Idestrom (1979) Female alcoholics, V. Morbidity. *Acta Psychiatr. Scand.* **60,** 199–213.

[79]D. W. Spain (1945) Portal cirrhosis of the liver: A review of 250 necropsies with reference to sex differences. *Am. J. Clin. Pathol.* **15,** 215.

[80]W. H. J. Summerskill, C. S. Davidson, J. H. Dible, G. K. Mallory, S. Sherlock, M. D. Turner, and S. H. Wolfe (1960) Cirrhosis of the liver: A study of alcoholic and nonalcoholic patients in Boston and London. *NEJM* **262,** 1.

[81] P. Wilkinson, J. N. Santamaria, and R. G. Rankin (1969a) Epidemiology of alcoholic cirrhosis. *Aust. Ann. Med.* **18**, 222–226.

[82] P. Wilkinson, J. N. Santamaria, and R. G. Rankin (1969b) Epidemiology of alcoholism: Social data and drinking patterns of a sample of Australian alcoholics. *Med. J. Aust.* **1**, 1020.

[83] N. Krasner, M. Davis, B. Partmann, and R. Williams (1977) Changing pattern of alcoholic liver disease in Great Britain: Relation to sex and signs of autoimmunity. *Br. Med. J.* **1**, 1497–1550.

[84] G. Pequignot, C. Chabert, H. Eydoux, and M. A. Courcoul (1974) Increased risk of liver cirrhosis with intake of alcohol. *Rev. Alcohol* **20**, 191.

[85] J. N. Hugues, G. Perret, G. Adessi, T. Coste, and E. Modigliani (1978) Effects of chronic alcoholism on the pituitary-gonadal function of women during menopausal transition and in the post-menopausal period. *Biomedicine* **29**, 279–283.

[86] D. J. Jones-Sumty, O. A. Parsons, and M. S. Fabian (1980) Familial alcoholism, drinking behavior, and neuropsychological performance in alcoholic women. *Alcohol Tech. Reports* **9(3,4)**, 29.

[87] J. S. Gavaler (1982) Sex-related differences in ethanol-induced liver disease: Artifactual or real? *Alcohol: Clin. Exp. Res.* **6(2)**, 186–196.

[88] D. Cahalan, I. Cisin, and H. M. Crossley (1969) *American Drinking Practices: A National Survey of Drinking Behavior and Attitudes,* Monograph No. 6, (Rutgers Center of Alcohol Studies, New Brunswick, NJ).

[89] D. Cahalan (1970) *Problem Drinkers.* (Josey-Bass, San Francisco, CA).

[90] D. Cahalan, and R. Room (1974) *Problem Drinking among American Men,* Monograph No 7, (Rutgers Center of Alcohol Studies, New Brunswick, NJ).

[91] W. B. Clark and L. Midanik (1982) Alcohol use and alcohol problems among U.S. adults: Results of the 1979 national survey, in *Alcohol Consumption and Related Problems* (National Institute on Alcohol Abuse and Alcoholism, ed., Alcohol and Health Monograph No 1, National Institute on Alcohol Abuse and Alcoholism, Rockville, MD, pp. 3–52.

[92] *American Psychiatric Association: Diagnostic and Statistical Manual of Mental Disorders* (3rd Ed.)(1980) Author, Washington, DC.

[93] J. Rimmer, F. N. Pitts, T. Reich, and G. Winokur (1971) Alcoholism: II. Sex, socioeconomic status, and race in two hospitalized samples. *Q. J .Stud. Alcohol* **32**, 942–952.

[94] M. P. Dawkins, and F. D. Harper (1983) Alcoholism among women: A comparison of Black and White problem drinkers. *Int. J. Addict.* **18**, 333–349.

[95] E. M. Corrigan, and S. C. Anderson (1982) Black alcoholic women in treatment. *J. Addict. Health* **3**, 49–58.

[96] M. B. Bailey, P. W. Haberman, and H. Alksne (1965) The epidemiology of alcoholism in an urban residential area. *Q. J. Stud. Alcohol* **26**, 19–40.

[97] J. B. Roebuck, and R. G. Kessler (1972) *The Etiology of Alcoholism: Constitutional, Psychological, and Sociological Approaches* (Thomas, Springfield, IL)

[98] G. Knupfer, R. Fink, W. Clark, and A. Goffman (1963) *Factors Related to Amount of Drinking in an Urban Community.* California Drinking Practices Study Report No 6, California State Department of Health, Berkeley, CA.

[99] D. Idleburg (1982) *An Exploratory Study of Treatment Outcomes in a 12 Year Follow-Up of Black and of White Female Alcoholics.* Unpublished Ph.D. dissertation, Washington University, St. Louis, MO.

[100] R. T. Trotter (1985) Mexican-American experience with alcohol: South Texas examples, in *The American Experience with Alcohol: Contrasting Cultural Perspectives* (L. A. Bennet, and G. M. Ames, eds.) Plenum, NY, p. 279.

[101] Technical Systems Institute: Final report: Drinking practices and alcohol-related problems of Spanish-speaking persons in three California locales (1977) (Author, Alhambra, CA).

[102] E. R. Padilla, A. M. Padilla, A. Morales, and E. L. Olmedo (1979) Inhalant, marijuana, and alcohol abuse among barrio children and adolescents. *Int. J. Addict.* **14,** 945–964.

[103] J. B. Page, L. Rio, J. Sweeney, and C. MacKay (1985) Alcohol and adaptation to exile in Miami's Cuban population, in *The American Experience with Alcohol: Contrasting Cultural Perspectives* (L. A. Bennet, and G. M. Ames, eds.), Plenum, NY, p. 315.

[104] National Institute on Alcohol Abuse and Alcoholism: Spanish Clients Treated in NIAAA-Funded Programs: Calendar Year 1977. Author, Rockville, MD, 1978.

[105] R. Caetano (1984) Self-reported intoxication among Hispanics in Northern California. *J. Stud. Alcohol.* **45,** 349–354.

[106] J. C. Weibel-Orlando (1985) Indians, ethnicity, and alcohol: Contrasting perceptions of the ethnic self and alcohol use, in *The American Experience with Alcohol: Contrasting Cultural Perspectives* (L. A. Bennett and G. M. Ames, eds.), Plenum, NY, p. 201.

[107] P. A. May (1989) Alcohol abuse and alcoholism among American Indians: An overview, in *Alcoholism in Minority Populations* (T. D. Watts, and R. Wright, Jr., eds.), Thomas, Springfield, IL, p. 95.

[108] J. Leland (1978) Women and alcohol in an Indian settlement. *Med. Anthro.* **2,** 85–119.

[109] S. J. Kunitz (1983) *Disease Change and the Role of Medicine: The Navajo Experience* (University of California, Berkeley, CA).

[110] P. A. May, K. J. Hymbaugh, M. Aase, and J. M. Samet (1983) Epidemiology of fetal alcohol syndrome among American Indians of the southwest. *Soc. Biol.* **30,** 374–387.

[111] J. C. Marsh and N. A. Miller (1985) Female clients in substance abuse treatment. *Int. J. Addict.* **20(6&7)**, 995–1019.

[112] M. Vannicelli and L. Nash (1984) Effect of sex bias on women's studies on alcoholism. *Alcohol: Clin. Exp. Res.* **8(3)**, 334–336.

[113] M. Vannicelli (1989) *Group Psychotherapy with Adult Children of Alcoholics: Treatment Techniques and Countertransference Considerations* (Guilford, NY).

[114] D. C. Henderson and S. C. Anderson (1982) Treatment of alcoholic women. *J. Addict. Health* **3**, 34–48.

[115] F. Duckert (1987) Recruitment into treatment and effects of treatment for female problem drinkers. *Addict. Behav.* **12**, 137–150.

[116] L. J. Beckman, and H. Amaro (1986) Personal and social difficulties faced by women and men entering alcoholism treatment. *J. Stud. Alcohol* **47(2)**, 135–145.

[117] C. Allan, and M. Phil (1987) Seeking help for drinking problems from a community-based voluntary agency. Patterns of compliance amongst men and women. *Br. J. Addict.* **82**, 1143–1147.

[118] B. M. Herr and H. M. Pettinati (1984) Long term outcome in working and homemaking alcoholic women. *Alcohol Clin. Exp. Res.* **8**, 576–579.

[119] B. Haver (1987a) Female alcoholics: III. Patterns of consumption 3–10 years after treatment. *Acta Psychiatr. Scand.* **75**, 397–404.

[120] B. Haver (1987b) Female Alcoholics: IV. The relationship between family violence and outcome 3–10 years after treatment. *Acta Psychiatr. Scand.* **75**, 449–455.

[121] B. Haver (1987c) Female Alcoholics V: The relationship between family history of alcoholism and outcome 3–10 years after treatment. *Acta Psychiatr. Scand.* **76**, 21–27.

[122] J. Macdonald (1987) Predictors of treatment outcome for alcoholic women. *Int. J. Addict.* **22(3)**, 235–248.

[123] L. Y. Silvia, G. T. Sorell, and N. A. Busch-Rossnagel (1988) Biopsychosocial discriminators of alcoholic and nonalcoholic women. *J. Subst. Abuse* **1**, 55–65.

[124] M. Vannicelli (1984) Barriers to treatment of alcoholic women. *Subst. Alcohol Actions Misuse* **5**, 29–37.

[125] H. B. Braiker (1982) The diagnosis and treatment of alcoholism in women, in *Special Population Issues, Alcohol and Health,* Monograph No. 4 (National Institute on Alcohol Abuse and Alcoholism, Rockville, MD) p. 111.

[126] L. J. Beckman and K. M. Kocel (1982) The treatment-delivery system and alcohol abuse in women: Social policy implications. *J. Social Issues* **38**, 139–151.

[127] L. Dahlgren and A. Willander (1989) Are special treatment facilities for female alcoholics needed? A controlled 2-year follow-up study from a specialized female unit (EWA) versus a mixed male/female treatment facility. *Alcohol Clin. Exp. Res.* **13(4)**, 499–504.

[128]B. L. Underhill (1986) Issues relevant to aftercare programs for women. *Alcohol Health. Res. World* **11(1)**, 46–48.

[129]L. Midanik (1983) Familial alcoholism and problem drinking in a national drinking practices survey. *Addict. Behav.* **8**, 133–141.

[130]B. W. Lex, S. E. Lukas, N. E. Greenwald, and J. H. Mendelson (1988) Alcohol-induced changes in body sway in women at risk for alcoholism: A Pilot study. *J. Stud. Alcohol* **49(4)**, 346–356.

[131]D. B. Abrams and G. T. Wilson (1979) Effects of alcohol on social anxiety in women: Cognitive versus physiological processes. *J. Abnorm. Psychol.* **88**, 161–173.

[132]D. B. Newlin (1989) Placebo responding in the same direction as alcohol in women. *Alcohol Clin. Exp. Res.* **13(1)**, 36–39.

[133]N. K. Mello (1983) Etiological theories of alcoholism, in *Advances in Substance Abuse, vol. 3* (N. K. Mello, ed.) JAI, Greenwich, CT, p. 271.

[134]N. K. Mello (1983) A behavioral analysis of the reinforcing properties of alcohol and other drugs in man, in *The Pathogenesis of Alcoholism, Biological Factors, vol. 7* (B. Kissin, and H. Begleiter, eds.) Plenum, NY, p. 133.

[135]B. W. Lex, M. L. Griffin, N. K. Mello, and J. H. Mendelson (1989) Alcohol, marijuana, and mood states in young women. *Int. J .Addict.* **24(5)**, 405–424.

[136]L. M. Birnbaum, T. H. Taylor, and E. S. Parker (1983) Alcohol and sober mood state in female social drinkers. *Alcohol Clin. Exp. Res.* **7**, 362–368.

[137]M. Woodside (1988) Research on children of alcoholics: Past and future. *Br. J. Addict.* **83**, 785–792.

[138]M. Russell, C. Henderson, and S. B. Blume (1985) *Children of Alcoholics: A Review of the Literature* (Children of Alcoholics Foundation, NY).

[139]C. Gilligan (1982) *In a Different Voice* (Harvard University Press, Cambridge, MA).

Effect of Regulation on Alcoholic Beverage Consumption

Regression Diagnostics and Influential Data

Jon P. Nelson

Introduction

Following the repeal of Prohibition in 1933, the task of regulating the distribution and consumption of alcoholic beverages was left primarily to the states. Each state established its own system of control, but certain common features were broadly shared. All states set a minimum legal drinking age, ranging from 18–21. All states enacted special excise taxes on alcoholic beverages and most placed restrictions on advertising, hours of legal sale, number and type of outlets, local "dry area" options, and so forth. Eighteen states have chosen to create state monopolies to control wholesale distribution and (except in Mississippi and Wyoming) retail prices of one or more beverage types.* In the remaining 32 states and the District of Colum-

---

*All control states limit the sale of spirits and wine to state-operated stores, but a number also permit private sale of beverages with less than a specified maximum alcohol content. This makes designation of control states somewhat arbitrary, especially for wine sales. Moreover, state stores in Oregon are operated by independent contract agents, and in Michigan, the bulk of retail sales occur in private-licensed package stores. As a result of prevailing pricing policies, these states are traditionally treated as control states.

bia, a licensing system has been adopted, whereby a state alcohol control board determines the number of wholesale and retail operations.

Presumably, the network of laws and regulations in this market influences, directly and indirectly, the level of consumption by state. Direct effects occur when consumption is barred by law or availability and informational restrictions raise the "full cost" of a beverage. Indirectly, there are several regulations that can alter market prices, including resale price maintenance, price affirmation and price posting laws, and dramshop liability laws.

Many of these regulations have recently been the subject of public scrutiny and debate. For example, between 1970–1976, 30 states reduced the minimum drinking age, but between 1976–1984, 27 of these states raised the age again.[1,2] In California, a number of communities banned the common site sale of alcoholic beverages and gasoline, whereas Kansas voters amended the state constitution to allow drinking in restaurants. The state of Iowa terminated its retail monopoly in 1987, but a similar proposal was defeated in Pennsylvania. A number of states have also increased the penalties imposed on persons convicted of driving while intoxicated, including higher fines, mandatory jail sentences, administrative license suspensions, and so forth.

The purpose of this chapter is to examine those economic and regulatory variables that are most likely to have a direct effect on the demand for alcoholic beverages, leaving indirect effects to be captured in the price variable. The study differs in several important respects from earlier studies. First, retail transaction prices are used in cross-sectional demand functions for beer, distilled spirits, and wine. Second, regression diagnostics suggested by Belsley et al.[3] are used to examine the coefficients for instability resulting from influential data. Third, the estimates for wine are unique since earlier investigators have been stymied by a lack of cross-sectional price data. In addition, empirical problems resulting from cross-border purchases, adjacent-state price competition, shipment-based consumption estimates, and specification uncertainty are discussed and dealt with.

In general, the chapter demonstrates that the own-price, income, and tourism variables are the most important demand determinants. Selected regulatory variables are also shown to be significant, and certain states must be treated as influential data points. "Beverage Prices and Consumption" describes the price and consumption data, and presents some descriptive measures comparing control and license states. "Model Specification" follows. "Empirical Results and Influential Data Analysis" examines various model specifications and summarizes the regression diagnostics. The final section discusses the effect on consumption of a doubling of the federal excise tax for each beverage.

Beverage Prices and Consumption

A number of econometric studies provide estimates of price and income elasticities of demand for alcoholic beverages.[4] A major problem in these studies has been the limited availability of data reflecting retail transactions prices for alcoholic beverages. Cross-sectional beer demand studies have used state taxes on beer as a proxy for price differences,[5,6] wholesale prices provided by manufacturers and other confidential data sources,[7-9] and average price estimates from the trade publication *Beverage World*.[10] In some preliminary regressions, none of these measures outperformed the retail price date discussed below and some could not be replicated for disclosure reasons.

Separate studies of the demand for wine in the U.S. are rare, especially cross-sectional studies. Shapouri's[11] study used pooled regional data and BLS price indexes to provide some indication of cross-sectional differences in wine demand. The most extensive study of wine demand is Pompelli,[12] which used the USDA 1977/78 National Food Consumption Survey data and the National Panel Diary Corporation data for 1979–1980. Price information was obtained from personnel records of the participants in the surveys. These data cannot be duplicated for other years.

Cross-sectional studies of the demand for distilled spirits have been far more common, owing to the availability of shelf price data by brand from surveys conducted by the Distilled Spirits Council of the United States (DISCUS). However, this organization has ceased publication of its Annual Statistical Review, and it appears that 1984 will be the last year for which these price data will be made available. A number of cross-sectional demand studies have used the DISCUS or similar data for single or multiple brands.[8, 13–17]

Other investigators have aggregated across beverages by converting each type of beverage to ethanol equivalent consumption.[18,19] This procedure is questionable on several grounds. First, it assumes that people consume these beverages solely for their absolute alcohol content and that the ethanol content of each type of beverage is constant across states. Second, in order to aggregate in this manner, the relative prices of beverages must be constant and must be represented by the price of one beverage.* This assumption, although plausible in an aggregate time series,[20] is questionable on a state-by-state basis. Third, the results reported below suggest significant differences in price and income elasticities by beverage. These differences cannot be recovered from studies that aggregate by ethanol content.

The price data used in the present study are obtained from the quarterly price survey Inter-City Cost of Living Indicators, published by the American Chamber of Commerce Researchers Association (ACCRA).** The ACCRA survey covers 59 goods and services, including three alcoholic beverages. City Chambers of Commerce participate in the survey on a voluntary basis, gathering local retail price data through telephone, letter, or in-person surveys. Regional coordinators review the data for consistency. The number of cities participating varies by quarter, but generally exceeds 225, thus producing a wide base of data on cities of all sizes in all geographic areas of the country.

Alcoholic beverage prices in the survey include the price per six-pack of beer (Schlitz™ or Budweiser™ brand) in 12 oz containers, the price per 750-mL bottle of Seagram's 7-Crown™ whiskey, and the price per 750-mL bottle of Paul Maisson™ Chablis wine. It is assumed that prices for these popular brands will track well with the mean price for each beverage type. The beer price used here is a city population-weighted mean price for the second and third quarters of 1982, whereas the spirits and wine prices are weighted mean prices for all four quarters of 1982. Cities that reported only once were excluded from the latter calculations. Alaska and Hawaii are excluded because of lack of necessary data.

Consumption estimates in the present study are based on shipment data reported by the leading industry trade publications (*see* "Data Appendix"). These data have been the subject of some criticism by Cook.[23] First, they exclude illegal and home production, but there is no evidence that such activities are presently significant. Second, wholesalers may underreport

---

*Wilkinson[19] avoids this problem by using data on sales tax rates and receipts for each state to calculate an average price per unit of ethanol. For 10 states, data were not available or arbitrary adjustments were made. This approach does have the important advantage of reflecting on- and off-premise sales.

**More extensive discussions of the ACCRA survey data can be found in Healy and Cox[21] and Hogan and Rex.[22] Because the ACCRA cost-of-living index does not include taxes, I used the broader based (Bureau of Labor Statistics) cost-of-living index for major metropolitan areas as a deflator for prices and income by state.

their sales in order to evade state taxes, thus biasing shipment data downward in high tax states. These illegal activities have been investigated by Smith[14] with generally inconclusive results as to their significance. Third, some residents of a state may obtain alcoholic beverages from an adjacent state if the price differences between the two states makes this activity worthwhile. Empirical issues associated with adjacent-state price competition are discussed later. Fourth, shipments made to a given state include sales made within that state to nonresident tourists. Empirical solutions to this problem are also discussed later.

An alternative data series for alcoholic beverage consumption has been derived from state excise tax data by Doernberg and Stinson.[24] Examination of these data reveal that they differ little from shipment-based consumption estimates. For beer, the simple correlation between shipment and tax-based consumption estimates is $r = 0.989$. The distilled spirits and wine data in Doernberg and Stinson are a mixture of industry shipment and tax-based estimates. A few states show significant differences for unknown reasons, but industry consumption data are highly correlated with Doernberg and Stinson's data ($r = 0.993$ for spirits and $r = 0.992$ for wine). The industry data has been chosen for reasons of comparability with earlier demand studies.

Various descriptive data for consumption and prices are displayed in Table 1. In order to reflect some degree of underage drinking, all per capita consumption estimates are for persons aged 16 and over.* It is assumed that beverage demand functions are homogeneous of degree zero in prices and income. Therefore, all price and income variables in this study are expressed in real terms by deflating by a cost-of-living index derived from the broadly based BLS family budget survey of fall 1981. This procedure, which is admittedly crude, produced significantly better demand estimates for spirits and wine. Previous studies that used undeflated prices and income variables may have found significant results for selected variables that happened to be correlated with state cost-of-living differences.

Table 1 shows that capita consumption of each beverage type is lower on average in control states compared to license states, especially for

---

*The distribution of individual per capita ethanol consumption is highly skewed. Moore and Gerstein[25] estimate that the heaviest drinking 5% of the population accounts for roughly 50% of total consumption, and that roughly one-third of the adult population in 1979 were abstainers. In order to account for state differences in the latter group, a religion variable was incorporated in various model specifications.

Table 1
Descriptive Data on Alcoholic Beverage Consumption and Prices (1982)

Variable	Mean	(S.D.)	Median	Range
Per capita beer sales (gal.)	32.21	(5.7)	31.89	23.07–45.94
Control states[a]	31.24	(5.6)	30.92	23.07–44.02
License states	32.67	(5.6)	31.95	23.73–45.94
Per capita spirits sales (gal.)	2.63	(1.1)	2.51	1.38–6.91
Control states[a]	2.34	(1.0)	2.18	1.38–5.95
License states	2.77	(1.1)	2.64	1.58–6.91
Per capita wine sales (gal.)	2.65	(1.5)	2.28	0.89–8.44
Control states[b]	2.23	(1.2)	1.85	1.04–4.72
License states	2.77	(1.6)	2.42	0.89–8.44
Real beer price ($ per 6-pack)[c]	2.80	(0.3)	2.78	2.27–3.68
Control states[a]	2.82	(0.2)	2.83	2.44–3.28
License states	2.79	(0.4)	2.74	2.27–3.68
Real spirits price ($ per 750 ml)[c]	6.90	(0.7)	6.83	5.52–8.40
Control states[a]	7.02	(0.6)	7.05	5.96–7.89
License states	6.84	(0.7)	6.80	5.52–8.40
Real wine price ($ per 750 ml)[c]	3.47	(0.4)	3.45	2.64–4.65
Control states[b]	3.47	(0.3)	3.41	3.04–4.36
License states	3.47	(0.4)	3.47	2.64–4.65

[a]Control states are AL, ID, IA, ME, MI, MT, NH, NC, OH, OR, PA, UT, VT, VA, WA, and WV.
[b]Control states exclude ME, MI, OH, OR, and VT from the above list.
[c]Conversion multipliers for real mean price per oz. of ethanol are ca. 0.31, 0.10, and 0.32 for beer, spirits, and wine prices, respectively.

spirits and wine. Comparing control states and license states, mean real prices per unit are about the same for beer and wine, but real spirits prices are higher on average in control states. The range of prices is always less in the control state group, which reflects the uniform pricing policy often adopted in these states.[26] Using the conversion multipliers, mean real prices per ounce of ethanol are highest for wine and lowest for distilled spirits.

Table 1 indicates that there are interesting differences between consumption and prices for control vs license states. The more stringent set of regulations typically found in control states will play an important role in the model specification to be discussed in the next section.

Model Specification

The single-equation demand model to be estimated separately for beer, spirits, and wine has the following general form:

$$\log Q_{ij} = a_i + b_i \log P_{ij} + c_i \log Y_j + d_i R_{ij} + f_i C_j + e_{ij} \quad (1)$$

where Q_{ij} is per capita consumption of the i-th alcoholic beverage in the j-th state, P is the real own-price, Y is real per capita disposable income, R is a set of regulatory variables affecting availability and information, and C is other economic, cultural and demographic variables thought to condition the consumption of a given beverage. The regression coefficients for the i-th beverage are given by a, b, c, d, and f, and e_{ij} is the error term. Conventionally, P and Y are the main variables that constrain the consumption opportunity set of all individuals. The R and C variables apply more selectively because of state differences in legal, cultural, or demographic conditions.

The dependent variable in Eq. (1) is mean per capita beverage consumption, denoted by *beer, spirits,* or *wine* for persons age 16 and above in the year 1982. The major economic variables consist of the mean real own-price (*price*) of beer, spirits, or wine for 1982 or selected quarters thereof, mean real per capita disposable income (*income*) averaged over the entire state population, and a proxy variable for state tourism activity (*tourism*). For obvious reasons, the expected coefficient signs on these three variables are negative, positive, and positive, respectively. Prices of substitute beverages are omitted from Eq. (1). Previous studies have found no consistent evidence on substitutability among alcoholic beverages. Correlation among beverage prices limits the ability to detect substitution relationships in the present study. For example, the correlation between beer and spirits prices is 0.609, between beer and wine, 0.685, and between spirits and wine, 0.699.

Beverages sold in adjacent state are potentially close substitutes for a home state's retail beverages. Since Wales'[16] initial discussion of the problem of adjacent-state price competition, several empirical solutions have been proposed. Smith[14] suggested the use of the lowest adjacent-state price expressed relative to the home state's own-price. Ornstein and Hanssens[8] used the same variable deflated by the geographic size of the home state. Smith's variable is correlated with the home state's own-price (for spirits, the correlation in the present study is 0.652), and deflating by size produces a highly skewed distribution. The use of the lowest adjacent-state price is also misleading, since there are only nine states that dominate all surrounding states by virture of lower spirits prices. For the majority of the states, with both lower and higher adjacent prices, the effect on consumption of interstate purchases is uncertain. However, as pointed out by Swidler,[26] adjacent-state price competition is expected to occur more frequently in those control states that practice uniform pricing within their borders. In these states, direct market forces cannot equalize transportation-adjusted prices and, as a consequence, interstate spirit purchases are more likely to have a significant effect on home-state consumption. In the present study, the effect of adjacent-state price competition is captured in a control-state dummy variable.

Six regulatory variables are considered in the model. The first is a dummy variable equal to one for control states (*control*). For spirits there are 16 control states and for wine, 11 (*see* Table 1). Control states typically have more limited availability of outlets, brand selection, hours of business, and so forth. These restrictions raise the full cost of spirits and wine. Because of uniform pricing, more interstate purchases are likely by residents of control states. Both of these effects reduce consumption and are expected to produce a negative coefficient sign on *control* for spirits and wine. This variable is also included in Eq. (1) for beer, with the expectation of a positive sign resulting from higher transactions costs for substitute beverages.

The second regulatory variable is the total number of outlets per capita (*outlets*). A larger number of outlets reduces transactions costs of beverages, and outlets should therefore have a positive coefficient sign. The specification employed here is total outlets per capita, which includes both on- and off-premise outlets. Control states have fewer outlets per capita and significantly restrict the number of off-premise outlets. Combining both types of outlets helps prevent a collinearity problem.

Various states limit Sunday sales of alcoholic beverages in off- or on-premise outlets. A dummy variable equal to one is included for those states that ban off-premise sale on Sundays (*sunoff*) for a given beverage. Ornstein and Hanssens[8] argued that, for convenience-of-purchase reasons, this variable influenced only beer consumption. A positive sign is expected for *sunoff* in the beer demand equation, and no relationship is expected for spirits and wine. Availability of alcohol is also influenced by the legality of sales in nonspecialty stores, such as grocery or drug stores (*store*). For beer and wine, *store* is a dummy variable equal to one if legal sale is permitted in grocery stores. For spirits, *store* is a dummy variable equal to one if legal sale is permitted in drug stores. Collinearity prevents a more complex specification. A positive sign is expected on *store*, reflecting a reduction in per unit transaction costs of shopping trips.

Some states limit the availability of beverage information by banning billboards or preventing price advertising on billboards or in printed media. This author includes a dummy variable equal to one if the state bans price advertising in printed media (*adban*). The expected coefficient sign is negative. On theoretical grounds, bans on price advertising should raise consumer search costs, therby lowering consumption and raising the mean and variance of prices. These effects are more likely to influence off-premise sales, but only total consumption is considered in the present study. Price advertising bans might also result in an increase in nonprice advertising, although there is little or no evidence of a positive relationship between alcoholic beverage advertising and aggregate consumption.[4]

The last regulatory variable is a dummy variable equal to one for states with minimum legal drinking ages (MLDA) of less than 21 (*age*). Previous studies have encountered difficulty in obtaining significant results for an age variable.[8,18] These authors suggest that drinking by persons less than 21 yr of age is simply not quantitatively important relative to total consumption or that the limited variability of age variables prevents cross-sectional examination. Use of a dummy variable has several potential advantages over previous studies. First, age laws are discrete and categorical in nature. Second, dummy variables do a better job of capturing the effect on consumption because of border crossing by underage youth from adjacent states. Third, states with a common drinking age may possess other common characteristics that are difficult to measure, such as operation of drinking establishments that appeal to youth. The exact specification of *age* was determined by proxy variable searches. For beer, *age* equals one if the MLDA is 19 or 20. For spirits and wine, *age* equals one if the MLDA is 20. It is not difficult to think of reasons why 18 or 19 yr-olds may not affect per capita consumption, including parental influence, limited experience, smaller drinking populations, and in the case of spirits and wine, the overwhelming importance of beer as the drink of choice amoung youth.

Previous demand studies have included a host of cultural and demographic variables, including climatic conditions, urbanization rate, population density, employment and occupation status, ethnic origin, race, religion, and age distribution measures. Only the latter two variables are considered here. Other sociodemographic measures tend to be highly correlated with prices or income. Two religious groups, Southern Baptists and Latter-Day

Saints, have proscriptions against the consumption of alcoholic beverages. Because the Latter-Day Saints are quantitatively important in only a few states, only one religious variable has been included in the model. It is the percentage of a state's population who report themselves to be adherents to the Southern Baptist religion (*Baptist*). The expected sign is negative for all beverages. In addition because the drinking preferences of youth are often thought to differ from the rest of the adult population, the beer demand equation includes a variable for the percentage of a state's population between the ages of 16–24. The expected coefficient sign for *youth* is positive, reflecting both legal and illegal drinking behavior.

Empirical Results and Influential Data Analysis

A number of studies of economic regulations employ state cross-sectional data. The natural experiment created by economic, political, and cultural differences among the states leads to a variety of outcomes with respect to the type, timing, or severity of regulations. However, state-level econometric studies are often forced to employ small samples, and this combined with the uniqueness of some states can create statistical problems associated with outliers and influential data. In the present study, the regression diagnostics suggested by Belsley, et al. (BKW)[3] has been used to delete groups of observations selectively from the sample of states. A range of regression estimates are reported for perturbations of both sample and regressor specifications of the model.

Table 2 shows the regression estimates for the model specification using samples of 49 and 47 observations. The smaller sample deletes the two observations with the largest (absolute value) studentized residuals, which is the least-squares residual divided by its estimated standard error. The results in this table can be summarized as follows: the demand for beer is price inelastic, with an uncompensated own-price elasticity of about -0.6. The income elasticity is between 0.2–0.4. Beer consumption is also positively related to higher levels of tourism, more outlets per capita, more Southern Baptist adherents, and lower legal drinking ages. When two outliers, New Jersey and Texas, are omitted, *adban* is significant and positive. This result, which is contrary to expectations, has also been obtained by Hoadley et al.[18] for billboards. Ornstein and Hanssens,[8] however, obtained mixed results for billboard and printed advertisement bans as did Wilkinson.[19] In general, the diversity of results suggests that there is no effect on consumption of advertising bans. A dummy variable for off-premise Sunday

Table 2
Regression Model Estimates for Alcoholic Beverage Demand

Variable	(2.1) Beer[a]	(2.2) Beer[b]	(2.3) Spirits[a]	(2.4) Spirits	(2.5) Wine[c]	(2.6) Wine[d]
Constant	0.903 (1.56)	2.297 (1.28)*	-5.931 (3.93)	-2.676 (3.35)	-6.853 (6.31)	-5.782 (5.98)
Price	-0.558 (0.17)*	-0.613 (0.14)*	-0.829 (0.37)*	-0.636 (0.32)*	-1.600 (0.63)*	-1.286 (0.59)*
Income	0.384 (0.17)*	0.202 (0.14)	1.056 (0.40)*	0.639 (0.35)*	1.157 (0.67)**	0.994 (0.63)
Tourism	0.113 (0.03)*	0.120 (0.02)*	0.250 (0.05)*	0.200 (0.05)*	0.187 (0.9)*	0.174 (0.09)*
Outlets	0.166 (0.03)*	0.160 (0.03)*	0.039 (0.08)	0.052 (0.06)	-0.057 (0.13)	-0.062 (0.12)
Baptist	0.033 (0.01)*	0.028 (0.01)*	-0.022 (0.02)	-0.025 (0.02)	-0.057 (0.04)	-0.077 (0.04)*
Control	0.051 (0.04)	0.027 (0.03)	-0.143 (0.10)	-0.197 (0.09)*	-0.147 (0.15)	-0.162 (0.14)
Store	-0.031 (0.06)	-0.029 (0.04)	-0.105 (0.10)	-0.101 (0.09)	0.262 (0.12)*	0.276 (0.11)*
Age	0.081 (0.03)*	0.063 (0.03)*	0.254 (0.11)*	0.128 (0.10)	0.129 (0.20)	0.106 (0.18)
Adban	0.024 (0.05)	0.068 (0.04)*	-0.033 (0.09)	-0.016 (0.07)	-0.200 (0.15)	-0.217 (0.14)
Sunoff	-0.026 (0.05)	-0.067 (0.04)*	0.050 (0.10)	-0.018 (0.08)	-0.121 (0.17)	-0.143 (0.17)
Youth	0.204 (0.29)	-0.047 (0.23)				
R^2	0.740	0.841	0.662	0.659	0.609	0.636
SEE	0.100	0.078	0.221	0.184	0.383	0.353

[a]Sample is 48 states and DC; [b]Deletes NJ and TX; [c]Deletes DC and NH; [d]Deletes DC and ND. *Statistically significant at the 95 percent confidence level, one-tailed test (standard errors in parentheses).

sale bans is also significant and negative in regression (2.2). Taking the results for *outlets* and *sunoff* together indicates that beer sales are positively related to convenience, but this does not carry over to grocery store sales in a significant way. The *control* variable has the expected positive sign, but is insignificant. The results for *youth* suggest that their drinking patterns do not differ significantly from the general adult population.

Regressions (2.3) and (2.4) show the estimates for spirits consumption. Demand is price inelastic, with an uncompensated own-price elasticity between -0.6 and -0.8. The income elasticity varies between 0.6–1.1. Spirits consumption is also positively related to tourism activity, and the spirits elasticities on *tourism* exceed similar estimates for beer and wine. Raising the legal drinking age will reduce spirits consumption, although the *age* coefficient estimate is sensitive to the sample specification. When the District of Columbia and New Hampshire are omitted, the *control* variable is significant and negative. New Hampshire has aggressively promoted the sale of alcoholic beverages to out-of-state customers, so its inclusion in the sample masks the effect of *control*. The *Baptist* variable has the expected negative sign, but is insignificant, as are the other regulatory variables.

The results for wine indicate an elastic demand, with an uncompensated own-price elasticity of -1.3 to -1.6. The income elasticity is about 1.0 -1.2. Both of these estimates are consistent with the increase in wine sales in recent years. Wine consumption is also positively related to *tourism*. Unlike beer and spirits, wine consumption is positively related to availability in nonspecialty grocery stores. Omitting the District of Columbia and North Dakota results in a significant, negative sign for *Baptist*. This relationship is apparently masked by other low consumption states such as North Dakota. The *control* variable for wine is negative, but insignificant. None of the other regulatory variables have an effect on wine consumption.

The results in Table 2 suggest a rather limited impact of regulatory variables on alcohol consumption. These results are suspect on grounds that other influential data points may obscure more precise estimates of regulatory effects. Tables 3–5 explore the possible impact of influential data in greater detail. These tables use a slightly simplified version of the model which focuses on the regulatory variables *outlets, control, age,* and *store* Because the number of data points generated by the BKW diagnostics is proportional to the number of parameters estimated, this simplification was necessary to produce a manageable number of observations for examination. The first regression in each table shows the results for the full sample of 49 observations. The second regression again deletes the two states with

Table 3
Influential Data Analysis for Beer Demands

Variable	(3.1)	(3.2)	(3.3)	(3.4)	(3.5)	(3.6)
Constant	0.793	1.740	2.003	2.494	2.108	1.231
	(1.51)	(1.33)	(1.27)	(1.31)*	(1.29)	(1.27)
Price	−0.607	−0.686	−0.667	−0.773	−0.638	−0.638
	(0.16)*	(0.14)*	(0.13)*	(0.14)*	(0.13)*	(0.13)*
Income	0.367	0.274	0.239	0.205	0.228	0.324
	(0.16)*	(0.14)*	(0.14)*	(0.14)	(0.14)	(0.14)*
Tourism	0.115	0.119	0.104	0.129	0.109	0.118
	(0.03)*	(0.02)*	(0.02)*	(0.02)*	(0.02)*	(0.02)*
Outlets	0.166	0.160	0.172	0.136	0.168	0.151
	(0.03)*	(0.03)*	(0.03)*	(0.03)*	(0.03)*	(0.03)*
Baptist	0.035	0.029	0.035	0.026	0.031	0.029
	(0.01)*	(0.01)*	(0.01)*	(0.01)*	(0.01)*	(0.01)*
Control	0.048	0.035	0.056	0.033	0.026	0.042
	(0.04)	(0.03)	(0.03)*	(0.03)	(0.03)	(0.03)
Store	−0.041	−0.039	−0.041	−0.044	−0.047	−0.046
	(0.05)	(0.05)	(0.04)	(0.04)	(0.04)	(0.04)
Age	0.086	0.082	0.100	0.073	0.071	0.088
	(0.03)*	(0.03)*	(0.03)*	(0.03)*	(0.03)*	(0.03)*
R^2	0.733	0.806	0.816	0.816	0.810	0.814
SEE	0.098	0.083	0.079	0.079	0.080	0.078

*Sample for regression (3.1) includes 48 states and DC; (3.2) deletes NJ and TX; (3.3) deletes NJ, TX, and AL; (3.4) deletes NJ, TX, and UT; (3.5) deletes NJ, TX, and NH; (3.6) deletes NJ, TX, and WI. Results not reported for deletion of CT, IA, and MS.

the largest studentized residual. However, as pointed out by Belsley, et al.[3] observations with large residuals are not necessarily the most influential data points. This is confirmed in the third through sixth regressions in the tables, which selectively delete four additional observations.

Table 3 displays the results for beer. The coefficients for *price, tourism, outlets, Baptist,* and *age* are stable given the sample perturbations. The price and income elasticities are all within the range of estimates in Table 2. However, the income elasticity is insignificant when either Utah or New Hampshire is deleted along with Texas and New Jersey. The instability in this coefficient may result from the deflator used to calculate real disposable income, which is not precisely calibrated for each and every state in the sample. The coefficient on *control* becomes significantly positive when

Table 4
Influential Data Analysis for Distilled Spirits Demand [a]

Variable	(4.1)	(4.2)	(4.3)	(4.4)	(4.5)	(4.6)
Constant	−5.940	−2.861	−2.996	−2.847	−3.395	−2.478
	(3.67)	(3.18)	(3.22)	(3.18)	(3.13)	(2.99)
Price	−0.817	−0.656	−0.612	−0.792	−0.649	−0.698
	(0.36)*	(0.31)*	(0.33)*	(0.33)*	(0.34)*	(0.29)*
Income	1.039	0.649	0.642	0.677	0.701	0.612
	(0.37)*	(0.33)*	(0.33)*	(0.33)*	(0.32)*	(0.31)*
Tourism	0.236	0.197	0.176	0.197	0.190	0.188
	(0.05)*	(0.04)*	(0.06)*	(0.04)*	(0.04)*	(0.04)*
Outlets	0.052	0.073	0.076	0.047	0.087	0.086
	(0.06)	(0.05)	(0.05)	(0.06)	(0.05)*	(0.05)*
Control	−0.042	−0.100	−0.099	−0.109	−0.073	−0.114
	(0.07)	(0.06)	(0.06)	(0.06)*	(0.06)	(0.06)*
Age	0.308	0.175	0.173	0.173	0.167	0.151
	(0.10)*	(0.09)*	(0.09)*	(0.09)*	(0.09)*	(0.09)*
R^2	0.643	0.631	0.492	0.637	0.641	0.671
SEE	0.216	0.181	0.183	0.182	0.178	0.170

[a]Sample for regression (4.1) includes 48 states and DC; (4.2) deletes DC and NH; (4.3) deletes DC, NH, and NV; (4.4) deletes DC, NH, and OK; (4.5) deletes DC, NH, and IA; (4.6) deletes DC, NH, and MO. Results not reported for deletion of NB.

Alabama is deleted. The low level of per capita beer consumption in Alabama masks the positive effect on beer demand of control state regulations.

Table 4 shows the results for spirits demand, with the *price, income, tourism,* and *age* coefficients displaying stability as well as significance. The price and income elasticities are within the range of estimates found in Table 2. The R^2 falls when Nevada is deleted along with the District of Columbia and New Hampshire, but the coefficient magnitudes in regressions (4.2) and (4.3) are similar. The *outlets* coefficient is significant when Iowa or Missouri are excluded, and both of these are states with relatively low spirits consumption. Comparing regressions (4.1) and (4.2) shows that the coefficient on *control* rises in significance and (absolute) magnitude when New Hampshire and the District of Columbia are excluded. *Control* becomes significant when either Oklahoma or Missouri are excluded additionally.

Table 5 shows the results for wine. The *price, income,* and *tourism* coefficients are fairly stable. However, the price and income elasticities are

Table 5
Influential Data Analysis for Wine Demand[a]

Variable	(5.1)	(5.2)	(5.3)	(5.4)	(5.5)	(5.6)
Constant	−8.346	−10.879	−13.244	−10.062	−8.604	−9.137
	(5.97)	(5.42)*	(5.42)*	(5.36)*	(5.61)	(5.34)*
Price	−1.938	−1.988	−1.710	−2.149	−2.187	−1.932
	(0.57)*	(0.52)*	(0.52)*	(0.53)*	(0.53)*	(0.53)*
Income	1.346	1.621	1.840	1.609	1.393	1.411
	(0.63)*	(0.57)*	(0.56)*	(0.57)*	(0.59)*	(0.57)*
Tourism	0.192	0.175	0.175	0.275	0.158	0.152
	(0.09)*	(0.08)*	(0.08)*	(0.11)*	(0.08)*	(0.08)*
Outlets	0.061	0.151	0.175	0.138	0.139	0.155
	(0.11)	(0.10)	(0.10)*	(0.10)	(0.10)	(0.10)
Control	−0.086	0.093	0.096	0.076	0.011	0.101
	(0.14)	(0.14)	(0.14)	(0.14)	(0.15)	(0.14)
Store	0.227	0.105	0.117	0.106	(0.110)	0.091
	(0.12)*	(0.11)	(0.11)	(0.11)	(0.11)	(0.11)
Age	0.175	0.182	0.341	0.177	0.045	0.192
	(0.19)	(0.17)	(0.18)*	(0.17)	(0.20)	(0.17)
R^2	0.567	0.643	0.674	0.629	0.646	0.624
SEE	0.388	0.348	0.336	0.346	0.344	0.338

[a]Sample for regression (5.1) includes 48 states and DC; (5.2) deletes IA and OR; (5.3) deletes IA, OR, and NB; (5.4) deletes IA, OR, and NV; (S.S) deletes IA, OR, and NH; (5.6) deletes IA, OR, and DC. Results not reported for deletions of FL, OK, VT, and WA.

larger than those found in Table 2. This may reflect the omission of the *Baptist* variable from the model. The *store* coefficient is significant and positive in regression (5.1), but insignificant when Iowa and Oregon are omitted in regression (5.2). The latter state permits wine sales in grocery stores and has a relatively high per capita consumption level of wine. Also, both *outlets* and *age* are significant when Nebraska is omitted. Nebraska has a MLDA of 20 yr, but relatively low per capita consumption of wine. Including Nebraska tends to mask the effects of other states with MLDA of 20 yr.

The estimates in Tables 3–5 indicate that states with relatively high (DC, NV, NH, NJ, OR, TX, WI) and low consumption levels (AL, IA, MO, NB, ND, OK, UT) can affect the model's stability. These observations lie outside patterns set by other data, and the range of estimates indicates the extent to which various regression model outputs are sensitive to these observations.

Table 6
Age of Inferences on Necessary Variable Coefficients

Variable		(6.1) Beer	(6.2) Spirits	(6.3) Wine
Constant	Ext. Bounds[a]	0.728, 0.969	−6.780, −5.110	−9.900, −5.320
	Tables 3–5[b]	0.793, 2.494	−5.940, −2.478	−13.244, −8.346
Price	Ext. Bounds	−0.613, −0.552	−0.875, −0.770	−2.050, −1.520
	Tables 3-5	−0.773, −0.607	−0.817, −0.612	−2.187, −1.710
Income	Ext. Bounds	0.349, 0.402	0.961, 1.140	1.010, 1.490
	Tables 3-5	0.205, 0.367	0.612, 1.039	1.346, 1.840
Tourism	Ext. Bounds	0.108, 0.120	0.229, 0.257	0.151, 0.227
	Tables 3-5	0.104, 0.129	0.176, 0.236	0.152, 0.275
Outlets	Ext. Bounds	0.162, 0.170	0.009, 0.081	−0.066, 0.071
	Tables 3-5	0.136, 0.172	0.047, 0.087	0.061, 0.175
Baptist	Ext. Bounds	0.032, 0.037		
	Tables 3-5	0.026, 0.035		
Control	Ext. Bounds	0.046, 0.053	−0.147, −0.038	−0.168, −0.066
	Tables 3-5	0.026, 0.056	−0.114, −0.042	−0.086, 0.101
Store	Ext. Bounds	−0.042, −0.030		0.226, 0.263
	Tables 3-5	−0.047, −0.039		0.091, 0.227
Age	Ext. Bounds	0.079, 0.089	0.245, 0.317	0.086, 0.219
	Tables 3-5	0.071, 0.100	0.151, 0.308	0.045, 0.341

[a]Minimum and maximum estimates from Leamer and Leonard's[27] program for Bayesian inference. Sample is 48 states and DC.
[b]Minimum and maximum estimates from Tables 3–5 for same sample.

As a check on the specification used in Tables 3–5, the model was also estimated using Leamer and Leonard's[27] extreme bounds inference procedure. The independent variables were divided into necessary variables (those included in Tables 3–5) and doubtful variables. The prior variance matrix was allowed to take on any value, which gives the widest interval of estimates obtained by including or excluding all possible subsets of the doubtful variables. The extreme bounds estimates for the necessary variables are shown in Table 6. Also shown are the range of estimates obtained in Tables 3–5 using the diagnostic procedures for influential data. The latter set of estimates therefore reflects sample uncertainty and the former set, specification uncertainty. The range of estimates resulting from sampling uncertainty can be obtained from Table 2.

In general, the extreme bound estimates are more robust than those obtained in Tables 3–5. This means that the uncertainty associated with the sample is generally greater than that associated with the regressor list, and Tables 3–5 do not overstate the precision of the estimates on these grounds.

Discussion

The results obtained in this study suggest that:

1. Alcoholic beverage demand is largely determined by the own-price, consumer's real income, and tourism activity within a state;
2. The strongest case for effective regulatory constraints can be made for legal drinking age and outlet controls; and
3. Some evidence was found of offsetting behavior in connection with state monopoly controls, that is, monopoly control tends to reduce consumption of spirits and raise beer consumption.

In 1982, federal excise taxes were $0.29 per gallon of beer, $0.17 per gallon of table wine, and $8.40 per gallon of liquor (80 proof). Pogue and Spontz[28] and Manning et al.[29] calculated that, on social cost grounds, taxes on alcoholic beverages should have been at least doubled. Assuming that the same increase would have been applied to each beverage, that income effects were negligible, and that the tax increase was fully passed through to consumers, a doubling of alcohol taxes would, on average, have increased real beer prices by 5.8%, wine prices by 1.0%, and liquor prices by 24.2%. The elasticity estimates in this paper indicate reductions in per capita consumption of 3.5%, 1.5%, and 19% for beer, wine, and spirits, respectively.

However, a strong case can be made for higher tax increases for beer and wine. Currently, these beverages have a much lower tax rate per ounce of ethanol compared to distilled spirits. From the point of view of mitigating social costs, it may be desirable to equalize these tax rates. From the point of view of raising revenue, higher tax rates on beer would be justified, because beer has a less elastic demand than wine and there is therefore less induced inefficiency.[30] Additional research is needed to determine an optimal tax structure for alcoholic beverages that fully accounts for social cost, revenue, and income distribution considerations.

Data Appendix

Description of Variables and Data Sources

Variable	Description, Units, and Data Sources
Beer	1982 beer consumption per capita, in gallons per person aged 16 and over. *Sources*: (a), (b).
Spirits	1982 distilled spirits consumption per capita, in gallons per person aged 16 and over. *Sources*: (b), (c).
Wine	1982 wine consumption per capita, in gallons per person aged 16 and over. *Sources*: (b), (d).
Price	Beer—city population-weighted mean price for second and third quarters of 1982, deflated by BLS cost-of-living index, in dollars per six-pack. Spirits and wine—city population-weighted mean price for all four quarters of 1982, deflated by BLS cost-of-living index, in dollars per 750-mL bottle. *Sources*: (e), (f), (g).
Income	1982 per capita disposable income deflated by the BLS cost-of-living index, in dollars per person. *Sources*: (g), (h).
Tourism	Beer—logarithm of hotels and motels (SIC 7011) per thousand persons, in numbers per thousand persons aged 18 and over. *Sources:* (b), (i). Spirits and wine—logarithm of the proportion of total state payroll accounted for by hotels and lodging places (SIC 70). *Sources:* (i), (j).
Outlets	Logarithm of total retail outlets per thousand persons, in numbers per thousand persons aged 18 and over. *Sources:* (b), (c).
Baptist	Logarithm of the proportion of a state's total population who are members of the Southern Baptist Convention. *Sources:* (k).
Control	Beer—dummy variable equal to one if state has monopoly control over retail distribution of distilled spirits. Spirits—dummy variable equal to one for 16 states with monopoly controls on retail distribution of spirits (*see* Table 1). Wine—dummy variable equal to one for 11 states with monopoly controls on retail distribution of wine (*see* Table 1). *Source:* (l).

Store   Beer and wine—dummy variable equal to one if retail sale is permitted in grocery stores. Spirits—dummy variable equal to one if retail sale is permitted in drug stores. *Source*: (m).
Age   Beer—dummy variable equal to one if MLDA is 19 or 20. Spirits and wine—dummy variable equal to one if MLDA is 20. *Source*: (n).
Adban   Dummy variable equal to one if price ads are banned in printed media. *Sources*: (l), (o).
Sunoff   Dummy variable equal to one if off-premise retail sale is banned on Sunday. *Source* (l).
Youth   Logarithm of the proportion of the population aged 16 and over who are 16–24 years of age. *Source*: (b).

Sources: (a) United States Brewers Association. *Brewers Almanac*, Washington, DC, 1984; (b) US Bureau of the Census. State Population Estimates, by Age and Components of Change: 1980 to 1984, Series P-25, No. 970, Washington, DC, June 1985; (c) Distilled Spirits Council of the United States. *Annual Statistical Review*, Washington, DC, August 1984 and September 1985; (d) *The Wine Marketing Handbook*, Jobson Publishing Corporation, NY, 1984; (e) American Chamber of Commerce Researchers Association. Inter-City Cost of Living Indicators, Indianapolis, 1982; (f) US Bureau of the Census. County and City Data Book, Washington, DC, 1983; (g) Family budgets. *Monthly Labor Review*, January 1980 and July 1982; (h) State personal income, 1969–85: Revised estimates. Survey of Current Business, August 1986; (i) US Bureau of the Census. Census of Service Industries, Washington, DC, 1984; (j) US Bureau of the Census. County Business Patterns, Washington, DC, 1984; (k) B. Quinn, et al. *Churches and Church Membership in the United States*. Glenmary Research Center, Atlanta, GA, 1982; (l) Distilled Spirits Council of the United States. Summary of State Laws and Regulations Relating to Distilled Spirits, Washington, DC, June 1983; (m) *The Liquor Handbook,* Jobson Publishing Corporation, 1983; (n) A. C. Wagenaar, *Alcohol, Young Drivers, and Traffic Accidents*. D. C. Heath, Lexington, 1983; (o) *Modern Brewery Age Blue Book*. Business Journals, Inc., Norwalk, CT, 1983.

References

[1] A. C. Wagenaar (1983) *Alcohol, Young Drivers, and Traffic Accidents* (Lexington Books, Lexington, MA).

[2] R. J. Bonnie (1985) Regulating conditions of alcohol availability: Possible effects on highway safety. *J. Stud. Alcohol* Supplement No. 10, 129–143.

[3] D. A. Belsley, E. Kuh, and R. E. Welsch (1980) *Regression Diagnostics: Identifying Influential Data and Sources of Collinearity* (John Wiley, NY).

[4] S. I. Ornstein and D. Levy (1983) Price and income elasticities of demand for alcoholic beverages, in *Recent Developments in Alcoholism, vol. 1* (M. Galanter, ed.) Plenum, NY, pp. 303–345.

[5] I. Horowitz and A. F. Horowitz (1965) Firms in a declining market: The brewing case. *J. Ind. Econ.* 13, 129–153.

[6] B. G. Weinstein (1983) *Optimal Liquor Regulaton.* Unpublished Ph. D. dissertation. University of Michigan, Ann Arbor, MI.

[7] T. F. Hogarty and K. G. Elzinga (1972) The demand for beer. *Rev. Econ. Stat.* 54, 195–198.

[8] S. I. Ornstein and D. M. Hanssens (1985) Alcohol control laws and the consumption of distilled spirits and beer. *J. Consumer Res.* 12, 200–213.

[9] S. O. Schweitzer, M. D. Intriligator and H. Salehi (1983) Alcoholism: An econometric model of its causes, its effects and its control, in *Economics and Alcohol: Consumption and Controls* (M. Grant, M. Plant, and A. Williams, eds.), Gardner, NY, pp. 107–127.

[10] N. D. Uri (1986) The demand for beverages and interbeverage substitution in the United States. *Bull Econ. Res.* 38, 77–85.

[11] S. Shapouri (1979) *The Demand for Wine.* Unpublished Ph. D. dissertation. Washington State University, Pullman, WA.

[12] G. K. Pompelli (1987) *Consumer Demand for Wine by Households in the United States.* Unpublished Ph. D. dissertation. University of California, Davis, CA.

[13] S. L. Barsby and G. L. Marshall (1977) Short-term consumption effects of a lower minimum alcohol-purchasing age. *J. Stud. Alcohol* 38, 1665–1679.

[14] R. T. Smith (1976) The legal and illegal markets for taxed goods: Pure theory and an application to state government taxation of distilled spirits. *J. Law Econ.* 19, 393–429.

[15] S. Swidler (1986) A reexamination of liquor price and consumption differences between public and private ownership states: Comment. *Southern Econ. J.* 53, 259–264.

[16] T. J. Wales (1968) Distilled spirits and interstate consumption effects. *Amer. Econ. Rev.* 58, 853–863.

[17] A. Zardkoohi and A. Sheer (1984) Public versus private liquor retailing: An investgation into the behavior of state governments. *Southern Econ. J.* 51, 1058–1076.

[18] J. F. Hoadley, B. C. Fuchs, and H. D. Holder (1985) The effect of alcohol beverage restrictions on consumption: A 25-year longitudinal analysis. *Am. J. Drug Alcohol Abuse* **10**, 375–401.

[19] J. T. Wilkinson (1987) *The Effects of Regulation on the Demand for Alcohol.* Unpublished paper. University of Missouri, Columbia, MO.

[20] D. Levy and N. Sheflin (1983) New evidence on controlling alcohol use through price. *J. Stud. Alcohol* **44**, 929–937.

[21] L. W. Healy and W. N. Cox (1982) Cost of living data: A guide to sources. *Federal Reserve Bank of Atlanta Economic Review* **67**, 44–50.

[22] T. D. Hogan and T. R. Rex (1984) Intercity differences in cost of living. *Growth and Change* **15**, 16–23.

[23] P. J. Cook (1981) The effect of liquor taxes on drinking, cirrhosis, and auto accidents, in *Alcohol and Public Policy: Beyond the Shadow of Prohibition* (M. H. Moore and D. R. Gerstein, eds.), National Academy Press, Washington, DC, pp. 255–285.

[24] D. G. Doernberg and F. Stinson (1985) *U.S. Apparent Consumption of Alcoholic Beverages Based on State Sales, Taxation, or Receipt Data* (National Institute on Alcohol Abuse and Alcoholism, Washington, DC).

[25] M. H. Moore and D. R. Gerstein, eds. (1981) *Alcohol and Public Policy: Beyond the Shadow of Prohibition* (National Academy Press, Washington, DC).

[26] S. Swidler (1986) Consumption and price effects of state-run liquor monopolies. *Managerial and Decision Econ.* **7**, 49–55.

[27] E. Leamer and H. Leonard (1983) Reporting the fragility of regression estimates. *Rev. Econ. Stat.* **65**, 306–317.

[28] T. F. Pogue and L. G. Spontz (1989) Taxing to control social cost: The case of alcohol. *Amer. Econ. Rev.* **79**, 235–243.

[29] W. G. Manning et al (1989) The taxes of sin: Do smokers and drinkers pay their way? *J. Amer. Med. Assoc.* **261**, 1604–1609.

[30] F. Ramsey (1927) A contribution to the theory of taxation. *Econ. J.* **37**, 47–61.

Family Treatment of Alcoholism

Dawn M. Gondoli and Theodore Jacob

Introduction

During the past two decades, behavioral scientists have become increasingly interested in family influences related to the etiology, maintenance, and treatment of alcoholism. For the most part, however, empirical research has been concerned with family variables related to the onset and course of abusive drinking, with few efforts aimed at developing and evaluating family oriented alcoholism treatment. Thus, a brief review of the general family interaction and alcoholism literature will be presented before discussing the theoretical, empirical, and clinical literatures that specifically address treatment issues.

The Family Interactions of the Alcoholic

Much of the existing literature relevant to families of alcoholics has focused on individuals within the family matrix. In contrast, studies that examine the family as a unit, either as an influence in the etiology and perpetuation of abusive drinking or as a system disturbed by the effects of alcoholism, are still largely absent.[1] This individual emphasis can be traced to traditions that defined alcoholism as a moral deficit or medical problem, as well as to the psychodynamic focus of early clinical and empirical reports.[2-4] The latter influence was most apparent in early descriptions of alcoholics' wives as "disturbed" personalities who sought to dominate or punish their spouses.[2-4] Later, environmental perspectives cast wives as "victims" whose disturbances were the result of the accumulative stress of living with alcoholics.[5-6] Nevertheless, this research focus was still individual rather than interpersonal; research linking marital interactions with abusive drinking has only begun to develop during the past two decades.

Most relevant to this developing interest in the interpersonal aspects of alcohol abuse, the late 1960s and early 1970s witnessed the emergence of several observational studies of the interactions of alcoholics and their families. As noted in Jacob and Seilhamer's[1] recent evaluation of this literature, this interaction perspective offers several possibilities for clarifying the association of family factors and alcohol abuse. First, descriptions based on empirical data can dispel myths and misinformation generated by reports gathered within clinical contexts and based on small, unrepresentative samples. Second, to the extent that interaction research can provide further understanding of affective interchanges, problem-solving styles and their effectiveness, dominance patterns, and parent–child socialization practices that are associated with drinking and nondrinking situations, it is increasingly likely that treatment and prevention programs will be founded on more substance and less supposition than currently seems to be the case.

A major advance in family interaction research pertaining to alcoholism was reflected in the programmatic studies by Steinglass and his colleagues. This research effort began with several studies that included observations of inpatient alcoholics during sober and intoxicated phases. Results of these investigations suggested that the affective and structural characteristics of relationships in these drinking "gangs" were dramatically altered during drinking periods. For Steinglass, these observations confirmed the significance of reciprocal effects involving alcohol and interpersonal interaction, and led to a preliminary model of alcoholism based upon family systems theory.[7,8]

Steinglass' research then moved on to assessments of marital pairs in an experimental treatment program during which couples were housed in

Family Treatment of Alcoholism

apartment-like settings where alcohol was freely available.[9] Results from this effort indicated that intoxicated behaviors were both more exaggerated and more restricted in range than interactions displayed during sober states. Furthermore, striking differences in patterns of interaction were observed between sober and intoxicated periods—differences that appeared to serve important "adaptive" functions for the couple. According to Steinglass, if alcohol effectively reduced tension or solved a problem, short-term family stability could be achieved, and as a result, the change from sober to intoxicated interactional states could serve to stabilize an unstable system. However, because the family's problems were chronic, the solution provided by alcohol was only temporary.

More recent work by Steinglass and his colleagues has involved exploration of the "life-history model of alcoholism," a model that emphasizes a macroscopic, longitudinal view of drinking patterns, and suggests that periods of sobriety and active drinking form a cycle in the lives of most alcoholics.[10] In contrast with the maintenance model, which describes rapid changes from sober to intoxicated states with associated changes in patterns of interaction, the life history model suggests that three important phases—dry, wet, and transitional—appear and reappear many times over a 20–30 yr period. A key implication of this broader framework is that the alcoholic family fails to progress along a normal developmental course characterized by greater complexity and differentiation.

Without question, the work of Steinglass has been a major influence in the study of family interaction within the alcoholism field. At the same time, it must be acknowledged that his work was based on small, highly selective samples that lacked normal control groups and were uncontrolled for possible confounds, such as the co-occurrence of other psychiatric disorders in the alcoholic or spouse. Moreover, the data used to generate early conceptual models were based on impressionistic clinical summaries, and Steinglass' later efforts did not directly assess the acute effects of alcohol on family interchanges. Taken together, these limitations raise questions about the stability and interpretability of obtained results.

During the past several years, a number of studies have reported on the marital interactions of alcoholics (*see* Jacob & Seilhamer[1]), three of which involved experimental drinking as part of the procedures.[11-13] In general, these efforts involved small sample studies offering provocative hypotheses and empirical findings, but were limited by their preliminary nature. Jacob et al.,[13] for example, reported alcoholic couples to be more negative and to display less problem-solving behavior than normal controls, and to exhibit more negative communication in drink vs no drink sessions. Confidence in these findings, however, is limited by a small sample and the absence of appropriate comparison groups.

Another early study conducted by Billings et al.[11] included alcoholic couples, distressed (nonalcoholic) couples, and normal controls. A major finding was that alcoholic and distressed couples engaged in less problem-solving and in more negative and hostile behaviors than nondistressed controls, but that alcoholic and nonalcoholic distressed couples were not significantly different from one another. Again, methodological shortcomings, such as minimal alcohol consumption during drinking sessions, and the failure to assess participants' psychiatric status, limits confidence in these results.

An experimental study by Frankenstein et al.[12] controlled the alcohol consumption of subjects by administering fixed doses prior to interaction sessions. Analyses indicated that couples demonstrated more positive interaction in the drink vs no drink situation, a finding that resulted primarily from the spouses' change between sessions. Additionally, the alcoholics talked more than their spouses when drinking, and also tended to express more problem-solving statements when drinking, whereas this cross-sectional effect was not found for spouses. Upon closer examination, it appears that discrepancies between the Jacob et al.[13] and Frankenstein et al.[12] studies may be attributed largely to design characteristics. Specifically, critical differences are apparent in the amount and administration of alcohol, the presence versus absence of alcohol during ongoing interactions, and the application of coding schemes to marital interactions (*see* Jacob and Seilhamer[1], for elaboration of these issues).

In an effort to address the limitations of these early drinking studies, Jacob and his colleagues initiated a multi-faceted research program involving families of alcoholics as well as psychiatric and normal control groups.[14–16] In contrast to earlier studies, this effort was characterized by rigorous selection criteria, a carefully designed experimental drinking procedure, and a comprehensive battery of observational and report procedures. Although a variety of data was collected and analyzed, several findings are of particular interest in the current context. Specifically, normal couples were found to have exhibited higher rates of congeniality and positivity than both groups of disturbed couples, whereas alcoholic couples were found to have displayed more negative behavior than normal or depressed groups. Further examination of these data revealed that, when the alcoholics were analyzed according to drinking style,[16] steady and episodic drinkers displayed significantly different patterns of marital interaction. Most importantly, in the drinking condition, steady drinkers and their wives exhibited a higher rate of problem-solving behavior, whereas episodic drinkers and their wives exhibited reduced levels of problem-solving behaviors. Overall, these data suggest that the marital interactions of the steady drinkers are consistent with the "adaptive consequences" model of Steinglass, in that alcohol consumption facilitated problem solving, a function vital to the preservation of the family system. In contrast, the interactions of the episodic drinkers may reflect a "coercive control" mechanism, whereby the alcoholic avoids conflictual issues by behaving in a hostile manner while drinking.

Family Oriented Treatment of Alcoholism

In a recent review, McCrady[17] identified three theoretical perspectives that underlie most models of family oriented alcoholism treatment: disease perspectives, which view alcoholism as a "family disease," family systems perspectives, which view alcoholism as an important organizing principal for family life and which focus on reciprocal relationships between alcohol and family interactional behavior, and behavioral perspectives, which view alcoholism as maintained by multiple systems of reinforcement, including the family.[17] In her review, McCrady also discussed the substantial gap between clinical and empirical bases of practice; namely, that although treatment approaches derived from family disease and family systems perspectives are the most widely used, these models suffer from a lack of rigorously controlled evaluation studies. In contrast, behavioral models are not as widely used in treatment settings, although the best controlled outcome studies have involved evaluations of this theoretical/clinical perspective.[17]

The remainder of this section will present an overview of the three treatment models described above. Following a brief description of the theoretical underpinnings for each model, empirical outcome studies will be reviewed. Because well-controlled evaluations are largely absent for the disease and family systems models, the majority of studies reviewed will focus on the outcomes of behaviorally-based treatment. In particular, the research programs of McCrady[18] and O'Farrell[19] will be highlighted. This section relies heavily on McCrady's[17] comprehensive review, and readers who desire a more extensive discussion of treatment models and empirical outcome studies are referred to her work. The chapter concludes with suggestions for future research.

Disease Models

Currently, there is widespread interest in disease models in alcoholism treatment settings, and an increase in family programming in treatment settings based on the disease perspective.[17] Contemporary disease models extend the concept of alcoholism from an individual disease to a disease that affects the entire family. The family disease is termed "co-dependence" and is characterized by symptoms such as investing self-esteem in controlling the alcoholic, experiencing anxiety and distortion around issues of intimacy and separation, and enmeshment in dysfunctional relationships.[20] Some family disease models also focus on the family as a system, and include adjustment of family equilibrium, roles, and communication in the treatment process.[21-22] Treatment programs derived from a family disease perspective generally provide separate rather than conjoint therapy for the alcoholic, spouse, and other family members. Treatment usually includes education about the disease concept of alcoholism and education about codependence. Family members are usually referred to self-help groups, such as Al-Anon or Adult Children of Alcoholics, and may participate in individual and group therapy. In addition, there has been an increase in inpatient alcoholism treatment programs that offer short-term residential family therapy.[17]

As already noted, empirical studies assessing the effectiveness of family disease models are largely absent. In her review of this literature, McCrady[17] found only three studies published during the past 10 yr that evaluated family disease oriented programs. Two of the studies evaluated the residential family therapy program at the Hazelden Foundation in Minnesota,[21-22] which offered short-term (about three days) residential treatment for family members. Described as a therapeutic community, the program emphasized Al-Anon concepts, such as detachment, attitude change, and self-help through the sharing of experiences. The program also encouraged client awareness of family systems concepts, such as family equilibrium, family roles, and communication. Thus, the program encouraged cognitive changes that help family members cope more effectively with the addicted family member's drinking or drug use.

Cognitive change was assessed using a 20 item self-report questionnaire administered before and after program completion. Results suggested that family members made the greatest changes in recognizing that they could not ensure abstinence of the addicted family member, that they were not responsible for the addicted member's use of alcohol or drugs, that all family members had to take primary responsibility for their own problems, and that the cause of substance abuse was less important than changing the behavior and its impact on the family. No data were presented regarding sample demographics, and no other outcome measures for the family were presented (i.e., adjustment in areas other than coping with drinking). Further, no data were presented regarding the influence of family treatment on the alcoholic's drinking or other adjustment.[21]

Laundergan et al.,[22] reported results of a six-month Hazelden follow-up, in which family members completed the 20-item questionnaire, as well as other questionnaires assessing their support group participation, improvements with personal communication, and dealing with feelings. Results indicated that frequent Al-Anon and Alateen attendance was associated with adopting new communication patterns, new ways of dealing with feelings, and maintenance of attitudes developed during treatment. Again, no data were presented regarding the impact of treatment on the addicted family member's functioning.

A third published study involved an evaluation of Al-Anon,[23] focusing on the relationship between length of time nonalcoholic wives participated in Al-Anon, and the frequency of their ineffective or negative coping with spouse drinking. Participants included 123 women attending Al-Anon groups in the Washington DC area. Results indicated that duration of Al-Anon membership was associated with less negative coping, and that total coping was more associated with length of spouse's affiliation with Al-Anon than length of husband's abstinence or length of husband's affiliation with AA. No data were presented regarding the impact of Al-Anon attendance on the drinking behavior or other adjustment of the alcoholic.

All three of these studies suffer from serious limitations. First, none of the studies involved treatment for the entire family, or assessed the effect of family treatment on the alcoholic's drinking status or other adjustment. Second, family member's adjustment was examined only in terms of their coping with the alcoholic's drinking. Finally, these efforts are seriously limited because of the lack of appropriate control or comparison groups, and their exclusive reliance on self-reports.

Family Systems Models

Family systems models form the second approach to family-involved alcoholism treatment. These models incorporate many of the core concepts of family systems theory, including organization, homeostasis, circular causality of events, and feedback loops. Central to these models is the concept of the alcoholic family system, conceptualized as an interactional group in which behavior is organized around alcohol.[24] In alcoholic families, certain interactional behaviors may be associated with intoxication. If interactional behaviors that arise during intoxication are adaptive for the family, then abusive drinking itself takes on a functional role of problem solving. Treatment, therefore, is directed toward understanding changes in the family's interactional behavior during the presence vs absence of alcohol, and in helping the family to achieve adaptive consequences without the prior necessity of alcohol.[24,25]

Although family systems models are apparently popular in the alcoholism treatment community, controlled outcome research in this area is virtually nonexistent. To date, only one controlled outcome study has been reported in the literature. McCrady and her colleagues compared individually oriented alcoholism treatment with couples-involved treatment with and without joint hospitalization as part of the treatment.[26,27] The couples therapy in this study was not strictly systems based, but was described as "broadly interactional in focus."[17] This study is particularly noteworthy because it is the only controlled evaluation of the efficacy of joint hospitalization for alcoholics and their spouses.

Participants in this study were 33 couples, each containing one alcoholic spouse who had been admitted to a private psychiatric hospital for alcoholism treatment. Participants were randomly assigned to one of three treatment conditions: couples therapy with joint hospitalization, couples therapy without joint hospitalization, or individual treatment for the alcoholic only. In the joint hospitalization group, the alcoholic and spouse lived together at the hospital for a portion of the alcoholic's hospitalization. During this time, the couple attended all activities and meetings together, and were provided feedback on their interactions, which were observed by the project staff. The couple attended weekly couples group therapy, focusing on communication, the effect of alcohol on the marriage, and relationship issues. In addition, the alcoholic and spouse each attended weekly individual therapy groups during and after hospitalization. In the second condition, alcoholics and their spouses attended the same therapy groups described above, but the nonalcoholic spouses did not reside at the hospital. In the individual therapy condition, only the hospitalized alcoholic attended a weekly therapy group; the spouse did not participate in treatment.[26]

Six-month followup data suggested that the two couple-involved groups had better outcomes than the individual therapy group in terms of a reduction in quantity and frequency of drinking.[26] At four yr followup, there were no statistically significant differences between the three groups, although trends did suggest better marital adjustment and better drinking status for the joint hospitalization group as compared to the couples therapy and individual treatment groups.[17,27]

A family systems approach was more directly applied in a study reported by Steinglass.[24] This study also incorporated a period of joint hospitalization for alcoholics and their spouses as part of a three-phase treatment program. During the first phase (two weeks prior to hospitalization), couples met three times a week for multiple-couples group therapy, followed by 10 d of joint hospitalization, during which alcohol was freely available. During this time, couples' interactions were observed and videotaped, and daily multiple-couples group therapy was conducted. The observational data were used as an aid in identifying changes in the couples' interactions during sober vs intoxicated states, and in designing specific treatment strategies for each couple. During the last phase, couples completed three wk of twice weekly couples group therapy, followed by six mo of group meetings conducted every six wk. Ten couples completed the program.

Although no statistical analyses were presented, descriptive data for eight couples were reported at six-month followup. Results indicated that outcomes for drinking status and martial functioning were equivocal. For example, although only five of the alcoholics reported decreases in drinking quantity, eight showed changes in patterns and contexts of drinking. In terms of marital functioning, seven couples showed improved communication. However, these changes were often associated with the perception that there were other behavioral difficulties to be addressed, and decreased satisfaction with other areas of the marriage.[24]

Thus, despite the incorporation of family systems concepts in many alcoholism treatment settings, well-controlled studies evaluating the effectiveness of this model are lacking. Although the program reported by Steinglass is unique in its direct application of systems concepts and availability of alcohol during hospitalization, outcome findings are limited because of a small sample, and more importantly, lack of appropriate comparison groups. On the other hand, McCrady's research (although better controlled) was not strictly systems based. As McCrady[17] noted in her review of this small literature, "The controlled studies to date have suggested little beyond demonstrating that intense couples-involved treatment is feasible and may yield better outcomes than individually oriented treatment. Careful outcome studies that examine the process of family systems oriented treatment and that compare the outcomes to appropriate control conditions are simply lacking" (p. 176).

Behavioral Models

Behavioral models are the third approach to family involved alcoholism treatment. Although behavioral models form a distinct treatment approach, there is considerable overlap between behavioral and family systems concepts. For example, behavioral models assume that there is an interdependence between marital interactions and drinking. Marital interactions are viewed as reciprocal—that is, the behavior of each spouse serves simultaneously as a cue and a reinforcer for the other's behavior, including drinking behavior. When the alcoholic spouse drinks, positive changes in couple interaction may occur, which in turn, reinforce abusive drinking. Therefore, recognizing changes in interaction that occur during sober and intoxicated states is an important treatment goal.[17] Numerous behavioral approaches also incorporate techniques of behavioral marital therapy (BMT) into the treatment program. Treatment derived from this approach generally has two related foci; changing alcohol-related interactional patterns that maintain abusive drinking or trigger relapse, and altering general marital patterns, such as increasing the frequency of positive, caring, reciprocal interactions, and improving communication and problem-solving skills.[17,28]

Another key assumption of behavioral models is that alcoholism is maintained by multiple systems of reinforcement, including the spouse and other family members. Because spouses are seen as vital sources of reinforcement, some behavioral approaches have stressed training the spouse in new coping skills that reinforce sobriety, or involving the spouse in therapy-relevant behavior, such as being present each time the alcoholic spouse takes disulfiram. However, because nonfamily systems of reinforcement are also important, behavioral models include individually oriented behavior change techniques for the alcoholic; for example, identifying cues for drinking, role-playing stressful situations that could result in relapse, and role-playing new behaviors, such as drink refusal.[17]

Most of the empirical research on BMT in the treatment of alcoholism has been conducted by two research groups—one headed by Timothy O'Farrell at the Veterans Administration Medical Center in Brockton, Massachusetts, and the other by Barbara McCrady at the Rutgers Center of Alcohol Studies, in Piscataway, New Jersey. The remainder of this section will focus on outcome studies from these two research programs.

O'Farrell et al.[19] have reported findings from their Class on Alcoholism and Marriage (CALM) project. The goals of project CALM have been the development of BMT procedures for newly abstinent male alcoholics and their spouses, and the careful evaluation of interactional vs behavioral couples group therapy.[19,28] Participants in this study were 34 male alcoholics and their spouses who had been married an average of 16 yr. Couples were randomly assigned to one of three treatment groups:

1. A behavioral marital therapy group, which included Antabuse contracts, and behavioral techniques to increase positive, reciprocal exchanges between partners, and improve communication and problem-solving skills;
2. An interactional couples group, which emphasized mutual support, sharing of feelings, problem-solving through discussion, and verbal insight from both therapists and other group members; or
3. A no couples treatment control.

Although long-term data have not yet been published, results have been presented for the period immediately after treatment.[19] Findings from this study indicated that couples in the BMT group showed significant improvement on overall marital adjustment and communication, that these improvements were significantly greater than no treatment controls, and that those changes tended to be greater than those found in the interactional group. Although all participants showed short-term improvement in drinking status, alcoholics in the BMT group reported significantly fewer drinking days than those in the interactional group.

The research program of McCrady and her colleagues has focused on identifying the active components of spouse-involved outpatient alcoholism treatment.[17,18] Participants in the Project for Alcoholic Couples Treatment (PACT) study were 45 alcoholics and their partners. Couples were randomly assigned to one of three experimental conditions:

1. Minimal spouse involvement (MSI), in which the spouse was present for all therapy sessions, but all interventions were directed toward teaching the alcoholic behavioral skills to achieve and maintain abstinence;
2. Alcohol-focused spouse involvement (AFSI), in which the alcoholic was taught the skills in the MSI condition, and the spouse was taught skills to reinforce abstinence, respond more effectively in drinking situations, and decrease behaviors that cued drinking; or
3. Alcohol-focused spouse involvement plus behavioral marital therapy (ABMT), which included all the skills of the AFSI condition, plus BMT techniques to increase the frequency of positive couple interactions, and improve communication and problem-solving skills.

Extensive measures on drinking behavior, marital satisfaction and communication, and psychological, interpersonal, and occupational functioning were administered at baseline, during treatment, and at 6-, 12-, and 18-mo followups.[17,18]

During treatment, there was a substantial dropout rate in the MSI condition, with only 67% of participants in this condition completing five or more sessions, and less than 50% completing treatment. In contrast, dropout rates for the other two conditions were less than 20%. When only those completing the treatment were compared, individuals in the MSI and ABMT conditions significantly decreased the frequency of drinking. Participants in the AFSI condition did not report comparable decreases in drinking.[17,18] Results from the longer term followups indicated that, in general, ABMT couples had the most positive treatment outcomes. For example, marital satisfaction was higher in the ABMT group, there were fewer marital separations, and more positive and less negative affect. Time trend analysis of relapse showed that participants in the ABMT condition gradually decreased their drinking over time following treatment, whereas those in the MSI only condition showed the more usual pattern of a gradual increase in drinking over time. According to McCrady and her colleagues, this pattern suggested that BMT had its primary impact during the posttreatment maintenance phase. Behavioral approaches seem to be associated with helping couples manage relapse episodes, thus providing motivation and encouragement for continued work towards long-term sobriety.[17]

In addition to the PACT project, McCrady has also been involved in the Butler Environmental Treatment of Alcoholism Project (Project BETA). Participants in this study were 229 alcoholics who were randomly assigned to one of three experimental treatment groups:

1. Individually-focused behavior therapy;
2. Behavior therapy with spouse or another significant other involved; or
3. Behavior therapy with spouse/significant other involved, and techniques to enhance occupational functioning.

Similar to the PACT project, extensive assessments were conducted on drinking status and interpersonal and occupational functioning.[17]

Data have been reported for 92 participants who have completed 12 months of followup. Of most interest to the current review, analyses have shown a pattern of gradual improvement in drinking status, similar to the results obtained in the PACT study. Again, time trends for the three groups were significantly different and showed an interesting "cross-over" effect—participants in the individually-focused condition had better outcomes for the first six months, but showed a subsequent decline in abstinent days throughout the followup. In contrast, participants in the two spouse-involved conditions showed smaller decreases in abstinent days over the first six months, but a gradual increase in abstinent days thereafter.[17]

Future Directions

This review has focused on three contemporary models of family oriented alcoholism treatment: family disease, family systems, and behavioral models. As noted, there is a substantial gap between the popularity of these models in clinical settings and the treatment outcome literature.[17] Disease and family systems models, although common in practice, suffer from a lack of controlled evaluation studies. In contrast, several well-controlled evaluations of behavioral models have been reported (e.g., McCrady, O'Farrell, and their respective colleagues), yet these models currently enjoy less popularity in treatment settings. Another gap exists between the developing alcoholism and family interaction literature and theoretical/clinical models of family-involved alcoholism treatment. Although the interaction literature is accumulating a substantial empirical base with particular relevance to treatment issues, these findings have yet to be applied to treatment models. Thus, basic treatment outcome research is needed for family disease and family systems oriented programs, and better communication and translation of findings is needed between treatment settings, empirical treatment outcome studies, and the more general alcoholism literature.

Future efforts should also include the longitudinal assessment of couples and families throughout the long-term process of recovery. The behavioral literature suggests that treatment that includes BMT produces better long-term, although not necessarily short-term, outcomes than interactional or individually oriented therapies.[17,18] In turn, it has been suggested that BMT is associated with helping couples cope more effectively with relapse, thus producing better long-term outcomes. However, these observations are still preliminary in nature and need replication before they can be accepted with confidence. Further, as McCrady[17] has noted, no treatment outcome studies have examined the actual process of long-term recovery. Future efforts might compare the process of recovery in couples with and without relapse, or across different treatment modalities.

Another area of study deserving greater research attention involves the issue of client–treatment matching for family oriented alcoholism treatment. Briefly, recent reviews of the alcoholism treatment literature[29] suggest that no particular treatment approach has been found to be consistently superior to any other. Furthermore, it has been suggested that this lack of consistency may be largely the result of the differential impact of different treatment approaches on particular alcoholism subtypes, and that outcomes would improve if these subtypes were matched with appropriate treatments.

The importance of client–treatment matching in alcoholism treatment has been supported by both the literature on alcoholism typologies and the general psychotherapy literature. Review of the alcoholism literature, for example, indicates that a large proportion of alcoholics can be grouped into two major subtypes, the first characterized by an episodic style of drinking, high levels of social impairment, and greater antisocial and hostile tendencies, and the second by a more continuous drinking style, less social impairment, and possibly passive or unassertive tendencies.[16,30,31] Of particular interest to the current review, Jacob and Leonard[16] have found that these two types of alcoholics appear to establish very different marriages, one characterized by negativity and less effective problem-solving ("episodic drinkers") and the other by increased stability associated with periods of heavy drinking ("steady drinkers").

The general psychotherapy literature indicates that there are parallels to the two alcoholism subtypes among patients with nonalcoholic psychopathologies. For example, Beutler and his colleagues[32,34] have described subgroups of nonalcoholic patients who rely on "externalizing" vs "internalizing" coping styles, the former characterized by acting out, impulsivity, inability to delay gratification, and active resistance to external demands, and the latter by tendencies toward anxiety, passivity, and withdrawal in response to stress. Most importantly, Beutler and his colleagues have suggested that a behavioral approach is more effective for externalizing patients than a broader, family systems oriented approach, and that the opposite pattern is true for internalizers.[33,35] If applied to the previously described alcoholism subtypes, these conceptualizations and findings suggest several treatment dispositions. For example, episodic drinkers, whose drinking behavior disrupts family functioning, might benefit more from behavioral approaches that focus primarily on individual behavior change. On the other hand, steady drinkers may benefit more from therapy that addresses the stabilizing function of alcohol on family process, i.e, family systems or interactionally-oriented therapy. Research that directly and systematically explores these possibilities is needed.

Finally, most existing treatment programs and outcome studies focus on marital, rather than family treatment. The lack of research on family treatment seems to be primarily the result of the lack of manualized family treatment programs. Treatment manuals facilitate evaluation research by enabling researchers to specify the appropriate intervention for a particular treatment condition, to measure the expected effects of that intervention, and to provide a clearly delineated model that can be subjected to replication by independent investigators. Most relevant to this interest, Gonzalez et al.[36] have developed a treatment manual for their Multiple Family Discussion Group (MFDG), an intervention for families and patients experiencing a chronic, disabling medical illness. Based on a family systems perspective, MFDG was developed to address family issues that are generic to chronic medical illness, including the stressors associated with the illness, and the changes in family structure and process that occur as family members cope with the illness. This model is noteworthy in two respects. First, it provides a generic view of chronic illness in the family that could be applied to alcoholism as well as other disorders, and second, it provides an excellent example of a manualized family treatment program that is open to evaluation and replication. Future efforts should focus on developing similar manuals for other family approaches for the treatment of alcoholism.

In summary, the past two decades have witnessed increased attention to family factors related to the etiology and perpetuation of alcoholism, and a rapid increase in family programming in alcoholism treatment settings.[17] Despite the relative lack of controlled treatment evaluation research, reviews of existing outcome studies show, rather consistently, a small but positive benefit of involving family members in alcoholism treatment.[17,37] Particularly encouraging, several research teams have recently initiated more programmatic efforts, which in time, should promote the development of accumulative findings and a better integration of clinical and empirical literatures. Hopefully, such efforts will strengthen the research base on which family treatment can be developed, and in so doing, provide greater insight into the family's role in understanding and treating alcoholism.

Acknowledgments

Preparation of this manuscript was supported by NIAAA Grant No AA03037, awarded to Theodore Jacob.

References

[1] T. Jacob and R. A. Seilhamer (1987) Alcoholism and family interaction, in *Family Interaction and Psychopathology: Theories, Methods, and Findings* (T. Jacob, ed.), Plenum, NY, pp. 535–577.

[2] S. Futterman (1953) Personality trends in wives of alcoholics. *J. Psychiatric Social Work* **23**, 37–41.

[3] M. Kalashian (1959) Working with wives of alcoholics in an outpatient clinic setting. *J. Marriage and the Family* **21**, 130–133.

[4] M. Lewis (1937) Alcoholism and family casework. *Family* **18**, 39–44.

[5] K. Jackson (1954) The adjustment of the family to the crisis of alcoholism. *Q. J. Stud. Alcohol* **15**, 562–586.

[6] T. Jacob and R. A. Seilhamer (1982) The impact on spouses and how they cope, in *Alcohol and the Family* (J. Harwin and J. Orford, eds.), Crown Helm, London, pp. 114–126.

[7] P. Steinglass (1975) The simulated drinking gang: An experimental model for the study of a systems approach to alcoholism, I. Description of the Model II. Findings and implications. *J. Nerv. Men. Dis.* **161**, 101–122.

[8] P. Steinglass, S. Weiner, and J. H. Mendelson (1971) A systems approach to alcoholism: A model and its clinical application. *Arch. Gen. Psychiatry* **24**, 401–408.

[9] P. Steinglass, D. Davis, and D. Berenson (1977) Observations of conjointly hospitalized "alcoholic couples" during sobriety and intoxication: Implications for theory and therapy. *Fam. Process* **16**, 1–16.

[10]P. Steinglass (1980) A life history model of the alcoholic family. *Fam. Process* **19**, 211–226.

[11]A. Billings, M. Kessler, C. Gomberg, and S. Weiner (1979) Marital conflict—resolution of alcoholic and nonalcoholic couples during sobriety and experimental drinking. *J. Stud. Alcohol* **3**, 183–195.

[12]W. Frankenstein, W. E. Hay, and P. E. Nathan (1985) Effects of intoxication on alcoholics' marital communication and problem solving. *J. Stud. Alcohol* **46**, 1–6.

[13]T. Jacob, D. Ritchey, B. H. Cvitkovic, and J. Blane (1981) Communication styles of alcoholic and nonalcoholic families when drinking and not drinking. *J. Stud. Alcohol* **43**, 466–482.

[14] T. Jacob, R. A. Seilhamer, and R. Rushe (1989) Alcoholism and family interaction: A research paradigm. *Amer. J. Drug and Alcohol Abuse* **15**, 73–91.

[15] T. Jacob and G. L. Krahn (1988) Marital interactions of alcoholic couples: Comparison with depressed and nondistressed couples. *J. Consult. and Clin. Psychol.* **56**, 73–79.

[16]T. Jacob and K. Leonard (1988) Alcoholic-spouse interaction as a function of alcoholism subtypes and alcohol consumption. *J. Abnorm. Psychol.* **97**, 231–237.

[17]B. S. McCrady (1989) The outcomes of family-involved alcoholism treatment, *Recent Developments in Alcoholism* (M. Galanter, ed.), *vol VII: Treatment Issues*. Plenum, NY, pp. 165–181.

[18]B. S. McCrady, N. E. Noel, D. B. Abrams, R. L. Stout, H. F. Nelson, and W. M. Hay (1986) Comparative effectiveness of three types of spouse involvement in outpatient behavioral alcoholism treatment. *J. Stud. Alcohol* **47**, 459–467.

[19]T. J. O'Farrell, H. S. G. Cutter, and F. J. Floyd (1985) Evaluating behavioral marital therapy for male alcoholics: Effects on marital adjustment and communication from before to after treatment. *Behav. Ther.* **16**, 147–167.

[20]T. Cermak (1989) Al-Anon and recovery, *Recent Developments in Alcoholism, vol VII: Treatment Issues* (M. Galanter, ed.), NY, Plenum, pp. 91–103.

[21]J. C. Laundergan and T. Williams (1979) Hazelden: Evaluation of a residential family program. *Alcohol Health Res. World* 13–16.

[22]J. C. Laundergan, M. R. Shroeder, and B. P. Barnett (1980) Family program client changes: A followup. *Alcohol Clin. Exp. Res.* 221.

[23]J. M. Gorman and J. F. Rooney (1979) The influence of Al-Anon on the coping behavior of wives of alcoholics. *J. Stud. Alcohol* **40**, 1030–1037.

[24]P. Steinglass (1979) An Experimental treatment program for alcoholic couples. *J. Stud. Alcohol* **40(3)**, 159–182.

[25]P. Steinglass (1977) Family therapy in alcoholism, *The Biology of Alcoholism, Vol 5. Treatment and Rehabilitation of the Chronic Alcoholic* (B. Kissin and H. Begleiter, eds.) Plenum, NY, pp. 259–299.

[26]B. S. McCrady, T. J. Paolino, Jr., R. L. Longabough, and J. Rossi (1979) Effects

of joint hospital admission and couples treatment for hospitalized alcoholics. A pilot study. *Addict. Behav.* **4,** 155–165.

[27]B. S. McCrady, J. Moreau, T. J. Paolino Jr., and R. L. Longabaugh (1982) Joint hospitalization and couples therapy for alcoholism: A four year follow-up. *J. Stud. Alcohol* **43,** 1244–1250.

[28]T. J. O'Farrell and H. S. G. Cutter (1984) Behavioral marital therapy for male alcoholics: Clinical procedures from a treatment outcome study in progress. *Amer. J. Fam. Ther.* **12,** 33–46.

[29]W. R. Miller and H. R. Kester (1986) Inpatient alcoholism treatment: Who benefits? *Amer. Psychol.* **41,** 794–805.

[30]C. R. Cloninger, M. Bohman, and S. Sigvardsson (1981) Inheritance of alcohol abuse: Cross fostering analyses of adopted men. *Arch. Gen. Psychiatry* **38,** 861–868.

[31]L. C. Morey, H. A. Skinner, and R. K. Blashfield (1984) A typolology of alcohol abusers: Correlates and implications. *J. Abnorm. Psych.* **93,** 408–417.

[32]L. E. Beutler (1983) *Eclectic psychotherapy: A systematic approach.* (Pergamon, NY).

[33]L. E. Beutler and R. Mitchell (1981) Pychotherapy outcome in depressed and impulsive patients as a function of analytic and experimental treatment procedures. *Psychiatry* **44,** 297–306,

[34]S. J. Calvert, L. E. Beutler, and M. Crago (1988) Psychotherapy outcome as a function of therapist-patient matching on selected variables. *J. Soc. and Clin. Psych.* **6,** 104–117.

[35]L. E. Beutler and J. Clarkin (1990) *Systematic treatment selection: Toward targeted theraputic interventions.* (Brunner/Mazel, NY, 1990).

[36]S. Gonzalez, P. Steinglass, and D. Reiss (1989) Putting the illness in its place: Discussion groups for families with chronic medical illnesses. *Fam. Process* **28,** 69–87.

[37]B. S. McCrady (1985) *Alcoholism, Clinical Handbook of Psychological Disorders* (D. H. Barlow, ed.), Guilford, NY, pp. 245–298.

Changing Drug Use Patterns and Treatment Behavior

A Longitudinal Study of Urban Black Youth

Ann F. Brunswick, Peter A. Messeri, and Angela A. Aidala

Introduction

This chapter will report changing drug involvements and treatment needs in a community representative sample of nonHispanic urban Black Americans. The study group has been followed for 20 years to date. Individuals in the study group were selected in the late 1960s because they were adolescents residing in the Central Harlem health district of New York City. The first section of the chapter includes a discussion of drug use patterns, focusing on changes that appeared as the sample moved from postadolescence (aged 18–23 yr) to young adulthood (ages 26–31). Discussion in the second section turns to drug treatment issues. Attention is directed there, specifically, to pathways into and outcomes of treatment for heroin abuse.

A careful analysis of patterns of substance use and treatment in specific subpopulations must precede policy discussions of treatment needs. It has long been established that those who use drugs are not a homogeneous population, nor can any overall similarity be found among addicts or those who develop problem drug use.[1-4] Particularly important are differences in the experiences of Americans who are urban, mostly poor, and Black vs other Americans, differences that may trigger different drug use and treatment behaviors. In addition, the importance of gender, age, and cohort-historical factors must be taken into consideration in any attempt to understand drug use patterns and the individual and social consequences of use.

A longitudinal, community representative study of an inner-city Black population is an important complement to research based upon national cross-sectional samples. Such research is also a necessary addition to studies of special samples of treatment populations. For a decade, data from the study reported here have been documenting the excess prevalence of drug use among Black Americans relative to white.[5-7] These higher drug use rates of Black people have been partially concealed in national surveys, i.e., underestimated, largely because of methodological artifacts. Those more likely to be using drugs were more often missing from households (homeless, nomadic, institutionalized) and, therefore, from studies based on households. In addition, the clustering of Black households in certain census tracts requires oversampling of those areas to obtain representative data. Data from school samples, of course, are subject to bias from differential absentee and dropout rates among minorities most at risk of drug use.[6,8] Regarding treatment behavior, an area representative study such as this provides subsamples for comparing life outcomes of treated and nontreated users, and, of course, nonusers, for analyzing the correlates of natural cessation of use and conditions that foster or retard entering treatment and/or attaining a state of abstinence. Such data are presented here because they are crucial for formulating population appropriate prevention and treatment strategies.

Formulating such strategies becomes even more urgent when considering the applicability of reliable information concerning drug use and treatment patterns to AIDS risk reduction programs. This is an issue on which more directly targeted information is being collected in the current cycle of this longitudinal research.

Patterns of Drug Use

One regularity that has been demonstrated consistently is the strong relationship of age to drug use initiation. Initiation occurs primarily during the teen years.[5,7,9,10] More recently, evidence regarding the abatement of drug use with the assumption of normative adult roles (regular employment, marriage, parenthood) in the life stage of the mid-20s has been reported.[10-12]

In approaching developmental and maturational issues in changing drug abuse patterns, age-related influences need to be disentangled from cohort-historical and period factors.[13,14] Although initiation and termination of drug use have been linked to particular life stages, the popularity or prevalence of individual substances is sensitive to period or historic effects. Recent, trend data, for example, show a marked decline in prevalence of marijuana use among adolescents and young adults.[15,16] Studies in addition to our own have shown a decline in heroin initiation among more recent cohorts of adolescents as they passed through the life stage of highest risk for drug involvement.[13,17]

Another critical consideration when analyzing changing patterns of drug use in adulthood is the disparate socioeconomic circumstance of Black Americans relative to white and their concentration in economically depressed, inner-city areas. Overall, Black males have nearly double the unemployment rate of whites.[18] The rate of joblessness for inner-city Black young males, specifically, approaches 50%.[19,20] With less opportunity for achievement in socially desirable channels, but with needs for competency and adult role attainment still in place, substance use for many urban Blacks does more than alter mood or provide escape. For many it serves essentially occupational functions, satisfying work role and economic needs.[5,6,21-23] We might, thus, hypothesize that the age and adult role relationship to cessation of drug use might operate differently in an urban Black population than what has been reported from predominantly white samples.

With these considerations in mind, the following questions were posed in this analysis comparing drug use patterns in a sample of urban Black Americans at ages 18–23 and at ages 26–31, the latter representing ages when adult roles presumably have been assumed:

1. To what extent does drug use initiation occur after the teen years?
2. To what extent do patterns of cessation occur in an urban Black sample at ages adult life roles typically have been assumed?
3. Is there evidence of a substitution process in changing drug preferences? Specifically, did another substance replace heroin as the marker of heavy drug use among the younger cohorts in this sample who did not initiate heroin use, or did the decline in heroin initiation herald a more general cohort decline in drug involvement?

For both theoretical and empirical reasons, gender-specific analyses of changing drug use patterns were performed. Gender differences also were the focus in our analysis of antecedents and consequences of drug treatment, considered in the second section of this chapter. Although longitudinal data based primarily upon white populations indicated that there has been increasing convergence in male and female patterns of drug and alcohol use,[24] important gender differences still remained in this sample regarding substances used, consequences of use, and the role of treatment in terminating drug use.[5-7, 21, 25, 26] These suggested that divergent gender norms of tolerance for drug use continued to be salient among Black populations.[27-29]

Methods

Source of Data

The data for this research come from the second and third waves of an ongoing prospective health study of nonHispanic Black adolescents begun in 1968. The study panel, about equally divided between males and females, numbered 668 and were ages 12–17 at first study. The panel was drawn from an area probability sample of households in Central Harlem (New York City) over two consecutive years (1967–1968) using a sampling ratio of 1 in 25 households each year. All age-appropriate adolescents in these households were drawn into study.

The first restudy similarly extended over two years, in 1975–1976, six to eight years after initial study, when the panel were ages 18–23. In that first restudy, 94% of the initial sample was located. For reasons of economy and sample homogeneity, interviews were sought only with those still living in the metropolitan New York City area. Completed interviews numbered 536, representing an 89% response rate among the surviving New York City sample, with similar rates of completion for males and females (Table 1).

The second restudy (Wave 3) was conducted in 1983–1984, seven to eight years after the prior wave of interviews, when panel members were ages 26-31 and approx. 15 yr had elapsed since the study began. This time, 91% of the prior wave's sample was located and the response rate based on the Wave 2 surviving New York City sample was 86 %, somewhat higher than that for females and lower for males (Table 1). Combined with 15 respondents who had not been available for their second interviews, a total

Table 1
Sample Completion

	Wave 2[a]			Wave 3[b]		
	Total, 601	Male, 308	Female, 293	Total, 479	Male, 239	Female, 240
Response rate (eligible sample only, including nonlocated)						
Interview completed	89%	90%	88%	86%	83%	88%
Refused	2	1	4	4	3	5
Not located	7	6	7	10	13	6
Never at home/nomadic	2	3	1	c	—	1
	Total, 668	Male, 351	Female, 317	Total, 536	Male, 277	Female, 259
Sample completion (including dead and moved out of area)						
Located and interview completed	80%	79%	82%	77%	72%	82%
Refused	2	1	3	4	3	5
Never home/nomadic	2	2	1	c	—	1
Dead	2	3	1	2	4	—
Armed forces	3	5	c	1	2	—
Other out of area/institutional	6	5	7	8	8	7
Not located	6	6	6	9	12	5

[a]Response and completion rates calculated on base of initial Wave 1 sample. (In addition, to compensate for 1-yr sampling in Wave 1 of 16–17 yr olds vs 2 yr for 12–15 yr olds, older and younger respondents are given differential proportional weights to adjust for their differences in selection probability while avoiding inflation of actual sample size. For complete description, see Brunswick, 1984).

[b]Response and completion rates calculated on base of Wave 2 sample only. In addition, 15 respondents were interviewed at Wave 3 who had not been available for second interview (12 males and 3 females, 7 "never home" and 8 "out of area," chiefly military) for total Wave 3 interviewed sample of 426. Since the study began, a total of 12% of the initial sample have moved out of the area, 4% are dead, 5% have refused reinterview, and 13% have not been located.

[c]Less than half of one percent. Because of rounding, percentages may not total 100.

of 426 interviews was completed at Wave 3. In the first two waves of study, the sample was 52% male and 48% female. At the third interview, the gender proportions shifted to 51% female and 49% male. Increased male loss was attributable to their higher loss through nonlocation (e.g., few males compared to females could be located through welfare rolls and Medicaid) and to their higher rate of deaths (by Wave 3, 6% of the initial sample of males had died compared to 1% of females). For both genders, cause of death was primarily from homicide or other violent causes. Through 1989, deaths accounted for 9% of the initial male sample and 2% of female. The male loss, furthermore, was concentrated disproportionately among older cohorts and heroin users. Generally, females regardless of cohort, had higher sample retention rates than males, and younger cohorts, regardless of gender, had better retention rates than the older. These facts reflect less on the survey methods and more on what is happening in the population from which the sample was drawn.

Overall, when those retained and lost to study were compared on a broad range of demographic, health, and drug use variables, only small differences appeared. Considered cumulatively, differences indicated opposing directions of sample loss among men and women. Male loss was greater among the more socially disorganized, but among females, the more upwardly mobile or "better-off" had a greater chance of being lost to study. The longitudinal sample, therefore, will overstate to a slight degree the experiences of relatively more advantaged Black males and less advantaged females.

Data Collection Procedures

At all study times, data have been collected through individual interviews conducted in the respondent's home by ethnic and gender-matched interviewers using a structured interview schedule consisting largely of closed-ended questions. Hypotheses, data collection, and analyses in this longitudinal study have all along been guided by a model emphasizing contextual factors, i.e., influences external to the individual, such as life situation and social background characteristics as well as broader cohort and period effects. This is appropriate in studying a disadvantaged population subgroup.[31,32] Thus, besides extensive measurement of drug use and health, the data set also included information about:

1. Family background characteristics;
2. Role attainment and living conditions;

3. Interpersonal influences; and
4. Psychosocial attitudes.

Together these comprised a multidomain ecological model of behavioral influences.[33–35]

Given the focus of this paper on drug use patterns, derivation of the drug use variables will be described here in greater detail. Life histories of drug use were obtained on both Wave 2 and Wave 3 interviews. (This information continues to be collected during the fourth wave of data collection just now in the field.) Respondents were asked whether or not they had ever used each of ten drugs or classes of drugs that were read to them one at a time: marijuana, cocaine, heroin, PCP, methadone, "uppers," "downers," "glue or some other inhalant," alcohol, and cigarets. PCP was inquired about differently at the two study waves: Wave 2 asked about acid or other psychedelics, whereas at Wave 3 PCP was specified as a separate substance. Interwave comparisons, therefore, will not be made with respect to PCP.

Multiple measures of onset were obtained as checks in establishing reliability of report on the timing of initiation into use of each drug (i.e., how old respondent was, how long ago it was, and what the major life activity was at time of first use). Usual frequency and the recency of last use were among other items of information obtained about each drug. On the basis of usual frequency, experimental use (once or twice) was distinguished from nonexperimental. Unless specifically noted otherwise, the term "user" and all analyses of use are restricted to nonexperimental users only. (*See* Table 2 for lifetime prevalence of drug use in the sample at Wave 3, ages [26–29,31–32].)

Findings: Patterns of Drug Use

To What Extent Does Onset of Substance Use Occur After the Teen Years?

A direct answer to our question is given by straightforward analysis of reported dates of drug use onset (Table 3). To improve reliability, note that this information was taken from the earlier interview if a respondent had reported use by that time. For alcohol, marijuana, and heroin, at least six in seven of all users had begun by age 19. In the case of cocaine, a somewhat extended range of onset occurred, that we interpreted as reflecting the more recent general diffusion of this substance through inner-city areas. Its earlier

Table 2
Lifetime Prevalence of Drug Use at Ages 26–31, in Percentages

	Total 426	Males 210	Females 216
Alcohol			
Experimental	1	2	1
Nonexperimental	96	95	96
Marijuana			
Experimental	8	5	11
Nonexperimental	80	87	74
Cocaine			
Experimental	8	7	8
Nonexperimental	46	52	40
Heroin			
Experimental	2	2	2
Nonexperimental	14	16	13
Other opiates			
Experimental	1	1	2
Nonexperimental	1	3	—
Uppers			
Experimental	5	5	5
Nonexperimental	8	11	4
Inhalants[a]			
Experimental	4	5	3
Nonexperimental	4	6	2
Hallucinogens[b]			
Experimental	16	21	11
Nonexperimental	11	16	7
Methadone			
Experimental	2	2	2
Nonexperimental	6	6	5
Downers			
Experimental	5	7	3
Nonexperimental	6	7	4

[a] "Nitrites and poppers" were asked about separately, and then combined with "glue or other inhalants." [b] Includes acid, PCP, and other hallucinogens.

history was as a hard drug linked with heroin, e.g., at second wave all heroin users had also used cocaine and heroin users at that time comprised half of all cocaine users. This linkage was considerably attenuated by Wave 3, and

Table 3
Age Specific Incidence: Age at First Use of Five Substances[a]

Age	Alcohol male,[c] 199[b]	Alcohol female,[c] 206	Marijuana male, 182	Marijuana female, 160	Cocaine male, 108	Cocaine female, 86	Heroin male, 33	Heroin female, 28	PCP male, 28	PCP female, 8
Under 12 yrs	20	9	[d]	[d]	•	•	•	•	•	•
12	31	19	12	2	•	•	6	•	•	•
13	39	28	18	8	2	2	12	6	•	•
14	45	41	34	19	4	5	26	18	•	•
15	63	56	50	33	13	8	51	41	7	•
16	79	75	64	55	20	18	62	70	10	•
17	88	84	82	67	36	28	84	73	26	•
18	96	92	93	79	63	47	92	85	49	•
19	•	96	96	87	70	59	[c]	91	65	10
20	97	97	97	93	80	68	97	97	78	40
21	98	97	98	96	84	76	100	100	84	•
22	•	98	98	97	87	83			91	70
23	99	•	99	99	88	89			94	•
24	99	•	100	•	89	92			[c]	90
25	100	•		•	95	95			[c]	90
26		•		•	98	97			97	100
27		•		•	100	99			100	
28+		100		100		100				
Median	15	15	16	16	18	19	15	16	19	22
Mean	14.7	15.3	15.4	16.6	18.7	19.3	15.8	16.2	19.2	22
SD	(3.44)	(3.02)	(2.50)	(2.57)	(3.13)	(3.22)	(2.11)	(2.01)	(2.75)	(2.38)

[a]Cumulative percentages based on nonexperimental users of each substance. [b]Eleven males and nine females reported never drinking or drinking only once or twice (experimental use). [c]No cases. [d]One-half percent or less. Source: Reference 7.

cocaine's increased popularity outside the ghetto was reflected inside it as well. This was a clear example of what we refer to as a period effect—cocaine use increased across all age groups and both genders.[14*] Still, more than half of cocaine users in this sample (70% of male users and 59% of female) had started use by age 19, and approx. nine in ten initiated use by age 23. The same timetable of onset appeared for PCP among males, while the very small group of female PCP users ($N = 8$) achieved the 90% onset rate by age 24. (This, of course, presupposes no initiation after Wave 3 and ages 26–31, a hypothesis we are testing in our current fourth wave of study at ages 32–37 years.)

Does Illicit Substance Use Abate by Ages at Which Adult Roles Are Assumed?

To answer this question, the proportion of lifetime (nonexperimental) users of five illicit substances who have continued use as adults, defined uniformly as age 26, was compared to analogous rates for the licit substances tobacco and alcohol.

For most substances, the great majority of those who ever became involved with the drug on more than an experimental basis were still using at age 26 (Table 4). For male users of marijuana and cocaine, approx. three-fourths continued use at an age when the putative influences of adult role responsibilities should have been at work exerting pressures toward cessation of substance use. Similarly, two-thirds of male PCP users were using the drug at age 26. For females, approx. 60% of lifetime users of marijuana and PCP, and 82% of cocaine users were using these drugs at age 26. Except for heroin and inhalants, rates of continued illicits use were not unlike the percentages of those who continued smoking cigarets and indulging in heavy alcohol drinking (defined as five or more drinks daily at least once a month).

Two substances showing substantial portions of lifetime users who discontinued use by age 26 were heroin and inhalants; 30% of male heroin users and 46% of female heroin users were continuing use. (Remember, however, that 37% of male heroin users had died or otherwise were lost to Wave 3 interview). None of the very few female users of inhalants and only a small proportion (30%) of their male counterparts were currently using inhalants (Table 4). Note that, although heroin use was approx. 25% less

*These data were collected in 1983 before the emergence of "crack" in 1985.

Table 4
Continuation of Drug Use at Age 26

Substance	Percentage of lifetime users continuing use at age 26			
	Females		Males	
Cigarets	83%	(139/168)[a]	85%	(124/146)
Heavy alcohol	60%	(34/57)[b]	77%	(65/84)
Marijuana	63%	(100/160)	75%	(137/182)
Cocaine	82%	(69/84)	77%	(83/108)
PCP	63%	(5/8)	68%	(19/28)
Inhalants	0%	(0/3)	31%	(4/13)
Heroin	46%	(13/28)	30%	(10/33)

[a]Percentage of nonexperimental users by Wave 3 who were currently using at age 26. [b]Heavy alcohol was percentaged on regular monthly or more frequent users of five or more drinks in a day.

prevalent among females than males (*see* Table 2), once involved with these drugs, females were somewhat more likely to continue use in adulthood, but this observation may have been biased by the substantial loss of male heroin users. It would be expected, however, that it would mirror what actually happens in heroin careers of Black men and women.

The reduction of drug use in the mid-20s observed in studies of predominately white samples is usually explained with reference to the role conflict between using drugs and the assumption of adult responsibilities that typically occurs at this age. To test the relevance of the "role conflict" hypothesis to an inner-city Black population, a logistic regression analysis was performed estimating the effect of being married and number of children on the probability of continuing, past age 26, regular use of marijuana, cocaine, and heavy drinking. Current or past marriage had an inhibiting effect on adult use of marijuana and cocaine for women. Marital status had a more modest effect on heavy drinking, although the direction of the relationship was in the opposite direction: ever married women, more so than those who had never married, tended to continue heavy drinking past age 26. For males, marital status had no effect on patterns of heavy drinking and/or marijuana or cocaine use. Neither males nor females evidenced a relationship between parental status and drug use cessation.[36]

The role conflict hypothesis was further tested in a separate study directed at distinguishing predictors of continued moderate adult use from heavy drug abuse. Most briefly, the role conflict hypothesis explained Black women's adult drug abuse, but not men's.[36]

Another way to examine patterns of continuing drug use into the adult life stage is to look at rates of current use among the entire study sample at ages 26–31 compared to ages 18–23. With respect to percent of current use (i.e., use within the year prior to interview), a modest decline on the order of 10% had occurred in marijuana use, no change in heroin, and for cocaine, a 33% increase in past year use for males and a doubling of the proportion of current users for females (Table 5).*

Is There Evidence of a Substitution Process in Changing Drug Use Patterns? Did Another Substance Replace Heroin as the "Hardest" Drug Used?

On the basis of its relatively recent introduction into the panoply of available substances, phencyclidine or PCP ("angel dust") was the most plausible drug to test as a possible substitution candidate. To determine a substitution effect, the comparability of these two substances on pharmacological (psychoactive) and normative (degree of social acceptability and acceptance) dimensions must be examined.

Considering the pharmacological comparison first, PCP appears to be an unsuitable candidate, given the different effects of heroin as a narcotic and PCP as an hallucinogenic. On the level of specific biological effects, to the extent that pharmacologic properties influence choice of psychoactive substances, the evidence does not support a hypothesis of substitution effects.

Considering the normative dimension, PCP was first examined as a marker of heavy drug involvement. On the basis of the number of other substances used (licit and illicit), PCP and heroin were equivalent. This can be seen in the number of substances (of a maximum of 12) that users of these two substances reported. Males who used heroin reported a lifetime nonexperimental experience with a mean of 6.72 substances, and PCP users a mean of 6.71. (Note that 9 individuals overlapped the two groups, i.e., used both substances, accounting for about a third of each group.) For females, heroin users reported a mean lifetime nonexperimental use of 5.67 substances and

---

*In an earlier article, Brunswick et al.[7] also examined frequency of substance use at the two life stages. Except for heroin, which showed a slight decline in reported daily use, reported frequencies were remarkably similar at the two life stages. Even if this conceals a considerable degree of individual changes in frequency, it properly reflects the absence of any overall direction in change; no systematic evidence of diminution in use appeared.

Table 5
Current Substance Use at Two Life Stages, in Percentages[a,b]

	Females, N = 212		Males, N = 199	
	Ages 18–23, current use	Ages 26–31, current use	Ages 18–23, current use	Ages 26–31 current use
Alcohol	79	89	83	82
Marijuana	47	42	73	64
Cocaine	14	29	27	36
Heroin	4	3	4	4

[a]"Current use" refers to use within year of interview. Table based on those interviewed at both Waves 2 (ages 18–23) and 3 (ages 26–31).
[b]Source: Reference.[7]

PCP users 7.25. As shall subsequently be noted, this reflects the fact that female heroin users historically were not known to engage in use of a wide range of substances. Finally, three women, who constituted 10% of female heroin users and 37% of PCP users, used both substances.

Further, although only 16% of all men in the sample had used as many as six of 12 substances or classes of substances queried about, among heroin users and PCP users, the proportions were 58% and 61%, respectively. Corresponding rates were 8% for lifetime use of six or more substances among the full sample of women, 44% among female heroin users, and 80% among female PCP users (Table 6). Note, however, that the case base for women PCP users is extremely small ($N = 8$), and thus, any inferences based on them would be fragile indeed.

One of the other consistently observed regularities of drug use involvement is that the harder the substance used, the more heavily that individual will be involved with so-called lighter substances.[5,13,37] Therefore, the substitution hypothesis was also tested by contrasting usual frequency of marijuana and cocaine consumption reported by groups of PCP and heroin users (Table 6). For males, heaviness of marijuana use, indicated by usual frequency of use, was somewhat greater among PCP users than heroin users. However, this was counterbalanced by the opposite difference in cocaine use. Almost half of male heroin users had used cocaine on multiple weekly occasions, compared to somewhat more than a third of PCP users. On balance, for men, PCP and heroin users' involvement in these two substances might be considered to be approximately equivalent.

Table 6
Substance Involvement: Heroin and PCP Users
(Wave 3 sample)[a]

Number of substances used (nonexperimentally)[b]
in cumulative percentages

		Females					
		Heroin N = 29		PCP N = 8		All N = 215	
		Lifetime	Past year	Lifetime	Past year	Lifetime	Past year
Number of substances used: At least	6	44	—	80	20	8	1
	5	73	22	100	90	17	5
	4	91	37	—	100	36	20
	3	100	58	—	—	73	31
	2	—	67	—	—	90	51
	1	—	88	—	—	100	91
		Males					
		Heroin N = 33		PCP N = 28		All N = 210	
		Lifetime	Past year	Lifetime	Past year	Lifetime	Past year
Number of substances used: At least	6	58	11	61	19	16	2
	5	100	30	90	64	30	11
	4	—	58	97	77	48	26
	3	—	64	100	90	81	37
	2	—	89	—	90	95	64
	1	—	97	—	97	100	92

(continued)

The comparison, once again, is more complex for the women. Female PCP users showed heavier involvement in both marijuana and cocaine than did the heroin users. PCP using females had triple the proportion of daily marijuana smokers compared to heroin users. When all frequencies of cocaine use up to multiple monthly occasions were combined, PCP users had almost twice as many regular cocaine users (90%) as appeared among fe-

Table 6 (continued)

	Females			Males		
	Heroin, N = 29	PCP, N = 8	All, N = 215	Heroin, N = 33	PCP, N = 28	All, N = 210
Usual frequency of marijuana use in percentages:						
Daily	12	40	17	28	39	21
Few times/wk	29	30	17	33	35	29
Few times/mo	21	10	20	17	13	18
Once a mo or less	18	20	20	22	13	19
Not regular user	21	—	26	—	—	13
Usual frequency of cocaine use in percentages:						
Daily	12	20	3	17	10	3
Few times/wk	38	30	9	30	26	10
Few times/mo	9	40	11	14	19	14
Once a mo or less	21	10	16	39	35	24
Not regular user	21	—	61	—	—	48

[a]Owing to rounding, percentages may not total exactly 100.
[b]Include 12 licit and illicit substances.

male heroin users (59%). The exceptionally small number of female PCP users makes these estimates highly unstable. Even so, they demonstrate that, on the dimension of degree of involvement in so-called "lighter" substances, PCP would seem to have assumed a role of "hard" drug and, thereby, comparable to heroin.

It must be noted here that, on the basis of the sheer number of users, heroin and PCP were not equivalent. PCP use, at least up to the ages and dates studied here, had not acquired the number of followers achieved by heroin. This was particularly the case among Black women.

Another approach is to examine differential patterns of heroin and PCP use across different birth cohorts. As measured at ages 18–23, heroin prevalence declined progressively from 24% among those born in 1952 ($N = 94$) to 3% of those born in 1956 and 1957 ($N = 159$).[13] When examining the heroin cohort phenomenon at Wave 3, the three oldest single-year cohorts (born 1952–1954) and the three youngest single-year cohorts (born 1955–1957) were combined to make dichotomous gender-specific contrasts in lifetime use rates at ages 26–31 yrs. Approximately 1 in 5 of both men and women among the older cohort (born 1952–1954) had used heroin nonexperimentally by time of the third interview; the comparable percentages for younger males and females (born 1955–1957) were 11% and 6%, respectively.[7] Thus, heroin use showed significant variation by birth cohort for both genders.

On the other hand, PCP use was significantly greater (at least double) among younger than older cohorts of both genders. Lifetime experience was 18% of younger male cohorts vs 8% of older, and 7% vs 1% among female younger and older cohorts, respectively. Even though data are based on only 28 male PCP users and eight female, gender-specific cohort tests were significant at $p = .02$ (Tau b) and at $p = .002$ when genders were pooled.[7]

These large cohort differentials would seem to support the hypothesis that a substitution effect occurred between PCP and heroin, with that specific replacement resulting from the intersection of historical period and maturational forces. Lower rates of PCP use among the older cohort might logically be explained by the fact that individuals in the older cohorts had completed adolescence and, accordingly, the time of greatest risk for initiating new substances by the time PCP had diffused as a drug of choice in inner-city Black neighborhoods. For a combination of social and historical reasons, heroin had become less attractive for the younger cohorts as they entered the period of greatest likelihood for drug use initiation.[38,39]

Thus, the intuitively appealing question of whether newly popular substances substitute for older ones that , for whatever reasons, become less fashionable is more complex than it might readily appear. If pharmacological equivalence is a prerequisite, PCP clearly fails as a replacement for heroin. If that dimension is less important, as appears to be the case, and the social situational aspects are more critical, then there is evidence for PCP's substitution for heroin among the cohorts included in this study. Relevant, too, is the fact that older and younger cohorts were not significantly different in the total number of illicit substances they had used. Among men, older and younger cohorts averaged 2.10 (SD 1.98) and 2.07 (SD 1.52) illicits, respectively. For females, older and younger averages were 1.62 (SD 1.42) and 1.38 (SD 1.24), respectively.

In closing this discussion of changing drug use patterns, over the seven year interval between postadolescence and the assumption of full adult roles at ages 26–31, and over the chronological time span 1976–1983, the basic theorem that drug patterns and cycles need to be considered "on an individual substance by substance basis" still prevails.[7,14] Over and above its pharmacologic character, the incidence and prevalence of any substance are responsive to historic normative factors pertaining to that substance's availability and acceptability and to user vulnerability. The latter has a clear relationship to life stage and the availability of resources for acting out appropriate social roles.

In sum, no evidence of a sharp drop in drug use at the adult age of 26, such as has been reported in largely white samples, appeared in this cross-section sample of urban Black Americans. Although rates of heroin initiation were responsive to a cohort effect so that younger cohorts initiated at a much lower rate than older, heroin use prevalence in the sample remained almost constant over the seven-year interval. The total number of illicit substances showed no significant difference by cohort. Prevalence of cocaine increased, irrespective of cohort, and at a more rapid rate among Black women than men. These findings have obvious implications for treatment needs. The second section of this chapter will now present a discussion of the influences on selection into treatment.

Treatment Behavior

Because of its homogeneously Black racial composition and its basis in a systematically drawn sample of dwelling units, this longitudinal study offers a view of treatment rarely permitted in other studies. What is known about treatment entry and effectiveness is almost entirely based upon treatment samples, comprised of drug users who voluntarily or perhaps under legal coercion have some contact with the drug treatment system. Evaluation of treatment consequences is most often determined by using a one group prepost experimental design. More elaborated quasi-experimental designs are sometimes used in which a "nontreated" comparison group is constituted from persons who enroll but do not participate, those who cut treatment short, or those who receive only a limited detoxification regimen.[40,41]

Yet, studies that draw conclusions based on reflexive or nonequivalent controls are subject to the criticism that apparent improvements in the treated group could arise because of nonrandom differences between the treated and nontreated groups. For example, persons entering treatment are typically at a low ebb in their lives and improvements in psychosocial functioning, therefore, might be attributable to a natural rebound from abnormally low states. Greater motivation and other personal or social resources may explain why persons who enroll and stay in treatment do better than those who fail to start or who drop out before completion of the program.

A more serious limitation is that any sample of persons drawn from treatment programs cannot be regarded as representative of all drug users. There is strong evidence that many drug users, heroin users included, pass through their entire drug using careers without any contact with treatment programs[2,42,43] and a substantial portion of heroin users return to a drug-free state without benefit of formal treatment.[26,44]

Because, in the past, virtually all treatment was related to heroin use, these analyses were confined to treatment's relationship to the dynamics of heroin careers. Given the community representative nature of the present data base, it was possible to systematically examine:

1. How treated users differed from nontreated users and the broader population from which they came;
2. What attributes or conditions facilitated or impeded treatment entry; and
3. What influenced cessation of drug use, with or without treatment.

A "natural history" approach was brought to these analyses. Natural history imagery emphasizes, e.g., that heroin use is a process that extends over time and space. The concept of a heroin "career" implies that there is an orderliness to heroin use or at least limited variation in the type of natural histories individual users experience.[45] First, a description of treatment experiences in the sample is presented, followed by a static comparison of treated heroin users with nontreated users and with the remaining nonheroin using sample. This descriptive material provides variable elements of different heroin careers, which will then be subjected to dynamic analysis. Using techniques that sociologists term event-history analysis, and biostatisticians term hazard or survival analysis, multiple factors that influence the likelihood of treatment entry, the timing of treatment entry, and the significance of treatment and other factors that move heroin careers to the state of abstinence will subsequently be examined.

A central issue in all of these analyses will be examination of gender differences. Findings already reported from this research[5,25,26] are at variance with other studies concerning gender differences in timing of treatment entry.[46,47] The influence of familial context as a possible explanation of gender differences in treatment experiences will also be examined.

Findings: Treatment Behavior

Treatment Histories

A total of 73 treatment episodes for heroin use was reported by 51 or about 10% of respondents at the second and/or third study waves. However, analyses of treatment experiences and comparisons between treated and nontreated users will be based on the Wave 3 study group, except as noted. The rationale here is that those careers are more complete and that what adult life outcomes might have been for the approx. one-third of male heroin users lost to the third interview cannot be assumed.

As previously shown, 16% of males and 13% of females interviewed at Wave 3 reported use of heroin on a minimum of three occasions (see Table 2). Heroin use typically was begun in middle adolescence and the average length of a heroin career through the third wave interview in 1983 (at ages 26–31) had lasted almost eight years for women (mean 7.66) and approx. six years (mean 6.23) for men. Care was taken to refer here to an end point of heroin abstinence as opposed to what cannot yet be identified as permanent cessation or the end of a heroin career, since relapse is an ever-present possibility. Nevertheless, just over two-thirds of users in the sample did not report use within a year of interview, and among those meeting this definition of abstainer, a majority had remained heroin free for three years or more. For women, twice as many treated (81%) as untreated (40%) had abstained for at least a year. However, for male heroin users, the difference—although smaller—was in the reverse direction, with a somewhat greater proportion of abstainers among the untreated (87%) than among the treated (61%).

When treatment episodes within heroin careers were considered, by ages 26–31, two-thirds of males (22/33) and 62 % of females (18/29) who had used heroin nonexperimentally had been treated at least once. For males, this represented an increase in treated heroin users, up from approx. half of male heroin users at ages 18–23. For females, the rate was constant compared to the prior study time seven years earlier.[5]

Most of the gender differences in treatment patterns observed through postadolescence[5,25] continued through the young adult stage. Males started treatment at a younger age than females, had briefer treatment episodes, and a greater number of them. These tendencies became even more pronounced by ages 26–31. This was especially apparent in the average length per treatment episode and the cumulative time in treatment. Females' individual treatment episodes averaged nearly 2$\frac{1}{2}$ years (29 mo) and males episodes averaged 4 mo; females' total time in treatment exceeded four years on average (51.5 mo) and males' total time was slightly more than half a year (6.6 mo). Indeed a small number of females had been in treatment continuously between interviews. This obviously was a function of the treatment modality utilized. Seven in ten of women's treatment experiences were in methadone maintenance facilities; barely 1 in 5 (19%) of males' experiences were. Males most frequently mentioned residential services (38%) and detox only (26%) as modality of treatment (Table 7, *see* pp. 284,285).

A series of questions were asked about reasons and motivations for entering treatment. Both men and women said that their own desire to stop using heroin was their primary motivation for entering treatment. In better than nine in ten treatment episodes, the individual reported that she/he chose the program rather than being assigned to it. The reasons heroin users themselves most often gave for seeking treatment emphasized their personal fears about becoming addicted, the consequences of heroin use for family responsibilities, and the influence of their families in encouraging them to discontinue use. An interesting gender difference among reasons given for seeking treatment related to the availability of drugs to the individual. Over half (55%) of women heroin users reported difficulty in obtaining drugs as one of the factors influencing them to seek treatment; less than 10% of males listed this as a reason (Table 7).

The following will be an examination of differences between treated and untreated heroin users and a comparison of both to the total sample. Contrast between treated and untreated within the drug using group is necessary to avoid confounding those differences with what appears between heroin users and nonusers *per se.*

How Do Treated Users Differ from Nontreated Users and from the Broader Population from Which They Come?

Treated and untreated heroin users were first compared regarding antecedent differences, such as early family experiences and attitudes and aspirations during adolescence. For this discussion, respondents who reported treatment status at either the Wave 2 or Wave 3 interview were examined, rather than restricting the examination to the Wave 3 sample. Thus, a potentially small but unknown number of individuals who reported heroin use but no treatment experience at Wave 2 interview, and who were subsequently lost to interview, of necessity were here classified among the "untreated," although they conceivably might have entered treatment at some later point.* A more serious consideration in interpreting these antecedent differences between treated and never treated heroin users was that these baseline measurements were obtained at varying points in heroin careers, and these differed according to treatment status. In the case of women, particularly, more than twice as many in the treated group (63%) than the untreated (25%) were already using heroin when the baseline measurement was taken. Male differences were modest on this score (Table 8). Thus, treatment groups were clearly not equivalent on this important variable, and this nonequivalence underscores the necessity to guard against making causal inferences from the data. Differences reported here can only be suggestive of some of the selection biases that might operate in distinguishing who does and does not enter treatment.

Antecedent Differences Between Treated and Not Treated

Nonetheless, our findings are strongly suggestive that both male and female heroin users who entered treatment differed in important ways from their untreated counterparts, well prior to entering treatment (Table 8). As discussed above, heroin users in general were more likely to be drawn from the older birth cohort. Cohort made a difference in treatment status, however, only for females, and a strong one, where 92% of the treated 23 female heroin users compared to 63% of untreated were born in the years 1952–1954.

Regarding family of origin and early family experiences, migration status again distinguished treated and untreated females, but not males. The families of *untreated* females had been in the North longer relative to treated

---

*Of the 15 male heroin users lost to Wave 3 reinterview, 11 had already previously been in treatment as reported on Wave 2; all of the four lost female heroin useres had been treated. Thus, except for four males who might have subsequently entered treatment, treatment status for all heroin users in the combined Wave 2 and Wave 3 sample was determined. The general patterns regarding antecedent differences between treated and nontreated heroin users shown in Table 7 remained unchanged when analysis was restricted to the Wave 3 sample only.

Table 7
Treatment Experiences[a,b]

No. treated	Females, (18)	Males, (22)
Percent treated:		
Based on full sample	8 (of 216)	10 (of 210)
Based on heroin users	62 (of 29)	61 (of 33)
Age first treatment:	(16)	(20)
14–16 yr	—	36%
17–18 yr	23%	18
19–20 yr	6	14
21–24 yr	59	9
25 yr	12	23
$\overline{X}$	21.5	19.7
(SD)	(2.9)	(4.5)
Total no. treatment episodes		
1	44%	36%
2	33	45
3+	23	18
Treatment modality per episode[c]		
(based on all episodes):	(28)	(42)
Methadone maintenance	70%	19%
Residential	24	38
Outpatient-drug free	6	13
Prison	—	4
Other/detox only	—	26
Goal of entering treatment[d]		
(based on all episodes):	(28)	(42)
To stop using	97%	77%
To cut down amount	3	21
Other	—	2
Reasons for entering treatment		
(based on all episodes):	(28)	(42)
Fear of becoming addicted	77%	98%
Family responsibilities made you want to get off drugs	82	73
Family/mate wanted you to	77	79
Drugs hard to get	55	7
Involuntary, assigned to program	5	9

(continued)

Table 7 (continued)

No. treated	Females, (18)	Males, (22)
Duration of treatment (in mo; based on no. episodes):	(28)	(35)
Less than 1 mo	37%	42%
1–2 mo	6	19
3–6 mo	13	25
7–12 mo	7	8
13–24 mo	—	6
More than 2 yr	37	—
$\overline{X}$	29	4
SD	(20.7)	(4.3)
Cumulative time in treatment (in mo, per individual):	(15)	(17)
1 mo	—	21%
2 mo	6%	—
3 mo	6	5
4 mo	—	16
5 mo	—	5
6 mo	17	5
7 mo	—	21
12 mo (1 yr)	—	10
13-24 mo (1-2 yr)	11	16
25-36 mo (2-3 yr)	—	—
37-48 mo (3-4 yr)	6	—
49-60 mo (4-5 yr)	22	—
61-72 mo (5-6 yr)	11	—
More than 6 yr	22	—
$\overline{X}$	51.5	6.6
SD	(42.7)	(4.8)

[a] Owing to rounding, percentages may not total exactly 100.

[b] Data combine second and third wave reports of third wave sample. In this and all subsequent tables, because of rounding, percentages may not total exactly 100.

[c] Two treated females and six treated males did not provide detailed treatment episode information.

[d] Each reason presented with yes/no answer alternative.

women and to the norm for the full female sample (Table 8). It is interesting to note that, contrary to theories emphasizing the significance of father absence or parental separation in the etiology of drug abuse, father's presence made no differences in the *male* sample. Treated and untreated male heroin users showed similar proportions, and both were quite like the full sample of males. Father's presence did differ by women's treatment status. Treated female heroin users twice as often had a father/stepfather present in the household (63%) as did untreated and even considerably more often than the female sample in its entirety.

Indicators of social involvement and other psychosocial measures during adolescence were examined for heroin users who subsequently entered treatment compared to those who did not. The direction of differences between treated and untreated on measures of peer influence diverged by gender. Subsequently, *treated female* heroin users spent more time alone (data not shown), scored lower on an index measuring peer influence on decisions (indicating poorer social networks during adolescence), and belonged to fewer organized groups/clubs. Subsequently *treated males* relative to untreated reported greater peer influence on decisions and spending more time with friends rather than alone or with family. However, they, too, belonged to fewer organized groups/clubs than untreated men. This anomalous direction of differences could be suggestive of differences in the nature and function of support networks among Black males and females, something Brunswick and Messeri have also examined in analyses of drug use and health.[48]

Treated of both genders attached greater importance to religion than untreated. The difference was more marked among males than females. Two psychosocial measures also produced inconsistent results across gender. Subsequently, *treated female* heroin users scored lower on self-esteem and on personal efficacy in adolescence than never treated users. Among males, the subsequently treated scored higher on personal efficacy but showed no real difference in self-esteem compared to their never treated counterparts.

Although some of the differences described did not meet the criterion of statistical significance, a general pattern was suggested. More consistently than males, female heroin users who subsequently became involved in formal treatment programs compared less favorably, i.e., seemed more disadvantaged in personal and social resources compared to their heroin using peers who never entered treatment. However, the caveat, should be repeated that, in interpreting these data, the absence of a control for onset of heroin use makes straightforward interpretation difficult.

Table 8
Antecedent Differences Between Treated and Untreated Heroin Users

	Female heroin users			Male heroin users		
	Treated (20)	Not treated (13)	All females[a] (260)	Treated (32)	Not treated (20)	All males (288)
Birth cohort						
Older (percent)	92	63	55	70	74	49
Birthplace, respondent, and mother						
Both born in North (percent)	38	47	30	30	17	27
Family structure						
Father or stepfather in the household (percent)	63	31[f]	46	52	47	49
Peer influence[b]						
Mean scale score	.166	.688	.351	.883	.217[e]	.498
Number of groups/clubs						
Mean scale score	0.08	0.25	0.49	0.14	0.44[d]	0.34
Self-esteem						
Mean scale score	8.50	9.62[f]	8.69	9.09	8.87	8.96
Personal efficacy						
Mean scale score	7.87	8.94	8.54	8.86	7.91[f]	8.91
Psychophysical symptoms[c]						
Average weighted score	18.78	12.50	14.01	13.62	12.08	8.91
Importance of religion						
Mean scale score (low score = more important)	2.23	2.88	1.90	2.00	2.57[f]	2.17
Heroin use at baseline						
(percent using)	63	25[d]	8	42	48	8

[a]Data shown are values obtained at baseline adolescent interview for respondents included in Wave 2 or Wave 3 sample. [b]Number of situations in which follow friends advice (rather than parental or make own decision) out of eight inquired above. [c]Based on nine-item scale. Average weighted score derived by dividing number of symptoms present by nine hundredths (.09). Intergroup differences in means (t-test) comparing treated and nontreated users for each gender. [d]$p \leq .05$. [e]$p \leq .01$. [f]$p \leq .10$.

Substance Use Histories of Treated and Nontreated Users

Considering females first, relative to untreated, treated female users had used heroin longer and more heavily than untreated (Table 9, *see* pp. 290, 291). Untreated users, however, were more likely to be current heroin users at time of the third interview and also to have used a greater variety of illicit substances in their lifetimes. This, it is inferred, relates to their younger cohort membership and the changing role of heroin use. Historically, it would appear that heroin using females did not use a wide variety of other illicit substances besides heroin. Other than their current use of heroin, however, untreated and treated female heroin users showed but slight differences in *current* substance use patterns. The one exception was in the very high rates of cigaret smoking among treated females (62% smoking at least one pack of cigaret a day) compared not only to untreated females, but also to cigaret smoking among males, regardless of their treatment status.

Contrasting patterns of substance use among treated and untreated male heroin users lend themselves to more ready summation. On every count, untreated male heroin users were less involved drug users—not only with respect to heroin (e.g., current male heroin users were drawn almost entirely from the pool of treated men), but in terms of their use of other substances, and not only in terms of current drug use, but lifetime experience as well (Table 9).

Substance use histories included questions about perceived problems from use of heroin and other drugs. The general pattern indicated that heroin users who entered treatment had experienced more problems associated with drug use—including drug dependency—either prior to entering treatment, following treatment, or both (i.e., data presented indicated problems anytime up to the third interview, ages 26–31). The differences were more compelling regarding males. Better than two-thirds of treated male users (69%) reported problems resulting from their drinking or taking drugs, compared to fewer than one in ten untreated (8%). This finding, of course, is highly consistent with the observed lesser heroin involvement of untreated males. Among females, about a third of the treated (37%) and a quarter of untreated (23%) considered themselves having had problems stemming from substance use (Table 10). This trivial difference (considering the small numbers in both groups) and the low problem rate (i.e., acute drug problems) among women who had ever entered treatment warrants special note. It could be inferred that critical events might instigate male treatment where women's entry may be motivated more by chronic or more enduring problematic life situations.

Turning to specific types of acute reactions to use, such as overdose, being in an accident, or getting arrested, treated heroin users of both genders, not unexpectedly, were more likely to have experienced such reactions than untreated. The single exception was the case of male arrest rates, which were comparable regardless of treatment status.

Finally, regarding anticipatory treatment behavior, three-quarters of those men who actually entered treatment one or more times indicated additional times they had thought about entering and the majority reported other times they had to wait to enter (53%) or were refused altogether (5%). About a quarter of treated females reported unsuccessful attempts at treatment entry. Untreated users reported no such experiences: i.e., no untreated user in this sample, male or female, had ever attempted to enter treatment (Table 10).

Family Formation

The relationship of child-bearing, child-rearing, and marriage to drug treatment is of interest, both as they influence treatment entry and retention and as they are affected by treatment experiences. When static comparisons were performed of treated and untreated heroin users at ages 26–31, important gender differences became clear and in ways that were not entirely predictable (Table 11). *Untreated female* heroin users were the most likely (84%) of the four gender/treatment groups to be currently living without either a spouse or mate. However, *untreated males* were those most likely (67%) to be living *with* spouse or partner. *Treated females* had their first child at a younger age than untreated (59% of treated compared to 23% of untreated women had a child by age 17) and had more children than untreated (39% of treated and 23% of untreated had as many as three or more children). At the same time, 85% of *untreated* vs 61% of *treated* women reported 4–8 pregnancies. This apparent inconsistency in untreated women's greater number of pregnancies but fewer births is resolved when it is considered that induced abortion rates were higher among the untreated, averaging two per woman, than among treated females, where the abortion rate was about one per woman as it was in the full female sample (Table 11).

Among males, *untreated* heroin users were more likely to have had children, and to have fathered a child before age 18, than either treated males or the entire male sample (Table 11). All untreated females were living with

Table 9
Treated vs Not Treated Heroin Users: Patterns of Substance Use

	Female heroin users		Male heroin users	
	Treated (18)	Not treated (11)	Treated (22)	Not treated (11)
Age first heroin use				
Median	15	16	15	17
X̄	15.8	16.8	15.6	16.3
SD	(1.74)	(2.33)	(2.04)	(2.27)
Usual frequency of heroin use				
Daily or near daily	62%	15%	63%	25%
Few times/wk	29	54	13	42
Few times/mo	5	23	8	17
Once a mo	—	—	13	8
Few times/yr	5	8	4	8
Duration of use of heroin				
Less than 1 yr	5%	—	—	33%
About 1 yr	—	8%	8%	25
2 yr	—	15	4	8
3–4 yr	24	15	13	17
5+ yr	71	62	75	17
X̄	8.2	6.8	8.0	2.7
SD	(4.20)	(4.43)	(4.64)	(3.03)
Recency last used heroin[a]				
Less than 1 mo	6%	20%	28%	—
Less than 2 mo	—	20	—	—
Less than 3 mo	—	—	—	—
3 mo–1 yr	13	20	11	13%
Over 1 yr	81	40	61	87
Number lifetime uses of heroin[b]				
X̄	2155	1244	2199	481
SD	(1622)	(1733)	(1855)	(883)
Current cigaret smoking				
Less than 1/2 pack/day[c]	24%	47%	37%	67%
1/2-1 pack/day	14	8	17	—
1+ packs/day	62	46	45	33

(continued)

Table 9 (continued)

	Female heroin users		Male heroin users	
	Treated	Not treated	Treated	Not treated
	18	11	22	11
Number other illicits used excluding heroin				
Lifetime $\bar{X}$	2.2	3.2	3.9	3.0
(SD)	(0.95)	(2.01)	(2.01)	(0.74)
Past yr $\bar{X}$	1.1	1.2	2.2	1.8
(SD)	(0.97)	(0.91)	(1.79)	(0.62)

[a]Relative to Wave 3 interview. Owing to missing values, females bases treated, 16, nontreated, 10; males = treated, 8, nontreated, 18.
[b]Estimated by multiplying number of yrs between first and last use by usual frequency of use. Does not take into account intermittent periods of nonuse, if any.
[c]Includes those who never smoked.

at least some of their children, but a quarter (26%) of treated females with children were not living with any of them. Among males, those who had been in treatment were also least likely to be currently living with any of their children (Table 11). Treated women were more satisfied than untreated with their relationships with their children, with the help they had in caring for their children, with their children's behavior, and even with their own performance as mothers. (No available data explain this difference.) Treatment status showed no differences among males regarding satisfaction with their relationships with their children, but treated male users gave themselves poorer ratings as parents than did untreated males.

Social Attainment

It is evident from preceding information that, during adolescence, heroin users who subsequently entered treatment differed from their non-treated counterparts on a number of prior characteristics. When socioeconomic measures were examined at ages 26–31, the same pattern indicating greater disadvantage of treated users was apparent: *untreated* users, regardless of gender, were better off (Table 12). For example, both male and female heroin users who had never entered treatment had rates of current employment and proportions on welfare, and for untreated males, median income level, indistinguishable from their full gender matched samples.

Table 10
Treated vs Not Treated Heroin Users:
Heroin and Cocaine Use Problems (in percentages)

Dependency	Females		Males	
	Treated (17[a])	Not treated (9)	Treated (19)	Not treated (8)
Heroin:				
Never felt dependent	55	82	33	89
Physical dependency	15	18	14	—
Emotional dependency	—	—	5	—
Both	30	—	47	11
Cocaine:				
Never felt dependent	80	100	76	100
Physical dependency	10	—	5	—
Emotional dependency	—	—	5	—
Both	10	—	14	—
Ever had a problem because of drugs or drinking				
Yes	37	23	69	8
No	63	77	31	92
Acute reactions-heroin:				
Overdose	6	—	43	11
Hospital	23	—	52	11
Not think straight	29	—	43	22
Feel crazy/suspicious, really down	21	11	43	22
In fight	39	—	33	—
Accident	7	—	5	—
Arrested	14	—	19	22
Acute reations-cocaine:				
Overdose	—	—	9	—
Hospital	—	—	19	—
Could not think straight	14	—	24	22
Feel crazy/suspicious, really down	29	11	38	22
In fight	24	—	14	—
Accident	—	—	—	—
Arrested	—	—	14	22

(continued)

Changing Drug Use and Treatment Behavior

Table 10 (continued)

	Females		Males	
	Treated	Not treated	Treated	Not treated
Dependency	17[a]	9	19	8
Ever thought about going for treatment but did not go:				
Yes	—	12	75	—
No	100	87	25	100
Ever tried but could not get in:				
Yes, had to wait	18	—	53	—
Yes, refused entry	9	—	5	—
No, neither	73	100	42	100

[a]Case base reduced because of respondents who did not provide details of drug related problems.

Only 9% of treated females and 12% of treated male heroin users were working compared to 54% and 58% of never treated females and males, respectively. Almost all treated females (86%) and half of treated males (55%) themselves were receiving welfare. Heroin users in general were marked by educational deficits; however, seven in ten treated users of both genders had failed to complete high school, a higher proportion than the 40% of female and 60% of male untreated users.

The final sections of the chapter follow, in which the methods change from static descriptive to process-oriented multivariate procedures captured by event history analysis.* Factors that influenced treatment entry and, then, an analysis of the significance of treatment among other factors that influenced cessation of heroin use are the problems that were formulated for this part of the analysis. The fact that, in this research, individuals with treatment experience came from a larger sample of heroin users, and they, in turn, were part of a still larger sample of similar individuals (i.e., drawn from

---

*This method is particularly appropriate with skewed dependent variables, such as treatment entry and heroin cessation, and it enables retaining the larger sample in the analysis, i. e., heroin users who never enter treatment and/or the full sample who never used heroin. Event-history analysis is especially useful where there is this problem of censored data.

Table 11
Drug Treatment and Family Life

	Female heroin users			Male heroin users		
	Treated	Not treated	All females	Treated	Not treated	All males
	(18)	(11)	(216)	(22)	(11)	(210)
Marital status						
Never married	52%	54%	51%	71%	33%	55%
Married (past)	5	15	7	—	—	3
Married now	9	8	21	8	25	23
Separated	9	8	7	4	—	3
Live w/partner	19	8	11	17	42	15
Live w/partner (former marriage)	5	8	3	—	—	1
No. children						
0	10%	—	29%	50%	25%	49%
1	33	31%	32	25	17	22
2	19	46	21	17	42	17
3	10	8	11	8	17	8
4	19	15	5	—	—	2
5	10	—	2	—	—	2
$\bar{X}$	2.3	2.1	1.4	.8	1.5	.9
(SD)	(1.59)	(1.05)	(1.27)	(1.01)	(1.09)	(1.21)
No. pregnancies						
None	10%	—	15%			
One	5	8%	19			
Two	24	8	20			
Three	—	—	12			

	(16)	(11)	(180)
Four	24	31	16
Five	9	23	7
Six	14	23	6
Seven	5	—	3
Eight	9	8	2
X̄	3.9	4.6	2.7
(SD)	(2.42)	(1.82)	(2.03)
No. abortions (based on % ever pregnant)	(16)	(11)	(180)
None	42%	23%	45%
One	32	—	26
Two	21	39	17
Three-Five	5	38	12
X̄	.9	1.9	1.0
(SD)	(.94)	(1.20)	(1.12)

	(16)	(11)	(153)	(11)	(8)	(107)
Age at first birth (of those w/children):						
15 or younger	21%	15%	11%	17%	—	3%
16–17	38	8	20	—	34%	13
18–19	5	54	25	17	11	24
Males 20–21	21	23	20	8	22	18
22 and over	17	—	24	58	33	42
X̄	18	18	19.6	22	21	21.2
(SD)	(3.15)	(2.27)	(3.45)	(4.75)	(4.55)	(3.55)

(continued)

Table 11 (continued)

	Female heroin users			Male heroin users		
	Treated (16)	Not treated (11)	All females (153)	Treated (11)	Not treated (8)	All males (107)
Proportion of children live w/respondent (of those w/children)						
All	68%	92%	92%	17%	33%	42%
Some	6	8	3	17	22	9
None	26	—	5	66	45	49
Satisfaction w/overall relationship (of those w/children):	(15)	(11)	(148)	(11)	(8)	(107)
Very satisfied	78%	23%	73%	50%	56%	67%
Fairly satisfied	6	54	20	25	22	17
Little/very dissatisfied	17	23	7	25	22	16
Self-rating as parent (of those w/children)	(16)	(11)	(153)	(11)	(8)	(108)
Very good	42%	23%	51%	25%	56%	49%
Average	53	77	47	58	44	43
Not so good	5	—	2	17	—	8
Want more help w/childcare						
Yes	36%	77%	46%			
No	64	23	54			
Frequently so angry at children lose control (of those living w/children)	(12)	(11)	(144)			
Very often	14%	—	3%			
Sometimes	29	62%	29			
Hardly ever	57	38	68			
Trouble with children[a] (of those living w/children)						
$\overline{X}$ stress score	1.0	2.6	1.6			
(SD)	(1.94)	(1.67)	(1.66)			

[a]Stress index for five problem areas: health, eating, sleeping, obeying and crying. Sum of five items each scored: a lot = 2, some = 1, hardly any = 0.

Changing Drug Use and Treatment Behavior

Table 12
Treated vs Not-Treated: Social Attainment[a]

	Female heroin Users			Male heroin Users		
	Treated (18)	Not treated (11)	All females (215)	Treated (22)	Not treated (11)	All males (210)
Current major life activity:[b]						
Working (only)	9%	54%	49%	12%	58%	55%
In school (only)	5	—	5	—	—	3
Work and school	—	—	9	—	—	3
School and looking for work	—	—	1	—	—	3
Looking for work (only)	19	15	12	46	17	21
Armed forces	—	—	—	—	—	2
Jail	—	—	—	12	8	6
Homemaker	52	31	21	—	8	*
Poor health, at home	14	—	3	12	8	4
Hanging out	—	—	1	17	—	3
Completed education:						
Less than high school	71%	40%	28%	72%	60%	33%
High school completed	5	—	16	—	10	19
Voc/tech (post high school)	19	40	15	—	10	12
College (any)	5	20	41	28	20	35
Household income:						
Under $5000	29%	31%	21%	8%	8%	9%
$5000–7449	29	15	15	13	—	5
7500–9999	18	23	8	8	—	8
10,000–14,999	12	15	12	17	8	15
15,000–19,999	—	—	11	21	33	19
20,000 or more	—	15	26	8	42	31
Refused answer	—	—	2	—	—	3
Do not know	12	—	4	25	8	10
Median income($)	6255	8250	12,500	12,500	17,500	17,500
Current welfare						
Do not receive	9%	62%	61%	37%	75%	77%
Yes, study subject	57	23	24	42	8	10
Yes, other household member	5	—	5	8	17	9
Yes, self and other	29	15	10	13	—	4

[a]Less than half of one percent.
[b]Because of rounding, tables may not always total exactly 100%.

the same universe with respect to race, SES, and inner-city locale), provides a quasi-experimental design with sufficient power for these multivariate analyses of treatment entry and of heroin abstinence.

This analytical strategy focuses on trajectories, choice points, and pathways within heroin careers. *Trajectories* denote quantitative descriptions of drug using careers and, in the present case, would include such variables as the timing of the onset of heroin use, duration and frequency of use, timing of temporary or permanent abstinence, and timing of treatment entry if it occurred. These parameters can be examined in their naturally occurring temporal sequences, so that more typical and less frequent courses that heroin careers are likely to take can be depicted. *Choice points* are critical events in the evolution of a heroin-using career, such as the decision to first experiment with heroin, the decision to enter treatment, and the decision to stop regular use of the drug. Note that the last two choice points may occur repeatedly during a heroin career. The idea of a pathway introduces an analytical element into this study of heroin careers. It constitutes the factors that systematically determine the occurrence or timing of choice points. Pathways into treatment refer to factors associated with and presumably influencing treatment entry. These are distinguished from pathways into heroin abstinence, which refer to multiple factors associated with the termination of heroin use, with or without treatment.

What Conditions Facilitate or Impede Treatment Entry?

Gender differences in age and duration of drug use prior to treatment entry had appeared in cross-tabular comparisons of the samples of young Black male and female heroin users. These seemed sufficiently different from what studies based on treatment samples had shown that more rigorous testing was warranted, which set in place appropriate controls for personal characteristics and patterns of use. Annual rates of treatment entry were formulated as the dependent variable for event history analysis of pathways into treatment. The basic design of the pathways analysis had been developed using data from the second study wave.[25]

In event-history analysis, the complexities of analyzing longitudinal data are handled by formulating the problem as a time varying phenomenon, i.e, in terms of period-specific probabilities of the occurrences of the event of interest—in this case, treatment entry. The event of treatment entry is termed the "hazard," and early vs late entry corresponds to different hazard rates. In effect, hazard rates are comparable to the proportions of current heroin users entering treatment each year among those heroin users who had not previously entered treatment. Such event-history models can be specified for analyzing how hazard rates of entry vary under differing conditions (the values of the independent variables). These themselves may be time varying, e.g., duration of prior use. (For a general discussion of event- history analysis, *see* [49,50])

The first such analysis used data from Wave 2, and revealed a strong and significant difference between young Black men and women in the Harlem sample in their timing of first treatment, relative to the length of exposure to heroin, with age and frequency of use controlled.[25] Men entered treatment at an earlier stage of their heroin careers than women.

The subsequent study, which added in data for the next seven years, extended the earlier analysis in several directions. First, patterns of influence on treatment entry were examined to see if they differed for events that occurred *before* and *after* the earlier observations (i.e., at ages 18–23 in calendar years 1975–1976). Second, several different formulations of the event-history variable for treatment entry were tested, i.e., both including and excluding detoxification and treatment in prison; combining all treatment experiences vs first-time treatment only. Third, variables of social support and status attainment were added because they could have represented systematic influences that impeded or facilitated treatment entry or further, could have helped to explain the observed gender differences.

Variables in the basic event history model (age, gender, frequency of use, duration of use, gender x duration, and prior treatment) were estimated before the introduction of social support and attainment variables. Constraints of sample size required that the latter be introduced one at a time after the basic set of variables. Estimates for these social context variables, thus, controlled for age, gender, and dimensions of use, but not for other social context variables. Each social context variable was tested for gender interaction before entry. If the interaction term proved significant, both the main and the interaction effects were estimated in the model.

Analysis of the model, which included the full span of study years and all treatment modalities (Table 13) demonstrated:

1. Replication of the findings from earlier analyses that females entered treatment only after using heroin at least two years, whereas men entered at a relatively constant rate.
2. Although age had a marginal effect in the earlier analysis, it now no longer played any role in increasing or retarding likelihood of treatment entry.

Table 13
Event-History Models: Treatment Entry[a]

Independent variables	First-time treatment		All treatment episodes	
	All modes of treatment	Exclusive of detox. and prison	All modes of treatment	Exclusive of detox. and prison
Baseline variables				
Age	−0.047	−0.017	−0.037	−0.014
Frequency of use	0.393[d]	−0.339[f]	0.326[d]	0.231
Gender (1 = male)	1.537[d]	1.271[f]	1.474[d]	1.308[d]
Duration (3 + y = 1)	1.697[d]	1.574[e]	1.741[e]	1.672[d]
Gender × duration	−1.883[d]	−2.061[e]	−1.944[e]	−2.233[e]
Prior treatment			0.715[d]	.544[f]
Additional variables[b]				
Lives with kids	−1.218[d]	−1.280[d]	−1.272[e]	−1.290[d]
Lives with kids × gender	1.567[d]	1.529[d]	1.241[d]	1.275[f]
Lives with mate	−.873[f]	−.904[f]	−.562	−.994[d]
Lives with mate × gender[c]	—	—	—	—
Mos. worked	−.044	−.056[f]	−.028	−.046
Mos. worked × gender	—	—	—	—
Number of illicit drugs used	0.018	−0.010	−.137	−.142
Illicit drugs × gender	—	—	—	—
Drop out	0.565[f]	0.388	0.355	0.291
Drop out × gender	—	—	—	—
Regular source of medical care	−0.059	−0.289	0.051	−0.094
Source of care × gender	—	—	—	—
Lives with parents	1.283[d]	1.414[d]	0.989[d]	1.108[d]
Parents × gender	−1.378[f]	−1.618	−1.046[f]	−1.147[f]

[a]Entries are regression coefficients. [b]These variables were entered singly, controlling for baseline variables. [c]Interaction terms with no values indicate that interaction effects were nonsignificant. [d]p < .05. [e]p < .01. [f]p < .1.

3. In models testing all treatment episodes, prior treatment increased the likelihood of entering treatment.
4. For women, living with children and living with a partner or spouse *retarded* treatment entry.
5. On the other hand, living with parents *increased* women's likelihood of entering treatment.
6. A male heroin user's decision to enter treatment showed less influence from these family network variables; living with a mate, however, did have a marginal effect on retarding their entering treatment.
7. The variables that evidenced *no effect* on increasing or retarding likelihood of entering treatment (all treatment episodes combined) included: completing high school, employment, number of illicit substances besides heroin used in a given year, and having a regular source of medical care.

The final question addressed by this event-history analysis was whether the social variables that significantly influenced treatment entry might explain the gender differences observed in the baseline model. For this, the main and gender interaction terms for the influence of duration of use in the basic models were compared to estimates of these coefficients obtained in models that included statistically significant social variables. Results indicated that the earlier findings remained substantially unchanged even after the inclusion of social variables. This invariance implies that the observed gender pattern of females delaying treatment entry occurred independently of the influence of the social context and attainment variables tested here.

What Influences Cessation of Drug Use, with or without Treatment?

A considerable body of empirical research over the last two decades has dispelled the belief that heroin use inevitably results in a permanent state of addiction; at least some subset of heroin users return to a drug-free state without benefit of formal treatment (*see* review in [2,51,52]). If periodic abstinence as well as lasting recovery from heroin abuse are now established phenomena, the same cannot be said for the role of treatment in ending heroin careers. In this community representative sample of inner-city Black Americans, it was found that more than half of male heroin users who had abstained from heroin for at least a year or more did so without going into treatment.[5] Thus, the analysis of treatment outcomes must be approached in a comparative perspective: Does treatment intervention reduce the duration of heroin careers relative to the length of careers preceding untreated abstinence? In this context, a time-varying phenomenon appropriate to the methodology of event-history analysis is being tested. Retaining the emphasis on specifying gender differences in drug-related behavior, the question is asked: Do male and female heroin users in the study sample differ in their reliance upon treatment as a means of ending their heroin careers?

Investigation of factors linked to abstinence as an event within heroin careers proceeded along lines followed for the analysis of treatment entry described above, as well as an earlier investigation of heroin abstinence within the study sample at ages 18–23.[26] Event-history methodology was applied to test the association between the annual probability of abstaining from heroin use and a number of independent variables, including treatment status. The focus was on abstinence events rather than "cessation," since the latter term suggests a more final and permanent state than can be assured at this stage in the longitudinal study. Individuals were considered to have abstained from heroin use if their most recent use occurred a year or more prior to the last interview in which heroin use was reported.

As in the analysis of treatment utilization, a model of baseline variables was first estimated, and then these variables were used as controls for estimating the effects of other factors. The baseline model was derived from earlier analyses, and included gender, prior treatment, and an interaction term for treatment x gender. Since, as was discussed in the first section of this paper, heroin use showed a clear cohort effect, a cohort variable was also included.

Table 14 shows the impact of variables tested as factors influencing duration of heroin careers in the event-history analysis. Prior treatment, gender, and an interaction between treatment and gender all were statistically significant. The fact that the interaction term for gender and treatment was significant signified that treatment has had a different effect on male and female abstinence rates. Among women, treatment made a large difference in annual abstinence rates; without treatment, males had higher abstinence rates than females. (Negative coefficients indicate low rates of abstinence and, hence, longer heroin careers.)

After adjusting for gender differences in age, frequency, and duration of heroin use, in each year following treatment entry, the odds that a woman heroin user would abstain increased more than six times over what they were for an untreated woman. Treatment intervention was clearly an important experience for reducing the length of young Black females' heroin careers. For males, the impact of treatment on the length of their heroin careers was

Table 14
Event-History Models: Abstinence

Variables	Regression coefficients
Baseline variables	
Gender (l = male)	.914[c]
Cohort (l = born in 1954 or earlier)	.914[d]
Frequency of use	.200
Prior treatment	2.196[e]
Treatment × gender	−1.984[e]
Additional variables[a]	
Drop out	−1.810[d]
Drop out × gender	1.492[c]
Regular source of care	−0.769[c]
Regular source of care × gender[b]	—
Live with kids	−0.066
Kids × gender	—
Live with parents	−0.156
Parents × gender	—
Live with mate	.328
Mate × gender	—
Number of mos. worked	.148[d]
Work × gender	−.128[c]
Number of illicit drugs used	−0.270[d]
Drugs × gender	—
Live alone	1.045
Mos. in Jail	.103
Negative life events	1.180
Negative life events × gender	—
Number of times involved with law	.413

[a] Effects of these variables were estimated one at a time after controlling for baseline variables.
[b] Interaction terms with no value indicate that interaction effects were nonsignificant.
[c] $p < .1$.
[d] $p < .05$.
[e] $p < .01$.

far less substantial. The effect of treatment for males (obtained by adding the main treatment coefficient to the interaction term: $/(2.196 + (-1.984) = .212$ was positive but of trivial magnitude. This indicated that the rates of abstinence that Black males achieved through treatment were but marginally greater than those arrived at naturally without treatment.

Regarding social context and attainment variables, the most influential were completion of high school and number of months worked in a calendar year. To a lesser extent, having a regular source of medical care and change in the number of illicit drugs used also influenced the probability of abstaining each year. Failure to complete high school was associated with lower rates of abstinence and, hence, longer heroin careers for *women*, but not men. Also for females, but not males, the larger number of months worked in a given year was associated with an increased probability of abstinence. That is, education and employment had deterrent effects—over and above treatment— for women but *not* for men. The absence of statistical significance for the interaction term for the other variables tested indicated that effects were similar for both men and women. Among variables that were not systematically associated with the probability of abstinence from heroin, after controlling for treatment, were indicators of different familial and household arrangements, and annual counts of negative life events.

Again, it was considered whether any of the social context or attainment variables might explain gender differences observed in the base line models. The absence of significant interactions indicated that gender differences in patterns of abstinence exerted themselves independent of any of the statistically significant social situational variables tested in these models.

Summary and Discussion

As its title implies, this chapter has had a dual focus: examination of changing drug use patterns and of behavior related to obtaining treatment for drug use. Change was examined over a particular period of time—with respect to developmental histories (life stage) and societal history. This analysis of change also has utilized a single sample, measured at three different time points, which was homogeneous with regard to ethno-racial and geographic group: nonHispanic Black Americans residing in the greater New York City Metropolitan area, who shared a common history of residing in Central Harlem when they were drawn into study 15 years before their third measurement.

Regarding drug use patterns, three hypotheses were tested. First, that incidence or initiation of use of established drugs of choice is virtually completed in the teen years, responding to developmental calendars. An exception to this regularity is the case of substances newly diffused through and accepted by the subculture after individuals' adolescent years. Findings supported these hypotheses. Marijuana and heroin, as established drugs of choice, showed few new recruits after age 19. PCP reflected the pattern of a recently diffused substance, not only in its more extended period of initiation, but also in its "cohort effect," i.e., differential rates of initiation (prevalence) among younger and older cohorts. Cocaine showed clear "period effects," i.e., equivalent impact regardless of cohort, resulting from its increased acceptance as a normative drug of choice, and thereby showing an extended initiation period. Notwithstanding these variations, which captured the interplay of cohort and period effects with developmental ones, virtually all initiation (at least 90% of lifetime, nonexperimental use) was completed by ages in the early 20s.

The second hypothesis was that diminution in involvement would occur at ages in the mid-20s—with the assumption of normative adult social roles, i.e., regular employment, marriage, child-rearing. In the aggregate, this hypothesis was not confirmed. Only two substances, inhalants and heroin, showed that fewer than half the lifetime (nonexperimental) users were continuing use at age 26. Heavy alcohol use, marijuana, and PCP showed somewhat fewer females than males continuing use. Women's continuing use rates, however, still were approx. three in five of lifetime users, compared to three in four male heavy alcohol and marijuana continuers. The male rate for continuing PCP was somewhat less than that, i.e., two in four who ever used still were using at age 26.

The third hypothesis postulated an aggregate substitution effect in patterns of heroin use being replaced by PCP use. Although distinctly not equivalent in pharmacological properties, examined as the marker of heavy drug involvement (i.e., numbers of other illicit substance used and heaviness of use of other illicit substances), PCP appeared to qualify as a replacement for heroin. Differences in the rates of use (prevalence) of heroin and PCP, especially marked among females, belie any simple substitution process, and it is well advised to recognize that each substance has its own pattern of use characteristics.

Overall, this analysis of changing patterns of substance use behavior confirmed that involvement in psychoactive substances continues even while the popularity of individual substances waxes and wanes in response to social norms and substance availability. A strict substitution or replacement theory is not appropriate, but rather distinct patterns of use that adhere to individual substances must be recognized. Substance use is truly a biopsychosocial behavior, and as used in the inner city, its social determinants can be assumed to outweigh individual so-called personality factors. Permitting speculation about the implications of these findings, the basic principle is called to mind that all people, explicitly or implicitly, need an organizing principle in their lives. Lacking alternatives in career, religion-ethos, and so on, that can satisfy basic needs for affiliation, belonging, and goal-oriented achievement, psychoactive escape routes are resorted to. Over and above this rationale for the consumption of drugs, in attempting to understand and ultimately to intervene in drug use behavior, the increasing utility of drug selling—distribution to provide income when alternative economic channels are blocked and when deterrent personal and/or social norms are absent—cannot be overlooked.

This analysis of continuing drug use among a community based sample of Black adults provided the foundation for discussing treatment issues. The analysis of treatment focused first on comparisons between treated and untreated heroin users and the broader population from which they both came. It was found that heroin users who entered into treatment were different from those who did not in antecedent and concurrent patterns of drug use, in adult attainments, and with respect to intraindividual supports, such as self-esteem and aspiration. Heroin users had heavy polydrug involvement, and male heroin users who have been in treatment were the most drug involved of all.

Treated heroin users, both male and female, were much more likely than the untreated to report having had problems from their drinking or drug habits. A considerable number of those who actually entered treatment indicated additional times they had thought about or attempted entry. No untreated user, either female or male, had ever attempted to enter treatment; very few had ever even thought about treatment for themselves. Nonetheless, 40% of never treated females and 87% of untreated males had ceased heroin use at least one year prior to interview. These differences suggest that heroin users are correct in their self-perceptions: those who enter treatment are those with more drug-related problems and with fewer resources to terminate use on their own.

This interpretation was corroborated by some suggestive evidence examining antecedent differences between heroin users who subsequently entered treatment and their untreated counterparts. Absence of control for timing of heroin use onset leaves some ambiguity in interpreting the baseline data (collected at ages 12–17). Nonetheless, a portrait emerged of the heroin user who subsequently became involved in formal treatment programs as one with fewer intrapersonal and social resources compared to his/her heroin using peers who managed their heroin careers, most often to the point of termination of use, without treatment intervention. The relative disadvantage of treated vs nontreated heroin users emerged again in comparisons of adult status attainments. For example, both male and female heroin users who had never entered treatment had rates of current employment and proportions on welfare, and for males, median income level, indistinguishable from their full gender matched samples. Treated users fared considerably more poorly.

The repeated emphasis above, that treated users compared less favorably to the untreated, was not intended to convey that treatment is a source of disadvantage or that treatment programs are inefficacious. When viewed as part of a natural history of heroin use, treatment entry represents an opportunity for individuals to acquire resources and skills needed for ending drug dependency—resources that clearly were not available to them in their natural environment. Thus, treatment is best conceptualized as a broader process of behavioral change, and of the imparting and acquisition of skills and resources that address personal and social deficits that go beyond drug use *per se*. Counseling to address intrapersonal problems (low self-esteem, learned helplessness, and so on) might be important, but equally so are programs that confront social inadequacies: literacy, job training, and job opportunities. Thus, the typical cutoff of supportive services to treatment clients once they have achieved detoxification should be reconsidered.[53]

Provision of services that go beyond addressing pharmacological dependence is also likely to motivate treatment entry, especially among heroin using adults. It was demonstrated that their own fears of uncontrolled drug dependency and a sense of inadequacy in meeting family obligations were reasons most often given by those seeking treatment. Programs that offer and deliver resources for more effective performance of adult roles are likely to accelerate treatment entry.

These analyses revealed differential patterns of heroin use and treatment behaviors for Black females and males. Females were less likely to become involved with heroin, reflecting differential gender norms, but once begun, they appeared to be more deeply involved, as suggested by their longer term of use and the longer lapse between females' onset of use and treatment entry. Once in treatment, however, they were likely to remain for an extended time and to stop using the drug. These gender differences in timing of treatment entry, and the role of treatment in terminating heroin use were firmly established and not explained by other factors in the more elaborated event-history models of influences on treatment entry and on abstinence. Netting out differences in age, frequency, and duration of heroin use, it was apparent that the benefits of treatment for abstinence were more evident for females than for males.

The fact that treatment was more instrumental in terminating Black women's heroin careers than men's is suggestive of the different social role needs of men and women that heroin involvement serves and that treatment programs, hopefully, will recognize. Furthermore, the fact that women's abstinence from heroin was clearly related to high school completion and employment whereas men's was not defies simple explanation. (*See* [36] for consistent findings and exposition of their meaning.) Might not these gender differences in treatment and abstinence pathways reflect the differential benefits from social institutions (school, job opportunities) for Black men and women?

Acknowledgment

This research has been supported by NIDA Grants No. 5-R01-DA0327 and 5-R01-DA05142, Ann F. Brunswick, Principal Investigator. The authors gratefully acknowledge the patient assistance of Michelle Gallant, Laura Kittross, Carla Lewis, and John Thompson in preparing this manuscript.

References

[1] P. Ferguson, T. Lennox, and D. J. Lettieri, eds. (1974) *Drug and Addict Lifestyles* (National Institute on Drug Abuse, Rockville, MD).

[2] B. Johnson (1977) The race, class and irreversibility hypothesis: Myths and research about heroin, in *The Epidemiology of Heroin and Other Narcotics* (J. D. Rittenhouse, ed.) National Institute on Drug Abuse, Rockville, MD, pp. 51–57.

[3] J. C. Marsh, M. E. Colten, and M. D. Tucker (1982) Women's use of drugs and alcohol: New perspectives. *J. Social Issues* **38** (2), 1–8.

[4] D. N. Nurco, I. H. Cisin and M. B. Balter (1981) Addict careers. I. A new typology. *Int. J. Addict.* **16** (8), 1305–1325.

[5] A. F. Brunswick (1979) Black youths and drug use behavior: An epidemiologic and longitudinal perspective on drugs used and their users, in *Youth Drug Abuse: Problems, Issues and Treatment* (A. Friedman and G. Beschner, eds.) Lexington, MA, pp. 443–492.

[6] A. F. Brunswick (1980) Social meaning and developmental needs: Perspectives on Black youth's drug use. *Youth and Society* **11** (4), 449–473.

[7] A. F. Brunswick, C. R. Merzel, and P. Messeri (1985) Drug use initiation among urban Black youth: A seven-year follow-up of developmental and secular influences. *Youth and Society* **17** (2), 189–216.

[8] L. N. Robins (1984) The natural history of adolescent drug use. *Am. J. Public Health* **74**, 656,657.

[9] D. B. Kandel (1978) Convergences in prospective longitudinal surveys of drug use in normal populations, in *Longitudinal Research in Drug Use: Empirical Findings and Methodological Issues* (D. Kandel, ed.) Hemisphere Press-John Wiley, Washington, DC, pp. 3–38.

[10] D. B. Kandel and J. A. Logan (1984) Patterns of drug use from adolescence to young adulthood: I. Periods of risk for initiation, continued use, and discontinuation. *Am. J. Public Health* **74**, 660–666.

[11] J. G. Bachman, P. M. O'Malley, and L. D. Johnston (1984) Drug use among young adults: The impacts of role status and social environment. *J. Pers. Soc. Psychol.* **47**, 629–645.

[12] K. Yamaguchi and D. B. Kandel (1987) Drug use and other determinants of premarital pregnancy and its outcome: A dynamic analysis of competing life events. *J. Marriage and Family* **49**, 257–270.

[13] A. F. Brunswick and J. Boyle (1979) Patterns of drug involvement: Developmental and secular influences on age at initiation. *Youth and Society* **11**(2), 139–162.

[14] P. M. O'Malley, J. G. Bachman, and L. D. Johnston (1984) Period, age, and cohort effects on substance use among American youth, 1976–1982. *Am. J. Public Health* **74**, 682–688.

[15] J. G. Bachman, L. D. Johnston, and P. M. O'Malley (1988) Explaining the recent decline in marijuana use: Differentiating the effects of perceived risks, disapproval and general lifestyle factors. *J. Health Soc. Behav.* **29**, 92–112.

[16] L. D. Johnston, P. M. O'Malley and J. G. Bachman (1987) *National Trends in Drug Use and Related Factors among American High School Students and Young Adults, 1975–1986.* National Institute on Drug Abuse, Government Printing Office, Washington, DC.

[17] J. A. O' Donnell, H. L. Voss, R. R. Clayton, G. T. Slayton, and R. G. Room (1976) *Young Men and Drugs—A Nationwide Survey,* NIDA Monograph No. 5. Government Printing Office, Washington, DC.

[18] US Bureau of the Census. *Statistical Abstract of the United States* (109th Ed.), Washington, DC, 1988.

[19] D. H. Swinton (1989) Economic status of Blacks 1987, in *The State of Black America 1988.* (J. Dewart, ed.) National Urban League, Inc., NY, pp. 129–152.

[20] K. Bradbury and L. Brown (1986) Black men in the labor market. *New England Economic Review* **March–April,** 32–42.

[21] A. F. Brunswick (1988) Young Black males and substance use, in *Young, Black, Males: An Endangered Species* (J. T. Gibbs, ed.) Auburn House Publishing Co., Dover, MA, pp. 166–187.

[22] B. D. Johnson, P. J. Goldstein, E. Preble, J. Schmeidler, D. S. Lipton, B. Spunt, and T. Miller (1985) *Taking Care of Business: The Economics of Crime by Heroin Abusers* (D. C. Heath, Lexington, MA).

[23] E. Preble and J. J. Casey (1969) Taking care of business: The heroin user's life on the street. *Int. J. Addict.* **4 (1),** 14–15.

[24] O. J. Kalant (1980) *Alcohol and Drug Problems in Women. Research Advances in Alcohol and Drug Problems, vol. 5.* (Plenum, NY).

[25] A. F. Brunswick and P. Messeri (1985) Timing of first drug treatment: A longitudinal study of urban black youth. *Contemporary Drug Problems* **2(3),** 401–418.

[26] A. F. Brunswick and P. Messeri (1986) Pathways to heroin abstinence: A longitudinal study of urban Black youth. *Advances in Alcohol and Substance Abuse* **5(3),** 103–122.

[27] V. J. Binion (1982) Sex differences in socialization and family dynamics of female and male heroin users. *J. of Social Issues* **38(2),** 43–57.

[28] M. E. Colten (1982) Attitudes, experiences, and self-perceptions of heroin addicted mothers. *J. of Social Issues* **38(2),** 77–92.

[29] P. B. Sutker (1981) Drug Dependent women: An overview of the literature, in *Treatment Services for Drug Dependent Women, vol. 1* (G. M. Beschner, B. G. Reed, and J. Mondanaro, eds.), National Institute on Drug Abuse, Washington, DC, pp. 25–51.

[30] A. F. Brunswick (1984) Health consequences of drug use: A longitudinal study of urban Black youth, in *Handbook of Longitudinal Research in the US, vol. 2* (S. A. Mednick, M. Harway, and K. M. Finello, eds.), Praeger, NY, pp. 290–314.

[31] C. Cordes (1985) At risk in America. *APA Monitor* **16 (1),** 9–11, 27.

[32] W. J. Wilson (1989) The underclass: Issues, perspectives, and public policy. *The Annals of the American Academy of Political and Social Science* **501,** 182–192.

[33] U. Bronfenbrenner (1979) *The Ecology of Human Development* (Harvard University Press, Cambridge, MA).

[34] A. F. Brunswick (1985) Health services for adolescents with impairment, disability, and/or handicap: An ecological paradigm. *J. Adolesc. Health Care* **6 (2),** 141–151.

[35] L. Kurdek (1981) An integrative perspective on children's divorce adjustment. *Am. Psychol.* **36,** 856–866.

[36] A. F. Brunswick, P. A. Messeri, and S. P. Titus (1990) Predictive factors in adult substance abuse: A prospective study of urban Black adolescents. Forthcoming.

[37] J. D. Miller, I. H. Cisin, H. Gardner-Keaton, P. W. Wirtz, H. I. Abelson, and P. M. Fishburne (1983) *National Survey on Drug Abuse: Main Findings 1982* (National Institute on Drug Abuse, Rockville, MD).

[38] J. Boyle and A. F. Brunswick (1980) What happened in Harlem? Analysis of a decline in heroin use among a generation unit of urban Black youth. *J. of Drug Issues* **10** (1), 109–130.

[39] P. Messeri and A. F. Brunswick (1987) Heroin availability and aggregate levels of use: Secular trends in an urban Black cohort. *Am. J. Drug Alcohol Abuse* **13**(1, 2), 105–129.

[40] S. B. Sells and D. Simpson (1980) The case for drug treatment effectiveness, Based on the DARP research program. *British J. Addiction* **75**, 117–131.

[41] D. Simpson and S. B. Sells (1982) Effectiveness of treatment for drug abuse: An overview of the DARP research program. *Advances in Alcohol and Substance Abuse* **2**, 7–29.

[42] L. N. Robins (1979) Addict careers, in Handbook on Drug Abuse (R. I. Dupont, A. Goldstein, and J. A. O'Donnell, eds.) Government Printing Office, Washington, DC, pp. 325–336.

[43] D. Waldorf (1983) Natural recovery from opiate addiction: Some social-psychological processes of untreated recovery. *J. Drug Issues* **13** (2), 237–280.

[44] D. Waldorf and P. Biernacki (1979) Natural recovery from heroin addiction: A review of the incidence literature. *J. Drug Issues* **9**, 281–289.

[45] S. Spilerman (1977) Careers, labor market structures, and socioeconomic achievement. *American J. of Sociology* **83**, 551–593.

[46] G. M. Beschner and K. G. Treasure (1979) Female drug use, in *Youth Drug Abuse*. (G. M. Beschner and A. F. Friedman, eds.) Lexington, MA: D. C. Health and Company, pp. 169–212.

[47] V. Klinge, H. Vaziri, and K. Lennox (1976) Comparison of psychiatric inpatient Male and female adolescent drug abusers. *Int. J. Addict.* **11** (2), 309–323.

[48] A. F. Brunswick and P. Messeri (1989) The role of substance use iealth decline: A longitudinal study of urban African Americans. Submitted for publication.

[49] N. B. Tuma, M. T. Hannan, and L. P. Groeneveld (1979) Dynamic analysis of event histories. *American Journal of Sociology* **84**, 820–854.

[50] J. D. Kalbfleisch and R. L. Prentice (1980) *The Statistical Analysis of Failure Time Data*. (Wiley).

[51] P. Biernacki (1986) *Pathways from Heroin Addiction*. Temple Univeristy Press.

[52] L. N. Robins (1974) *A Follow-up of Vietnam Drug Users, Interim Final Report, Special Action Office for Drug Abuse Monograph*, Series A, No. 1. Government Printing Office, Washington, DC.

[53] A. Allison and R. L. Hubbard (1985) Drug abuse treatment process: A review of the literature. *Int. J. Addict.* **20** (9), 1321–1345.

Using Incentives, Lotteries, and Competitions in Work-Site Smoking Cessation Interventions

Steven W. Malone and Leonard A. Jason

Introduction

Smoking cessation interventions have been most frequently based on individual-level and group-level conceptualizations. In this chapter, several advantages of a larger-scale perspective will be reviewed. In addition, some of the most promising smoking cessation interventions that employ incentives, lotteries, and competitions will be reviewed. These types of interventions are believed to have the most potential for changing organizational norms regarding smoking. In the final section of this chapter, several issues will be reviewed that are particularly important for organizational change agents, including assessing environmental factors that influence smoking behaviors and evaluating methods of increasing participation rates in smoking cessation programs.

Interventions at the Individual and Group Levels

In several recent review articles,[1,2] work-site smoking cessation interventions were categorized into four categories; bibliotherapy, physician advice, multicomponented behavioral cessation groups, and incentive programs. Below, the overall effectiveness of the first three types of interventions will be briefly reviewed, and in a later section, incentive programs will be reviewed.

Bibliotherapy is an example of a smoking intervention conceptualized at an individual level. Bibliotherapy programs have several unique strengths, including low cost and the potential to reach large numbers of people. In the studies reviewed by Klesges and Cigrang[1] and Klesges et al.,[2] participation rates in bibliotherapy programs were 26%. Average sample size was only 111, 86% of the studies did not use biochemical verification, and dropout rates were high at 47%. Posttest cessation rates were 31%, and followup cessation rates were 26%.

Having physicians provide clients with brief stop-smoking messages during physical or screening examinations is another example of individually oriented interventions or mass-individual interventions. All four studies in this category had large sample sizes (average $n = 5356$), and dropout rates were lower than in bibliotherapy approaches (29%; reported in two out of four studies). The most impressive statistics were the 78% average participation rates. Followup cessation rates were 12%. Unfortunately, only one study used biochemical verification.[1,2]

Multicomponent behavioral group cessation programs occur at the group level. These programs usually include self-monitoring, stimulus control, and the development of alternative behaviors, with other popular components being aversion training, nicotine fading, nicotine gum, stress management, social support, coping strategies, and cognitive restructuring.[3] Reviews[1,2] noted that these studies reported average sample sizes of 68, average participation rates of 43%, and average dropout rates of 24%. Posttest cessation rates were 33%, and followup cessation rates were 20%. Ten of 15 studies used biochemical verification.

Increasing Participation Rates

In order to impact the work-site-wide smoking rates, interventions need first to increase participation rates. To underscore this, assume that 20 smokers participate in a smoking cessation intervention. If the cessation rate is quite high at 40%, eight smokers will have quit. Yet if the participation rate is only 20%, then only 20 out of 100 smokers participated, and the overall impact on the work-site-wide smoking rates is only 8%.

Theory articulating stages of the smoking process might help to develop interventions that increase participation rates. Smoking cessation interventions have typically commenced when people were ready to take the first step toward quitting smoking. Two stages within the smoking habit[4] have seldom been addressed—the stage that involves smokers who are continuing to smoke, and the stage where smokers are contemplating quitting smoking. Those who continue to smoke might be encouraged to contemplate quitting smoking, and those who contemplate quitting smoking could be encouraged to take the first step toward quitting smoking. The challenge is how to design programs so that they maximally involve smokers in the change process, taking into consideration that they are probably starting out at very different stages in the quitting process. Later in this chapter, several strategies for increasing participation rates will be reviewed.

Relapse

Many of the studies reviewed in the previous section reported deterioration between posttest cessation rates and followup cessation rates. Clearly, many individuals were able to make a quit effort, but far fewer were able to maintain the behavior change.

One way to address the relapse problem is by examining how cognitions affect relapse. Marlatt and Gordon[5] hypothesized that ex-smokers who believed that a slip indicated they could not control their behavior were more likely to return to smoking. Several studies confirmed the effect of these attributions on eventual smoking status.[6,7] Unfortunately, greater understanding of the role of cognitions in the relapse process has resulted in treatment programs with higher smoking cessation rates in only one out of many studies.[8]

Motivation has been identified as another critical variable in understanding the relapse problem. Recent ex-smokers may know what coping skills to use when tempted to smoke, but they might not be motivated to practice those skills. Psychologists have tended to overemphasize information and skill building in smoking cessation programs, and to underemphasize the importance of motivation.[9] Several investigators have tried to heighten motivation within their interventions by, for example, using formal commitment procedures and contingency contracting.[10,11]

Several investigators have used social support to help smokers maintain abstinence. Social support within cessation groups has been found to at least temporarily bolster cessation rates.[12] Spouse support has been associated with long-term higher cessation rates.[13,14] Unfortunately, the effects of coworker support on quitting smoking has been less clear. Naturally occurring coworker support does not appear to impact cessation rates,[15] nor do attempts to bolster support in work-site cessation groups through buddy systems, meeting with partners, and partner support manuals.[16,17]

Work-site smoking cessation programs that have employed motivation and support strategies have not yielded higher cessation and maintenance rates. Perhaps the problem is that these programs have enhanced motivation and social support for 1 h a week for 8 wk, but continual smoking cues in natural environments can dwarf any procedures conducted within these types of time-limited groups.

Organizational Factors

Some of the best strategies in increasing participation and in reducing relapse may begin by recognizing the role of organizational variables. Allen and Kraft[18] stated that they had made some progress in developing individual motivation techniques [in changing health behaviors] but ... paid too little attention to the forces of the cultures in which the individual lives." They described the rationale behind individual interventions as similar to going into a school of fish and asking one or two of the fish to turn around and swim in the opposite direction. They saw cultural norms as slowly, but eventually overcoming most initial changes in health behavior. Thus, they concluded that a supportive cultural environment was essential for the maintenance of new health behaviors.

Temptations to smoke can be prompted by work-site structures and norms. Perhaps a recent ex-smoker can only take breaks in a smoky cafeteria. In this situation, the norms in a smoking cessation group might promote smoke-free lifestyles, but a conflicting organizational norm would promote smoking. Allen and Allen[19] saw work-site cultures as significantly affecting the success or failure of worksite health programs. They saw these cultures as changed through "...cultural influence mechanisms such as rewards, social recognition, training, orientation, communication, and information systems."

Behavioral psychologists could become involved in norm setting interventions by helping to design environments that reinforce desirable behaviors. As an example, smoking cessation groups could develop into ongoing influences that help develop new group standards and customs.[20] When an entire setting gets behind a particular change effort, and many individuals are caring about the people who are trying to quit, then organizational forces have been tapped. This chapter will provide examples of interventions that have attempted to accomplish these types of changes.

Rationale for Offering Material Reinforcers

Different types of reinforcers and reinforcement schedules could affect how many smokers participate in smoking cessation interventions. The greatest impact of reinforcers might be on participation rates,[21] because of the ability of reinforcers to arouse the interest of potential participants.

Reinforcements represent one method to change social norms. Reinforcers fulfill Koop's[22] admonition to be instructive and persuasive when promoting health. Reinforcers promote the desirable behavior, encourage voluntary behavior, and can engender a game-like and lighthearted atmosphere.

Reinforcers are unlike the naturally occurring benefits for quitting smoking, which are not certain to occur and are delayed. Consequences that most effectively increase behaviors are certain, immediate, and clear; these, of course, are the characteristics of incentives. Reinforcers might be more able to counteract the effects of withdrawal symptoms. Seen in this light, reinforcers represent a bridge between the short-term costs of quitting smoking and the long-term benefits of quitting.[23]

Reinforcers that are seen as "bribe" money might not be effective. The extrinsic motivation (e.g., incentives) should not be large enough to justify the response of not smoking. Will use of an extrinsic reward damage intrinsic motivation? If given a reward for an activity that a person enjoys, the person is less likely to engage in that behavior when the reward is withdrawn. Smokers, however, do not enjoy quitting smoking; consequently, because the intrinsic motivation is not initially present, the extrinsic reward will not undermine intrinsic motivation.[24]

To increase the probability that people view reinforcers in the most positive manner, the rationale for them should be clearly communicated to all employees. The reinforcer may serve at first to catch the attention of potential participants. Once participating, people might be told that reinforcers are a bridge to the long-term benefits of being smoke-free. The reinforcers can help individuals join the program, and then the program might provide the individuals with the support to remain abstinent. On the other hand, in some cases, the rewards might be enough in themselves to help smokers make a decision to quit and remain smoke-free.

The same reinforcers could have different effects in different worksites, since reinforcers "are part of a very complex web of forces ... not controlled by change agents. ... A contingency may be ineffective not because the reinforcer is itself too small or insignificant, but rather because it is administered in such a manner as to fly in the face of more powerful reinforcers..."[20] Layoffs or bitter union-management relations might negate otherwise effective reinforcers for quitting smoking.

Extreme care needs to be exercised in determining what reinforcers might work in which particular settings.[20] Time off from work, choice of job assignment, or choice of vacation time might be feasible and potent. These types of reinforcers, however, might be difficult for a setting to implement. On the other hand, money is widely valued, and it might appeal to a wide range of people. Money can be delivered in easily specified units allowing for clear operationalizations and replications.

A number of cessation group programs have refunded deposits of participants contingent upon quitting smoking.[11,25] For instance, Bowers et al.[26] collected $50–300 per group participant depending upon income. These funds were repaid 30% post-quit day, 20% for abstinence 1 mo later, 20% for abstinence 2 mo later, 20% for abstinence 3 mo later, and 10% for abstinence 6 mo later. Biochemical verification showed 43% of participants were smoke-free at the 6-mo mark. This was significantly greater than the 14% who were smoke-free 6 mo later in a group program where monies were repaid contingent only on group attendance as opposed to abstinence.

The literature on use of incentives suggests several things. First, higher amounts of money and more frequent dispensing of reinforcers produce higher cessation rates.[24] Even with other health behaviors, Warner and Murt[27] found that larger rewards had a greater impact than smaller ones, and repeated reinforcement was preferable to one-time incentives. In several studies, financial reinforcers increased cessation rates for 6 wk and then rates fell.[10,25,28,29] This effect was probably because reinforcers were often not dispensed after 8 wk.[25,28] With more long-term and continuing use of reinforcers, a few studies have showed high cessation rates lasting 6 mo.[11,26]

Reinforcement Programs

In this section, three different types of reinforcement programs will be reviewed. For each type of reinforcement program, studies without control groups will first be reviewed, followed by a review of studies with quasi-experimental or true experimental designs that do include control groups. The first reinforcement programs to be reviewed involve incentives, where individuals obtain reinforcers for being smoke-free.

Incentives

Uncontrolled Studies

A number of uncontrolled studies of work-site smoking interventions suggest that incentives can be effective. Shephard and Pearlman[24] cited 15 work-site smoking interventions that used incentives. Across these interventions, the average 1-yr abstinence rate was 52%, and when total abstinence was the desired behavior, 63% of participants were abstinent after 1 yr. Participation rates also appear to be very high as evidenced by the work-site-wide smoking reduction; 53% of the employees at these 15 companies smoked before the incentive programs, and afterwards, available data indicate that 27% smoked.

Several studies they reviewed are worth mentioning. In an ambulance company,[30] all employees were offered $5/mo if they did not smoke at work, and at Christmas time, employees bonuses matched the amounts they had already received for not smoking. Participation rates were extremely high (75%), as were cessation rates (58%). Another incentive program was conducted at Speedcall Corporation where all nonsmoking employees received $7 weekly for not smoking. Out of 36 total employees, the number of smokers decreased from 24 to 11.[24]

At Intermatic Company, each employee could wager up to $100 that he or she would not smoke for 1 yr. Those who won their bets also had $1000 divided among them. In a similar program conducted the next year, those who won their bets had the chance to win a free trip to Las Vegas. About 120 smokers participated, with 46% remaining abstinent for 1 yr.[20,24]

At another work-site, any participant who remained smoke-free for a year received a week's vacation or a week's pay. Two months after the quit date, 12 of the 14 participants were still abstinent. Twelve months later, only 36% of the participants were still abstinent as verified by carbon monoxide readings.[30,31] Perhaps if incentives were offered more frequently, the success rate would have been higher.

Controlled Studies

Windsor et al.'s[32] study involved about 19% of the smoking work force. One-year quit rates were 5% for those who received an American Lung

Association smoking cessation manual, whether or not they additionally received $25 after 6 wk and another $25 after 6 mo of not smoking. Others received self-help manuals and were taught deep breathing exercises in a 20-minute meeting, and 19% of these subjects were smoke-free for 1 yr. When the two $25 incentives were added, however, 1-yr abstinence rates dropped to 10%. This incentive may have failed to increase cessation rates because the incentive was small, frequency of administration was low, and receipt was delayed in time and received impersonally through the mail.

Malone[33] conducted a smoking cessation intervention at two work-sites. Both companies sponsored the American Lung Associations group-format cessation program. At one randomly chosen site, participants received $200 in incentives given on 13 occasions in units of $10 and $20 over a year's period of time. Although only 5% of smokers participated, 12-mo continuous cessation rates were high at 50%. In the condition where incentives were not offered, except for a rebate of the $25 entry fee, the cessation rate was also high (44%). These participants also had carbon monoxide assessments each month for 6 mo. Being regularly assessed on the carbon monoxide machine could be an incentive in itself.

This observation is supported by Scott et al.'s[34] intervention, which consisted of bibliotherapy and biochemical assessments (feedback on physiological states served as an incentive.) Twenty-nine nurses participated, of which half were assigned to the intervention. Nurses in the treatment condition practiced nicotine fading and had daily carbon monoxide testing for 3 mo, gradually fading to unannounced weekly assessments through 12 mo. The attrition rate was only 14%. At the 12-mo mark, 33% were abstinent (continual abstinence was 17%). The sharpest increase in relapses occurred between 3–6 mo, coinciding with the reduction in daily therapist contact and carbon monoxide assessments.

Rand et al.[35] offered employees $4 twice per week after carbon monoxide assessments verified their being smoke-free. Initially, cessation rates were higher, but after six mo of this reinforcement schedule only 6% were smoke-free. This may be because "subjects were carefully admonished that the project was not a formal stop-smoking program." Also, social and organizational support were minimized by conducting all treatments within the same work-site.

Summary

The uncontrolled case studies appear more successful than the controlled studies, and the one controlled study with high cessation rates[34] had low participation rates. Still, it is believed that in time, controlled studies will also show that incentives add to the impact of work-site smoking interventions. Incentive programs provide the immediate, certain, and clear reinforcements that many recent ex-smokers need. Conversely, the disadvantage of incentive programs is that people may be seen as quitting smoking just for money.

It is important to monitor possible second-order negative effects of using incentives. At one work site,[33] only 1 out of 89 nonparticipants resented management giving participants money. However, in another incentive program many unsuccessful participants were bothered by the "one cigaret and you're out" aspect of the incentive program.[33] Perhaps incentive programs need to provide more opportunities for participants to recycle into the program after a relapse.

Lotteries

Lotteries, another type of reinforcement program, are where smoke-free individuals get the chance to win a lottery prize. Lotteries have been accompanied not only by other smoking cessation components, but often by other incentive programs as well.

Uncontrolled Studies

Sorman[36] offered both incentives and a lottery, inducing 27% of all employees (probably over 70% of all smokers) to try to quit smoking for 1 yr. Ex-smokers could receive a $200 reward as well as lottery chances for vacation trips. As a result, 31% of the participants quit cigarets for the 1 yr.

At Dow Chemical,[37] employees earned a lottery ticket for each month they did not smoke, with a year-end prize being a $3,600 fishing boat. Each participant could have a sponsor, and every month the participant was smoke-free the sponsor won a lottery ticket with the prize being a second fishing boat. Also, $50 was raffled four times during the year. Participation rates were good (24%) and self-reported cessation rates 1 yr later were outstanding (76%). As a result, work-site-wide smoking rates were decreased by 18%.[37]

Stacknik and Stoffelmayr[38] offered employees 20 smoking cessation group meetings over 7 mo. At each meeting, $20 was awarded by lottery to a successful participant. The intervention occurred at three work sites, and from 47–70% of all smokers enrolled in the program. Cessation rates were extremely high (80–91%) 6 mo after the program ended.[36]

Cummings et al.[39] had smokers join their program in pairs. Pairs of ex-smokers were eligible for a lottery prize of $250 after 2 wk, and a lottery prize of $500 after three months. Participation rates were 14% and end of program quit rates were 36%. Participants remained smoke-free in part so that they would not let their partners down, since both were ineligible if one were to relapse.

Controlled Studies

Smoking interventions by Jason's team[40,41] have used mass media messages. The first of two interventions integrated media-based resources with self-help programs and work-site social support. A Chicago television station broadcast promotional ads, and then on each news broadcast for 20 d, it aired a segment on volunteers who quit smoking. Segments were coordinated with the American Lung Association's self-help manual, where smokers quit in 20 d. These self-help manuals were distributed in work sites, and twice a week for the 20 d that employees attended support groups at the work-site. Although the group intervention was initially successful in enhancing quit rates, at a 12-mo followup, there were no longer any significant differences between those who received the self-help materials and media vs those who received groups, self-help materials, and media.[40] This study did not use lotteries, but in a second media study, in order to reduce relapse, lotteries were used in 38 work sites. The intervention was again coordinated with the television station's broadcasting of a smoking cessation series. In the experimental condition, following the 20-d program, employees at half the companies received monthly support groups and lotteries. At the end of the program, 42% of group participants and just 16% of those provided only with the manual plus the televised program had quit smoking. At a 12-mo followup, cessation rates for group participants were significantly higher than for non-group participants (26 vs 16%).[41]

Summary

Even more than incentive programs, lotteries can capture the imagination of employees and create excitement over the smoking intervention programs. We see one advantage of lotteries being their ability to affect participation rates. They are a useful promotional tool because rather than spreading limited funds across all participants, each participant can be motivated by the prospect of winning a concentrated lump of money. Because of the limited number of studies conducted in this section, we can only speculate that these types of reinforcements hold much promise.

Competitions

Programs using competitions generally have one group compete against another in a good-natured, friendly rivalry. Participants in competition programs might focus less on the prize and more on the comradery of the team. Team participants who are tempted to smoke might exercise self-control in order not to let the team down. More than one type of competition or other incentive programs are often included with competition programs, so that smoke-free participants on losing teams often still receive material reinforcers.

Controlled Studies

Klesges et al.[42] recruited four banks into a competition, with a fifth bank serving as a control group. The bank presidents publically challenged one another, and employees attended group sessions on company time. Buttons reading "I'm in the healthy competition" were distributed to increase social support, and feedback on the progress of each work-site was displayed at each setting. Prizes to benefit both smokers and nonsmokers were awarded to the bank with the highest participation rate ($100), and to the bank with the largest reductions in carbon monoxide levels at posttest ($250). A final prize went to the bank with the greatest abstinence rate at the 6-mo followup (i.e., a dinner catered by the employees of the losing bank). Participation rates in the program were exceptionally high (88%), yet few people quit smoking after 6 mo (14%).

In a second study, Klesges et al.[43] recruited 136 smokers in eight work-sites to participate in a smoking cessation intervention. Four work-sites were randomly assigned to either formal competition or to no competition. Participation rates were about 48%. At the end of the 6-wk program, competition subjects had higher quit rates (39%) than those in the no competition condition (16%). Six months later, the cessation rate in the competition condition was reduced to 18%, so that there were no longer significant differences between conditions.

Malone[33] provided employees with incentives totaling $70 over 6 mo, given in units of $10 after carbon monoxide verifications were conducted. In addition, two competitions were run. The group adding the most members soon after the orientation meeting won a group prize of $40. In addition, 6 mo later, the participants in the most successful group received a choice of three prizes. Six months later, 54% were continuously smoke-free, and 12 mo later, 48% were smoke-free. The same smoking cessation group without the incentives and competitions was conducted at another manufacturing plant, resulting in a cessation rate of 18% at 6 and 12 mo. Most participants reported that the group support and the competitions had a greater effect on quitting than did the incentives.

Jason et al.[44] conducted a 20 d cessation programs using the American Lung Association's self-help manual, and after the 20 d program, employees were offered incentives, lotteries, and competition. Employees received $10 for attending each of the 14 meetings held over the following 6 mo. Employees were paid one dollar a day for each day of abstinence for 6 mo after the initial 3 wk. Those who were smoke-free for the last 2 mo of the program participated in a lottery. Also, teams of three smokers competed to see which team had the largest numbers of days absent, with the winning team receiving $300. Finally, gifts were provided to nonsmoking coworking buddies for supporting the participants quit efforts.

This program had an extremely high participation rate; 84% of smokers participated. Over 50% of the participants said they would not have tried to quit if the program had not been offered. As a result, 1 yr after quitting the cessation rate was 36%, significantly more than the 16% cessation rate at the control site. Continual abstinence was also significantly different (21% vs 5%). Most important of all, work-site-wide smoking reductions were significantly different 1 yr later (32% vs 13%). Process evaluations by participants were informative. Helpfulness of various components were rated on a 1:4 scale, with 1 being "a lot" helpful and 4 being "not at all" helpful. The group was rated most helpful at 1.4, with buddies and competition teams both rated at 2.1, the manual rated at 2.3, and the incentives rated at 2.4. Even though far more money was spent on the incentives than on the competition teams, it is important to note that participants rated the competition teams as more helpful than the incentives.

Summary for Competitions

In the Klesges et al.[42,43] studies, competition programs were the only reinforcers used and cessation rates were low. However, when competition programs were combined with either incentive programs or lottery programs, cessation rates were significantly increased. To be effective, then, competitions may need to be accompanied by other reinforcement programs. This provision may alleviate a potential problem of having some individuals quit smoking but not gain any material reinforcement.

Summary of Reinforcement Programs

The case studies reported by Shephard and Pearlman[24] showed great promise for influencing work-site-wide smoking rates. Unfortunately, these case studies lacked control groups, lacked biochemical verification, had small sample sizes, seldom collected enough baseline and followup data on participation rates and cessation rates, and did not use companies as the unit of analysis. Controlled studies that began addressing some of these methodological issues did not evidence the same impressive results.

Klesges and Cigrang[1] and Klesges et al.[2] reviewed seven reinforcement programs, only three of which were controlled studies. The average followup cessation rate was 46%, and when the study by Stacknik and Stoffelmayr[38] was excluded, the average followup rate was 26%. Participation rates were 61%. Currently nine controlled studies, summarized in Table 1, exist that employ experimental designs and biochemical verification. Average participation rates are 37%, posttest cessation rates are 45%, and followup cessation rates are 26% after 9 mo. Average followup cessation rates in comparison conditions are 13% after 9 mo. These participation rates seem higher than those of multicomponented groups without material reinforcers, but this is difficult to evaluate because many multicomponented group programs have not reported participation rates, although based on studies that did report rates, it is likely that many of these other programs had very low rates. Cessation rates reported in Table 1 are roughly equivalent to those reported by Klesges et al.[2] of multicomponented groups without material reinforcers. However, only 67% of the studies compiled by Klesges et al.[2] entailed biochemical verification, whereas all the studies in Table 1 used biochemical verification, so a comparison of these summaries may be skewed by unverified and potentially inaccurate data. In total, studies reviewed here support the hypothesis that incentives, lotteries, and competition programs heighten the impact of smoking cessation interventions.

A few studies[33,44] have given participants choices about which type of reinforcement program and what specific rewards they might have. This may be important in helping participants to choose the most potent reinforcer for them. Several studies[37,41] have also included sponsors of participants in incentive programs. This provision reduced concerns that nonparticipants might have resented the special resources given to participants.[45]

In future studies of programs using reinforcers, process evaluations need to play a more significant role. Currently, how and why incentives are

Table 1
Summary Statistics on Controlled Studies Using Incentives, Lotteries, and Competitions

	N	Participation rates	Dropout rates	Posttest cessation	Followup cessation	Months post-quit	Work force reduction
Incentives							
Windsor et al.[32]	387	19%	10%	20%	10%[a]	12	2%[b]
Malone[33]	44	5%	14%	82%	50%	12	3%
Scott et al.[34]	26	NR[c]	14%	75%	33%	9	NR
Rand et al.[35]	58	NR	36%	65%	6%	6	NR
Lotteries							
Jason et al.[41]	419[d]	29%	17%	42%	26%	12	6%
Competitions							
Klesges et al.[42]	107	88%	9%	21%	16%	6	7%
Klesges et al.[43]	136	48%	7%	31%	12%	6	9%[b]
Malone[34]	40	12%	13%	83%	48%	12	5%
Jason et al.[44]	95	84%	0%	49%	36%	12	32%
Averages	146	41%	13%	52%	26%	9	9%

[a]This condition involved bibliotherapy, a brief counseling session, and a small incentive. The second condition, a bibliotherapy program plus incentives program, is not listed here.
[b]Estimated from paticipation and cessation rates. May be slightly inaccurate depending upon how dropout rates are calculated.
[c]Not reported.
[d]38 work sites.

effective are matters of speculation. Perceptions of employees about each reinforcement program, and differences in perceptions across those programs, could help in designing more effective combinations of reinforcement programs.

More research needs to assess the singular and multiple effects of incentives, lotteries, and competitions upon work-site-wide smoking reductions. Future studies might examine each reinforcement program in isolation and in combination. Such research would help appreciably in better understanding the effects of these interventions.

Ideally, research that randomly provides different interventions to different settings, with each condition having adequate sample size, is needed. Such research would solve the unit of analysis problem. In addition, biochemical confirmation needs to be reported in studies. Finally, investigators should mention the percent signing up for the programs, the percent completing the program, and abstinence rates at 1-yr followup points. Data on work-site rates also needs to be more regularly reported.

Organizationally directed smoking interventions that employ incentives are likely to catch the attention and imagination of employees. This excitement may be needed by participants in order to counteract the discouragement of past unsuccessful efforts to change and the discomfort of withdrawal symptoms. Innovative programs might help the smoker look beyond these types of irritants in order to realize the rewards associated with smoke-free lifestyles. The final section of this chapter suggests ways to develop more specific concepts and hypotheses about how organizational issues affect smoking interventions.

Organizational Issues

Four topics will be reviewed in this section: organizational influences, stepped care, marketing to employees, and cost-outcome analyses.

Organizational Influences

A typology of organizational influences on smoking interventions might help us understand why individuals decide to make quit efforts, and why some individuals have long-term success. By understanding these organizational influences, interventions might be individually tailored so that they will have a better chance of succeeding in a particular setting. When incentives are part of the cessation interventions, it becomes even more important to assess these influences. It is possible that employees will be suspicious of incentive programs when the organizational climate is marked by recent layoffs, bitterness toward management, or unfair management practices.

Organizational influences do affect participation and cessation rates in smoking cessation programs. These environmental influences help account for the high variability that often exists in these cessation rates at different work sites.[1,2] For instance, Sloan and Gruman[46] found that employees who felt more supported by their supervisors were more likely to participate in a smoking cessation intervention. When incentives, lotteries, and competitions are implemented, there is no question that organizational dimensions will affect the program's efficacy, and the actual program will have effects on the organizational climate. Only more transactional measurement procedures can begin to capture these types of complicated organism-environment changes.

Several investigators have developed questionnaires to assess work-site environments. Moos[47] developed the Worksite Environment Scale to assess people's subjective perceptions of their environments. Their work assumes that environments have unique "personalities,"[48] and 10 subscales are used to tap three dimensions (relationships, personal growth, system maintenance) of organizational climate. Participants' perceptions of their work-site vs hypothesized perceptions of their ideal work-site environment can be compared. Moos[47] has administered the scale to enough work-sites to provide norms for different types of industries. Comparing a particular setting to these norms might provide an investigator with unique information about the setting where a behavior change initiative is about to be launched.

Another promising questionnaire is Hofstede's[49,50] Organizational Culture Scale, containing three subscales (degree of inequality of power, degree people feel threatened, individualism), which might also be used to measure social norms. Allen and Allen[19] have assessed three factors that they see as central to initiating and sustaining changes in organizational cultures:

1. Employees see themselves as working towards common goals;
2. A positive culture; and
3. A sense of belonging.

These types of scales have rarely been used in the evaluation of work-site smoking cessation programs. The next generation of interventions might see these types of higher level analyses as more critical and central to the overall objective of understanding the change processes within a particular setting.

An important organizational dimension is the smoking restriction policies. Currently, our understanding of restrictions is quite limited; this is surprising given that 77% of companies have smoking restrictions.[51] Partial restrictions may not weaken smoking habits, but instead they may cause people to adjust by smoking more in other situations.[52] Even total bans may not significantly affect smoking rates.[53] However, when combined with other interventions and presented in a certain way, restrictions might be more effective in helping individuals quit smoking. Restrictions might be accompanied by education about active and passive smoking, by offering cessation and reinforcement programs, and by adopting hiring policies that favor nonsmokers. In any event, these types of policies do need to be assessed in order to determine their possible influences on the success of work-site smoking cessation programs.

Other organizational dimensions, which are more objective and more specific to smoking interventions, might affect smoking interventions. A number of organizational variables, shown in Table 2, have been identified as critical in work-site smoking interventions.[54] Investigators need to assess these types of variables more regularly when implementing interventions, because any of these variables could potentially affect receptivity for and effectiveness of a wide range of programs.

Stepped Care

Organizational objectives to reduce work-site-wide smoking rates might best be accomplished by offering a series of smoking interventions or more extended interventions where recycling opportunities are possible. It is clear that most smokers have made past quit efforts, and most have had periods of abstinence. The two key factors are how to motivate individuals to make another quit effort, particularly when they might not feel confident given their past failures, and how to make quit efforts more successful in the long-term. Short, brief programs emphasize new efforts in quitting, but what might be needed are more long-term supports to help quitters maintain abstinence. Smoking cessation interventions might offer multiple programs, from bibliotherapy to multicomponented reinforcement programs. A series of programs might have synergistic effects; those unlikely to participate or quit in one intervention might do so in another self-selected intervention. In addition, over time, an individual not successful in a minimal program might opt for a more comprehensive intervention, particularly if the participant has seen other employees in the more comprehensive intervention succeed.

Table 2
Organizational Characteristics
Potentially Influencing Work-Site Smoking Cessation Programs[54]

1. Size of work-site
2. Current work-site smoking policies
3. Degree of management support for program
4. History of health promotion efforts in the work-site
5. Sex ratio of employees
6. Job stability and turnover
7. Union management relations
8. Percent of smokers in the work-site
9. Growth-oriented vs consolidating climate organization
10. Rank and sociometric standing of primary contact person
11. Socioeconomic level of employees

We need more research on who participates and who quits in cessation groups. It is possible that different types of interventions might need to be offered to different groups of smokers. Older and heavier smokers might be more likely to participate in group programs. Younger and less addicted subjects are more likely to quit smoking and remain smoke-free.[55,56] Although it is too soon to make recommendations, if broad programs were offered, and individuals with certain characteristics were more unsuccessful with particular types of programs, the knowledge base for matching individuals to programs would be enhanced considerably.

Offering a series of smoking cessation interventions individualizes the program, thereby giving employees a feeling of ownership about the program. This sense of ownership can be encouraged through individualized marketing of the smoking cessation interventions and by allowing participants to make choices within the smoking cessation interventions.[16]

Marketing Considerations

Marketing concepts and social communication theory might help investigators design more effective interventions. As an example, marketing concepts can be used to help tailor interventions to audiences. Parkinson,[57] for instance, emphasizes that smoking cessation interventions should be convenient. Smoking cessation groups held on company property are more convenient than those held off grounds, groups held during company time are more convenient than those held after company time, and interventions

Work-Site Smoking

not requiring group attendance may be more convenient than those that do. Also, as discussed earlier, incentives, lotteries, and competitions have within them marketing components that increase participation rates.

Personal selling is one marketing consideration. If personal selling is implemented by a supervisor, and the subordinate feels the supervisor will be disappointed if he or she does not participate, then this type of influence is likely to have negative or at best mixed results. More positive selling strategies probably occurred in the Cummings et al.[39] study where one participant requested another to participate together.

One of the most visible marketing strategies involves promotional campaigns. To structure promotional campaigns, in-depth information on audiences is needed. For example, Prochaska and DiClemente[4] found that individuals were at different stages of smoking. Different promotional strategies might be developed for people in these different stages. Cummings et al.[39] found that participants were more likely than nonparticipants to acknowledge smoking-related symptoms (e.g., coughing, shortness of breath, and loss of stamina). This finding suggests that recruitment campaigns should emphasize short-term benefits of quitting, such as no longer coughing and having more stamina and better wind, rather than the long-term benefits. By regularly asking smokers in the targeted company why they wish to quit smoking, promotional messages might become more individualized to that work site, and thus these messages might become more believable and effective.

The way in which the promotional material is displayed is critical to the campaign. For example, one should be able to read posters from more than several feet away. Professional-looking posters convey a message about the quality of the program. Using two or more mediums to broadcast the same message has synergistic effects.[58] Having variations of the same message presented by posters, messages on payroll checks, articles in company papers, and memos from presidents might be very effective. Recruiters should present multiple, believable messages to audiences a sufficient number of times in order for all the employees to see the information, and for the campaigns to become a topic of conversation for the work force. Of course, incentives are an excellent way to accomplish some of these goals.

Promotional campaigns can also be used to provide feedback on change efforts to both participants and nonparticipants, feedback being a potentially powerful means of changing behavior.[59] After a specific intervention is completed, and after consent is obtained, feedback about the success of individuals and groups might be publically posted. This type of feedback is particularly important and useful when competitions are being instituted in the setting. Interviews detailing how participants quit smoking might be publicized in the company paper, and quotes could be publicized on posters. This form of modeling and vicarious learning could induce more people to participate.[16]

Cost-Outcome Analyses

Cost-Benefit Analyses

Cost-benefit analyses list both costs and benefits of interventions in monetary terms. These analyses show if eventually the monetary benefits of interventions outweigh the initial costs. Kristein[60] offered the most reasonable analyses when he concluded in 1980 dollars that, several years after employees quit smoking, companies save $336–601 annually per employee. In 1990 dollars, adjusting these figures with 5% annual inflation rates, companies will save $532–979 annually when employees quit smoking. Unfortunately, none of the many line items Kristein identified were based on actual data; all data were estimated. Fielding[61] adapted Kristein's figures and similarly estimated that each average smoker incurred $200–500 (1990 dollars: $269–670) more than nonsmokers to companies.

Warner et al.[62] acknowledged the theoretical analyses conducted by Kristein[60] and others, but concluded that very limited empirical data existed on cost-benefit ratios of work-site smoking cessation programs. Actual data from individual companies were critical for helping companies of similar characteristics anticipate the financial parameters of smoking cessation services.

Cost-Effectiveness

An example of a cost-effectiveness ratio is determining that a smoking cessation program cost $200 per quit smoker. The first step psychologists might take in cost-outcome analyses would be to construct cost-effectiveness analyses. These analyses are easier to construct than cost-benefit analyses, since the benefit or outcome is left in behavioral terms. Cost-effectiveness analyses may not help executives establish goals, but once the goal of reducing workforce smoking rates is established, cost-effectiveness analyses can help executives determine the preferable means for reaching their goal.

The most complete cost-effectiveness analysis for smoking cessation was constructed by Altman et al.,[63] who assessed bibliotherapy, a cessation group, and a contest for 22 prizes including a trip to Hawaii. Cessation rates, assessed 4–11 wk after quit day, were 21% for bibliotherapy, 22% for the contest, and 35% for the group. Cost-effectiveness per quit smoker was assessed as $235–399 for the class, $129–236 for the contest, and $22–144 for the bibliotherapy. The cessation group was least cost-effective, and the bibliotherapy group most cost-effective.

Similar studies are needed in work-site smoking cessation interventions. Additional studies might not only provide critically needed data, but also establish standards for constructing cost analyses. Currently, Vladeck[64] notes "one can ensure that any service will be cost-effective, compared to others. One need only write the standards, requirements and reimbursement methods in the right way...." Adoption of common standards is vitally needed within cost-outcome analyses.

Conclusion

It is believed that smoking cessation interventions that employ incentives, lotteries, and competitions hold great promise for work-site smoking cessation programs. Millions of individuals have quit smoking over the past 20 yr. Those that are remaining tend to be the more addicted, and to have had more difficulty in quitting. Because the majority of adults are employed, work settings would be a key site for reaching the millions of individuals who are still addicted to cigarets. The key question is how to motivate more of these employees to make quit efforts and have long-term successes in maintaining abstinence.

Already, incentives, lotteries, and competitions are beginning to be associated with higher participation rates and higher cessation rates in worksite smoking cessation interventions. More research is needed to provide converging lines of evidence for their effectiveness. Clearly, launching these types of interventions is not simple. It is believed that different settings will have differential receptivity to work-site smoking cessation interventions. Only by having a better sense of the ecological domains within which interventions are situated will the move to the next generation of more potent interventions be possible. It is with this spirit that the need to conduct more thorough organizational assessments prior to launching all types of worksite interventions has been emphasized.

References

[1] R. C. Klesges and J. A. Cigrang (1989) Worksite smoking cessation programs: Clinical and methodological issues, in *Progress in Behavior Modification* (M. Hersen, R. M. Eisler, and M. Miller, eds.) Sage Publications, NY.

[2] R. C. Klesges, J. Cigrang, and R. E. Glasgow (1989) Worksite smoking modification programs: A state-of-art review and directions for future research. *Curr. Psychol. Res. Rev.* **6**, 25–56.

[3] E. Lichtenstein (1982) The smoking problem: A behavioral perspective. *J. Consult. Clin. Psychol.* **50**, 804–819.

[4] J. O. Prochaska and C. C. DiClemente (1980) Stages and processes of self-change of smoking: Toward an integrative model of change. *J. Consult. Clin. Psychol.* **51**, 390–395.

[5] G. A. Marlatt and J. R. Gordon, eds. (1985) *Relapse Prevention: Maintenance Strategies in Addictive Behavior Change* (Guilford, NY).

[6] S. Curry, G. A. Marlatt, and J. R. Gordon (1987) Abstinence violation effect: Validation of an attributional construct with smoking cessation. *J. Consult. Clin. Psychol.* **55**, 145–149.

[7] K. A. O'Connell and E. J. Martin (1987) Highly tempting situations associated with abstinence, temporary lapse, and relapse among participants in smoking cessation programs. *J. Consult. Clin. Psychol.* **55**, 367–371.

[8] V. J. Stevens and J. F. Hollis (1989) Preventing smoking relapse, using an individually tailored skills-training technique. *J. Consult. Clin. Psychol.* **57**, 420–424.

[9] K. D. Brownell, G. A. Marlatt, E. Lichtenstein, G. T. Wilson (1986) Understanding and preventing relapse. *Am. Psychol.* **57**, 765–780.

[10] H. A. Lando (1977) Successful treatment of smokers with a broad-spectrum behavioral approach. *J. Consult. Clin. Psychol.* **45**, 361–366.

[11] R. A. Winett (1973) Parameters of deposit contracts in the modification of smoking. *Psychol. Rep.* **23**, 49–60.

[12] B. D. Etringer, V. R. Gregory, and H. A. Lando (1984) Influence of group cohesion on the behavioral treatment of smoking. *J. Consult. Clin. Psychol.* **52**, 1080–1086.

[13] H. C. Coppetelli and C. T. Orleans (1985) Partner support and other determinants of smoking cessation maintenance among women. *J. Consult. Clin. Psychol.* **53**, 455–460.

[14] R. Mermelstein, E. Lichtenstein, and K. MacIntyre (1983) Partner support and relapse in smoking cessation programs. *J. Consult. Clin. Psychol.* **51**, 465, 466.

[15] J. M. Malott, R. E. Glasgow, H. K. O'Neill, and R. C. Klesges (1984) The role of co-worker social support in a worksite smoking control program. *J. Appl. Behav. Anal.* **17**, 485–495 (1984).

[16] D. B. Abrams, J. P. Elder, R. A. Carleton, T. M. Laster, and L. M. Artz (1986) Social learning principles for organizational health promotion: An integrated approach, in *Health and Industry: A Behavioral Medicine Perspective* (M. F. Cataldo and T. J. Coates, eds.), Wiley, NY.

[17] R. E. Glasgow, R. C. Klesges, and H. K. O'Neal (1986) Programming social support for smoking modification: An extension and replication. *Addict. Behav.* **11**, 453–457.

[18] R. A. Allen and C. Kraft (1984) The importance of cultural variables in program design, in *Health Promotion in the Workplace* (M. P. O'Donnell and T. H. Ainsworth, eds.), Wiley, NY, p. 71.

[19] R. A. Allen and J. Allen (1987) A sense of community, a shared vision and a positive culture: Core enabling factors in successful culture based health promotion. *Am. J. Health Promot.* 1, 40–47.

[20] P. Suedfeld (1982) Environmental factors influencing maintenance of lifestyle change, in *Adherence, Compliance and Generalization in Behavioral Medicine* (R. B. Stuart, ed.), Brunner/Mazel, NY, pp. 125–144, 165.

[21] R. A. Winett, A. C. King, and D. G. Altman (1989) Health Psychology and Public Health: An Integrative Approach (Pergamon, Elmsford, NY).

[22] E. Koop (1987) Worksite smoking interventions. Presentation given at the annual meeting of the Society for Behavioral Medicine. Washington, DC.

[23] L. W. Fredericksen (1985) Using incentives in worksite wellness. *Corp. Comment* 2, 51–57.

[24] D. S. Shephard and L. A. Pearlman (1985) Healthy habits that pay off. *Business and Health* 2, 37–41.

[25] R. Paxton (1981) Deposit contracts with smokers: Varying frequency and amount of repayments. *Behav. Res. Ther.* 19, 117–123.

[26] T. G. Bower, R. A. Winett, and L. W. Fredericksen (1987) Nicotine fading, behavioral contracting, and extended treatment: Effects on smoking cessation. *Addict. Behav.* 18, 181–183.

[27] K. E. Warner and H. A. Murt (1984) Economic incentives for health. *Annu. Rev. Public Health* 5, 107–133.

[28] R. Paxton (1980) The effects of a deposit contract as a component in a behavioural programme for stopping smoking. *Behav. Res. Ther.* 18, 45–50.

[29] F. L. Spring, J. F. Sipich, R. W. Trimble, and D. J. Goeckner (1978) Effects of contingency and noncontingency contracts in the context of a self-control-oriented smoking modification program. *Behav. Ther.* 9, 967,968.

[30] G. M. Rosen, and E. Lichtenstein (1977) An employee incentive program to reduce cigarette smoking. *J. Consult. Clin. Psychol.* 45, 957.

[31] S. W. Malone (1989) *Using Incentives and Rewards in Worksite Smoking Interventions.* Unpublished doctoral dissertation, Virginia Polytechnic Institute, Blacksburg, VA.

[32] R. A. Windsor, J. B. Lowe, and E. E. Barlett (1988) The effectiveness of a worksite self-help smoking cessation program: A randomized trial. *J. Behav. Med.* 11 (4), 407–421.

[33] S. W. Malone (1990) Using reinforcers in worksite smoking interventions. Paper presented at the annual meeting of the American Psychological Association, Boston, MA.

[34] R. R. Scott, D. M. Prue, C. A. Denier, and A. C. King (1986) Worksite smoking intervention with nursing professionals: Long-term outcome and relapse assessment. *J. Consult. Clin. Psychol.* 54, 809–813.

[35] C. S. Rand, M. L. Stitzer, G. E. Bigelow, and A. M. Mead (1989) The effects of contingent payment and frequent workplace monitoring on smoking abstinence. *Addict. Behav.* **14**, 121–128.

[36] K. Sorman (1979) This quit-smoking program works. *American Lung Association Bulletin* **1**, 747–741.

[37] B. H. Ellis (1979) How to reach and convince asbestos workers to give up smoking, *Progress in Smoking Cessation: International Conference on Smoking Cessation* (J. Schwartz, ed.), American Cancer Society, NY.

[38] T. Stacknik and B. Stoffelmayr (1983) Worksite smoking cessation programs: A potential for national impact. *Am. J. Public Health* **73**, 1395, 1396.

[39] K. M. Cummings, R. Hellman, and S. L. Emont (1988) Correlates of participation in a worksite stop-smoking contest. *J. Behav. Med.* **11** (3), 267–277.

[40] L. A. Jason, C. L. Gruder, L. Bruckenberger, T. Lesowitz, J. Belgredan, B. R. Flay, and R. B. Warnecke (1987) A 12-month follow-up of a worksite smoking cessation intervention. *Health Educ. Res.* **2**, 185–194.

[41] L. A. Jason, T. Lesowitz, M. Michaels, C. Blitz, L. Victors, L. Dean, and E. Yeager (1989) A worksite smoking intervention involving the media and incentives. Paper presented at the annual meeting of the American Psychological Association, New Orleans, LA.

[42] R. C. Klesges, M. M. Vasey, and R. E. Glasgow (1986) A worksite smoking modification competition: Potential for public health impact. *Am. J. Public Health* **76**, 198–200.

[43] R. C. Klesges, R. E. Glasgow, L. M. Klesges, K. Morray, and R. Quale (1987) Competition and relapse prevention training in worksite smoking modification. *Health Educ. Res.* **2**, 5–14.

[44] L. A. Jason, S. Jayaraj, C. Blitz, M. Michaels, and L. Klett (1990) Incentives and competition in a worksite smoking cessation intervention. *Am. J. Public Health* **80**, 205, 206.

[45] C. S. Orleans, and R. H. Shipley Worksite smoking cessation initiatives: Review and recommendations. *Addict. Behav.* **7**, 1–16.

[46] R. P. Sloan and J. C. Gurman (1987) Participation in workplace health promotion programs: The contribution of health and organizational factors. Paper presented at the annual meeting of the Society for Behavioral Medicine, Washington, DC.

[47] R. H. Moos (1986) *Work Environment Scale: Manual* (Psychologists' Press, Palo Alto, CA).

[48] K. Heller, R. H. Price, S. Reinharz, S. Rigerm, and A. Wandersman (1984) *Psychology and Community Change*, 2nd Ed., (The Dorsey Press, Homewood, IL).

[49] G. Hofstede (1980) *Culture's Consequences* (Sage Publications, Beverly Hills, CA).

[50] G. Hofstede (1980) National cultures in four dimensions. *International Studies of Management and Organizaiton* **13**, 46–73.

[51] J. E. Fielding and P. V. Piserchia (1989) Frequency of worksite health promotion activities. *Am. J. Public Health* **79**, 16–20.

[52] T. W. Meade and N. J. Walde (1977) Cigarette smoking patterns during the working day. *Br. J. Prev. Soc. Med.* **31**, 28.

[53] I. M. Rosenstock, A. Stergachis, and C. Heaney (1986) Evaluation of smoking prohibition policy in a health maintenance organization. *Am. J. Public Health* **76**, 1014,1015.

[54] U. S. Department of Health, Education, and Welfare. The health consequences of smoking: Cancer and chronic lung disease in the workplace. A report of the Surgeon General (DHHS Pub. No. 85-50207). U. S. Department of Health and Human Services, Public Health Service, Office of the Assistant Secretary for Health, Office on Smoking and Health, Rockville, MD.

[55] R. E. Glasgow, R. C. Klesges, L. M. Klesges, and G. W. Somes (1988) Predictors of participation and outcome in a worksite smoking control program. *J. Consult. Clin. Psychol.* **56**, 617–620.

[56] R. C. Klesges, K. Brown, R. W. Pascale, M. Murphy, E. Williams, and J. A. Cigrang (1988) Factors associated with participation, attrition, and outcome in a smoking cessation program at the workplace. *Health Psychol.* **7**, 575–589.

[57] R. S. Parkinson (1982) *Managing Health Promotion in the Workplace: Guidelines for Implementation and Evaluation* (Mayfield Publishing, Palo Alto, CA).

[58] M. L. Ray (1982) *Advertising and Communications Management* (Prentice Hall, Englewood Cliffs, NJ).

[59] M. R. Goldfried (1980) Toward the delineation of therapeutic change principles. *Am. Psychol.* **35**, 991–996.

[60] M. Kristein (1983) How much can business expect to profit from smoking cessation. *Prev. Med.* **12**, 358–381.

[61] J. E. Fielding (1984) Health promotion and disease prevention at the worksite. *Annu. Rev. Public Health* **5**, 237–265.

[62] K. E. Warner, T. M. Wickizer, R. A. Wolfe, J. E. Schidroth, and M. H. Samuelson (1988) Economic implications of workplace health promotion programs: Review of the literature. *J. Occup. Med.* **30**, 106–112.

[63] D. G. Altman, J. A. Flora, S. P. Fortmann, and J. W. Farquhar (1987) The cost-effectivness of three smoking cessation programs. *Am. J. Public Health* **77**, 162–165.

[64] B. J. Vladeck (1984) The limits of cost-effectiveness. *Am. J. Public Health* **74**, 652,653.

The Etiology and Consequences of Adolescent Drug Use

David W. Brook and Judith S. Brook

Introduction and General Review of Literature

This chapter focuses on the etiology and consequences of drug use from an interactional perspective. In the first part of the chapter, the interrelation of risk and protective factors as they affect adolescent drug use is discussed. Next, the childhood factors relating to adolescent drug use are discussed. The third part of the chapter addresses issues pertaining to the consequences of drug use. The chapter highlights recent advances in these areas and promising extensions in current research, prevention, and treatment.

Over the past decade, there has been increased attention paid to research into the complex interactions and predispositions resulting in adolescent drug use. At the same time, the adverse consequences of drug use and abuse on many areas of adolescent growth and development, including physiological and neuropsychological functioning, have become clearer. Although 20 yr ago illicit drugs were viewed by some as mind-expanding or emotionally growth-stimulating, now most workers in the field agree that recent research has revealed the multiple perils of adolescent drug use, especially heavy drug use and abuse. In particular, the contributions of interactions of risk and protective psychosocial factors, both in childhood and adolescence as they relate to adolescent drug use, have been thoroughly investigated. Such risk and protective factors can interact across domains of the parent–child relationship, child or adolescent personality, parental child-rearing practices, sibling interactions, peer relationships, and environmental and community structures and surroundings. In studies of such intrafamilial interactions, the roles of family members have been clarified, and data have been integrated from a number of disciplines concerning pathways leading to adolescent drug use. This chapter will deal with these research efforts at understanding the complex etiology of adolescent drug use from a developmental, epidemiological viewpoint, and will then examine some recent work concerning the consequences of such drug use.

In some past research investigations, data was often collected atheoretically, either because of lack of a clear framework or theory, difficulty in integrating data from several disciplines, or problems with research design, measurement, data collection, or statistical analysis. Recently, it has become more evident that a longitudinal, prospective design, utilizing a familial developmental theoretical approach emphasizing interactions provides one useful means of avoiding both atheoretical confusion and a piecemeal approach in data analysis and interpretation. This integrated, interactional approach also uses recently developed, sophisticated statistical techniques to evaluate interactional effects. In order to deal with some of these effects, an approach referred to as Family Interactional Theory has been developed. Such a data-based theoretical approach makes use of recently developed sophisticated statistical techniques to aid in appropriate evaluation of data, usefully integrates material from many disciplines, and has heuristic value for future research and greater understanding of adolescent drug use. Several other theoretical frameworks have proven to be of considerable utility in the study of drug use.[2-5]

A modern integrated theory that views drug use as part of a set of "problem behaviors" was first proposed by Jessor and Jessor.[2] According to the Jessors, problem behavior also included sexual promiscuity and delinquency, and occurred during the transitional developmental period of adolescence. Problem behavior, which led to difficulties for adolescents, families, and for society, was marked by such personality characteristics as increased deviance and tolerance of deviance, decreased emphasis on academic achievement, less adherence to religion, greater criticism of society, and more

Etiology and Consequences

emphasis on independence. For these adolescents, parents were less important than peers, and had less control and less influence than peers. Peers were important for support and as models for drug use. Concurrent characteristics also included more sensation-seeking and less conventionality, decreased school achievement, and less church attendance, compared to nonproblem behavior adolescents. According to Jessor,[6] the correlates of drug use are similar to those of general problem behavior.

In 1975, Kandel[7] identified four sequential stages of adolescent drug use, ranging from legal to illegal drugs, as follows:

1. Beer or wine
2. Cigarets or hard liquor
3. Marijuana
4. Other illicit drugs, including heroin and other opiates, cocaine, and amphetamines.

Kandel distinguished those adolescents who would probably progress from one stage to the next. Those who would be most likely to use hard liquor were identified by the presence of peer sociability, delinquency, and parental drinking, whereas likely marijuana users were marked by particular beliefs and personality traits and by drug-using peers. Marijuana was considered to be a "gateway" drug, since its use was usually seen in those adolescents who used other illicit drugs. Adolescents using other illicit drugs showed a poor parent–child relationship, psychological distress, and peer modeling of drug use.[4]

Brook and her colleagues have examined the differential factors related to stage of drug use and frequency of use, and they found that family factors were more related to stage than to frequency, whereas peer and personality factors were related both to particular stages of drug use and frequency of use.[8] Frequency of drug use was indirectly affected by personality and family factors mediated by peer group characteristics, but stage of drug use was independently affected by peer, family, and personality factors. To put it in a different way, peers influenced the occasions and timing of drug use, whereas personality and family factors had more influence on which particular drug the adolescent was likely to use.

Brook and her colleagues also investigated the interrelationships between family relations, peer influences, and personality attributes, looking at domains of causal influences and their interactions using a psychosocial developmental approach.[9,10] This interactional approach, which is a basic part of Brook's Family Interactional Theory, hypothesizes that a warm, relatively conflict-free, parent–adolescent mutual attachment relationship enables the parents to convey their version of society's values to their offspring through internalization, leading to increased adolescent identification with the parents. In other words, a certain kind of mutual attachment leads to increased identification with the parents, and internalization of their more conventional values and behavior, which is then manifested by the adolescent's conventional attitudes and behavior. Adolescent conventionality, in turn, serves to diminish the influence of peers compared to that of parents, and protects the adolescent from associating with drug-using peers.

Some investigators have used a family systems approach to study intrafamilial interactions. For example, Cooper, et al.[11] have studied intrafamilial communications and the psychosocial development of adolescents, and found that both connectedness to others and individuality are important for the adolescent's development of role-taking skills and identity. These investigators pointed to the importance for the adolescent of a "secure base," provided by a sense of connectedness, for outside exploration, as well as "individuated family relationships, characterized by separateness," allowing the adolescent to develop an individual view.

A number of other investigators have used an interactional approach, including Labouvie and McGee,[12] Magnusson,[13] Zucker and Gomberg,[14] and Bentler and Newcomb.[15] Some of these researchers have examined the latent behavioral variables and interactions affecting drug use using causal modeling by means of a statistical technique called (acronymically) LISREL, and they have been able to specify some of the complex causal factors involved.[3,16]

In studying the etiology of drug use, three areas in particular have received considerable attention: personality, family, and peer factors. In the personality area, three subsets—attitudinal unconventionality, emotional distress, and aggression/acting out—have been found to be implicated in drug use and abuse. Adolescents who reject dominant social norms are likely to initiate and sustain drug use. Such adolescents have an orientation to sensation-seeking[17-21] and are tolerant of deviance. Emotional distress has been found to be related to drug use and abuse in the clinical literature, even though there is some inconsistency in the research literature.[16,22,23] In a study by Swaim and colleagues,[24] of the variables they used to measure emotional distress, only anger had a direct if modest link to adolescent drug use. Furthermore, psychopathology appeared to bear an insignificant or very small relation to lesser degrees of use.[25] In fact, some researchers found that, in certain adolescent populations, experimental users of marijuana and other illicit drugs were in better psychological health than either heavy users or a subgroup of abstinent nonusers[26] (Block, personal communication, 1989).

The third subset, aggression/acting out behavior, is characterized by adolescent aggression, impulsivity, and rebelliousness, and has been consistently found to be related to adolescent drug use. Aside from the family, the peer group commonly serves as a major socialization influence on the adolescent's drug behavior. The strong association between friends' drug use (modeling) and self-drug use is well-documented (for reviews, see[27]). A dual process of selective association and socialization by peers appears to explain best how peers influence adolescent drug use.[28] There is also evidence in the literature that initiation to drug use, movement into recreational use (light or moderate), and progression to abuse seem to be influenced most directly by peer factors.[29]

Socialization within the family as it concerns drug use centers on two aspects of the interpersonal influence: (a) modeling, and (b) child-rearing practices. The modeling effects of parental drug use behavior on adolescent drug use are well-documented, although such effects vary depending on the drug in question (for review, see[30,31]). Child-rearing practices also constitute a principal means by which parents affect the drug use of their offspring, with each of the two major parenting dimensions of warmth and control exerting a distinctive influence on the overall quality of the parent–child relationship. The research of J. Brook and colleagues has focused on the warmth aspect, that is the attachment relationship between the parent and child as it affects the child's drug use. The nature of mutual attachment between parent and child has been explored through such variables as parental support, communication, responsiveness, affection, and the child's identification with the parent. Many of these variables are particularly potent in their inverse association with drug use when adolescents have formed an attachment to conventional or traditional parents.[32] The control dimension of parenting has also been found to be of importance in the etiology of drug use by adolescents.[33] Our research has revealed that the attachment relationship was consistently more important than the control dimension in insulating the adolescent from drug use.

A number of authors, including Kaufman[34] and Needle, et al.,[35,36] have studied intrafamilial risk factors for adolescent drug use, such as parental divorce or paternal drug use. Coombs and Coombs[37] have examined the familial manipulation of drug users, and the role of ethnicity has been examined by Kaufman and Borders.[38]

Recent work has taken a broader view of the family, and investigators have also looked at sibling influences on adolescent drug use. A number of mechanisms to account for sibling influences have been hypothesized, including differential treatment of siblings by parents and sibling rivalry. The important impact of parent–sibling interactions in adolescent drug use has also been studied.[10,39] Dunn, et al.[40] have examined parent–sibling interactions overall in child and adolescent development.

Brook, et al.[41] have identified three pathways of sibling influence on adolescent drug use. In the first pathway, the older brother's personality influenced the younger brother's personality via the hypothesized Personality Influence Mechanism, through identification and modeling, resulting in similar attitudes, values, and behavioral approaches. Their studies showed a strong association between the two brothers' tolerance of deviance and deviant behavior, in the direction noted. These unconventional attitudes in the younger brother were then expressed in his use of drugs.

Genetic factors played a role in the second causal pathway between the two brothers' personalities. In this pathway, the Genetic Temperamental Connection, both brothers inherited similar temperamental or psychophysiological characteristics or reaction patterns. This general area has been explored by Coccaro, et al.,[42] who have studied the psychobiological aspects of personality and personality disorders. Probably the two mechanisms described above worked in concert, with the older brother's personality influencing the younger brother's personality simultaneously in both ways.

The third pathway of causal influence was more indirect, since the two brothers' personalities were connected and mediated by the sibling relationship. In this mechanism, the Environmental Reactive Mechanism, the sibling relationship was disturbed, leading to increased intrapsychic distress and a lack of responsibility in the younger brother; that is, a troubled sibling relationship led to mutual withdrawal and decreased attachment between the brothers, intrapsychic distress manifested as anxiety, and lessened responsibility. A sibling relationship marked by a stronger mutual attachment with more nurturance, satisfaction, and identification, and less conflict and jealousy, resulted in decreased inner conflict and less psychic distress in the younger brother. This kind of nonconflictual sibling attachment was also related to more conventional attitudes and behavior, more responsibility, and less drug use in the younger brother.

The parental interactions and each sibling's relationship with both parents also influenced the sibling relationship, and adolescent drug use as well, although parent–child interactions and parental child-rearing techniques both also influence adolescent drug use.

The present authors[1] have developed a complex integrated developmental data-based model, which formulated the causative influences and interactions of several "domains" of behavior leading to adolescent drug use. Each behavioral domain was composed of several personality or behavioral attributes, which were derived either by analyzing the intercorrelations of measures for such attributes, or by the use of factor analysis. Causal connections between pathways were tested using multiple hierarchical regression analyses. Bentler, Newcomb, and associates at UCLA made use of the LISREL program to examine similar interrelationships.[15,43]

The integrated developmental model allowed a more thorough understanding of the complex psychosocial interactions and direct and indirect pathways, which played a role in adolescent drug use (Fig. 1). Using the data-based model revealed, for example, that the parental trait of conventionality was related to mutual parent–child attachment and the internalization of parental values, which were connected with greater adolescent conventionality. Causality emerged strongly, direct or indirect, along the path indicated. Greater adolescent conventionality was related to less peer drug use and less adolescent drug use. The model showed the effects on drug use of protective factors that could mitigate the negative effects of untoward environmental stimuli during growth and development. These effects were derived from these authors' research over the past 20 yr looking at children and adolescents raised at risk for drug use who have not used drugs. Such protective factors included the personality traits characteristic of conventionality, which subsumes lack of rebelliousness, greater responsibility, and high academic achievement.

Childhood Factors Related to Adolescent Drug Use

The integrated developmental model works mutually and reciprocally, for instance between parents and children, with feedback effects acting as

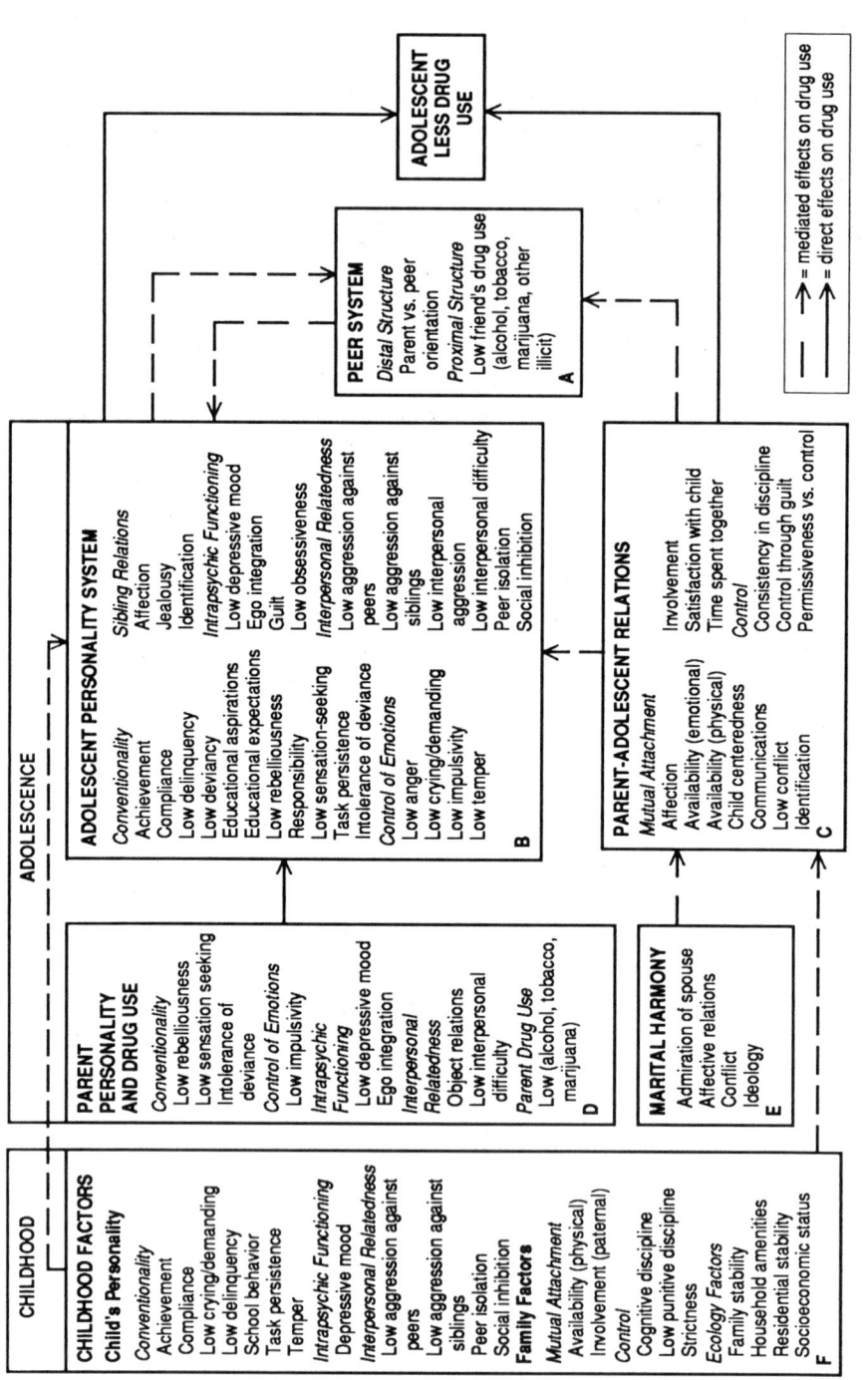

Fig. 1. Hypothesized developmental integrated model. Domains A–E were assessed during adolescence in both the Father and Mother Studies. Domain F was assessed during childhood in our Mother Study only (Brook et al., in press).

influences in both directions. The data reveal that, not only do the parents influence the child through parental personality and parental child-rearing practices, but also the child's characteristics affect the parent–child relationship. This in turn has effects on the adolescent's personality, which in its turn affects the parent–adolescent relationship. An example of this mutual reciprocal interaction is seen in the finding that childhood aggression predicts less mutuality in the parent–adolescent relationship, which is related to adolescent unconventionality and ultimately to a greater likelihood of more adolescent drug use.

The reciprocal relationship between parent and child attributes has been studied by a number of investigators. For example, Yarrow, et al.[44] found that different child attributes elicited different parental behaviors. Similar reciprocity can be found in every intrafamilial interaction. As concerns drug use, Kaufman and Kaufmann[45] noted that the parents of drug-abusing children, especially the mothers, were emotionally enmeshed with their children, so that parental feelings were largely determined by the child's behavior and by the closeness of the parent–child relationship.[34] The main implication of dyadic reciprocity such as this is that careful study is warranted when examining measures of each family member's behavior, since any measure can be influenced by each member of the dyad or by both simultaneously.

An illustration of the way in which the interplay of family interactions influences behavior may be seen in families marked by parental marital discord. A firm attachment to one parent can counteract the effect of the risk factor of marital discord on later drug use. Such a firm attachment to one parent can also mitigate the effects of a disturbance in the child's relationship with the other parent. Similarly, the effects of sibling risk factors for drug use, such as jealousy or lack of affection, can be lessened by a secure parent–child relationship with one parent. Other risk and protective factors also interact in this way to influence the end result of more or less drug use. The influence of sibling drug use (a risk factor) is lessened by nondrug-using peers (a protective factor). High parental affection leading to high mutual affection and identification with the parent (a protective factor) offsets the influence of low marital harmony (a risk factor).

As noted above, although there are many studies that have focused on the adolescent precursors of drug use, there are only a few major studies that have focused on the childhood antecedents of adolescent drug use. The first was a study of Black children who were first seen at six years of age and then again at ages 16–17.[46] Some early behaviors, particularly shy/aggressive behavior, had long-term consequences. The second prospective study was by Block and his colleagues.[47] Their findings indicated that, although there were some sex differences, a number of childhood factors were associated with later drug use for both boys and girls. Such antecedents included emotional lability, disobedience, lack of calmness, and aggression. Aggressiveness has not only been found to relate to drug use, but to a number of clinical syndromes, such as conduct disorders, attention deficits, and hyperactivity.[48] Taken together, studies by Block, by Kellam, and by Kaplan indicated that childhood personality attributes were important for a more complete understanding of drug use and certain types of clinical syndromes.

Brook and Cohen have been involved in a longitudinal study that examined the childhood precursors of later drug use. The goal was to examine childhood and adolescent intrapersonal and interpersonal short- and long-term influences on drug use, employing latent variable structural equation modeling. The study covered a period of over ten years, from childhood (ages 5–10) through middle and late adolescence (ages 16–21). The sample was interviewed at three points in time during the ten-year period. (T1 in childhood; T2 and T3 in early and middle to late adolescence). The measures included the following: Aggression and Parental Sociopathy at T1; Self Drug Use, Peer Drug Use, and Unconventionality at T2 and T3.

As regards the analyses, three-wave longitudinal latent variable models were employed to analyze the data using LISREL.[49] Because of space limitations, this discussion of the findings is limited to childhood aggression because of its importance in terms of later drug use. As shown in Fig. 2, the study delineates a number of pathways by which childhood aggression may affect adolescent drug use. Such aggression seemed to have an impact on T3 drug use in three ways.

First, aggression affects T2 drug use, which in turn is associated with the use of drugs at T3. In short, early aggression is a contributor to the stability of later drug behavior. Childhood aggression is also associated with a later developing orientation (unconventionality), which in turn is predictive of later drug use—a pathway that is independent of the earlier drug stability route. Moreover, low aggression is associated with two interacting factors (data not presented). Individuals who are low in drug use and high in conventionality at T2 are particularly protected against drug use at T3. These pathways may explicate mechanisms accounting for the ear-

Etiology and Consequences

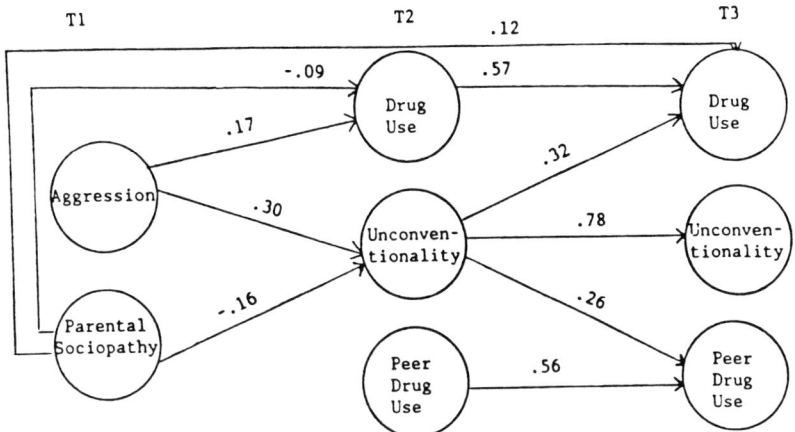

Fig. 2. Final structural model: childhood predictors of adolescent drug use. (Note: All coefficients are presented in the standardized metric and all effects are age adjusted.)

lier findings of Block and colleagues that early aggressiveness is related to later drug use.

The area of genetic influences on family interactions, and hence on drug use, referred to earlier as the Genetic Temperamental Connection, needs further exploration. This new field, the behavioral genetics of family behavior, promises exciting findings in the future. It is important not to confound a biological predisposition with the resultant behavior.[50] Significant research is also under way in the related area of the psychobiology of personality disorders by Siever and his colleagues.[51] These areas must be considered separately, particularly with regard to the question of direct genetic influences on substance use.[52] Adoption studies have shown the increased prevalence of alcoholism among adults adopted in childhood whose biological parents were alcoholics over that in adopted adults whose biological parents were not alcoholics. Alcoholism or heavy drinking in the adoptive parents played only a small role in this regard.[53,54]

One might speculate that a risk-diathesis interactional model explains these and similar findings. A genetically transmitted (probably autosomal and polygenic) predisposition, perhaps based on disturbances in metabolic or neuroreceptor functioning, or both, results in a vulnerability to alcoholism, or other substances of abuse. This diathesis depends for its phenotypic expression both on complex interactions with the psychosocial risk factors discussed in this chapter, as well as on interaction with the pharmacological effects of the abused substances. The relative importance of individual risk factors, hypothetical genetic diatheses, or pharmacological drug actions probably varies from factor to factor, drug to drug, and from one population cohort to the next, as does the nature of action of these influences, acting directly or indirectly, mediated by psychosocial factors. More evidence is needed to show the applicability of this model to all substance use and abuse, and indeed, to a wide range of psychiatric disorders.

Environmental or contextual factors can also have significant risk-protective effects on intrafamilial processes. In general, sociodemographic factors are not highly related to drug use patterns. Regional differences in rates of illicit drug use and abuse are readily apparent with higher rates in large urban centers. Drug availability, low perceived risk, and low disapproval of drug use are also important predictors in drug use and abuse. Other environmental variables include crime, neighborhood poverty and decay, and a lack of community support structures. Further research into the ways in which environmental factors influence drug use will undoubtedly yield clinically useful knowledge and a broader perspective about the psychosocial interactions leading to drug use. Moreover, investigators in recent times have not only studied the multiple influences on drug use, but have begun to look at specific categories and patterns of alcohol and drug use by adolescents according to such differential factors as gender, ethnicity, personality, parent/peer relations, and the like.[3, 5, 55-58] In sum, although much is known about the etiology of drug use, there is one area in particular that reflects needed emphases to accelerate the development of research in adolescent drug use. Research is needed to distinguish the causes of heavy drug use and drug abuse and to distinguish among different substances in this regard.

The Psychosocial Consequences of Marijuana Use

Having presented a review of the etiologic factors involved in adolescent drug use, a discussion of the consequences of adolescent drug use will now be presented. The findings regarding the consequences of drug use, with the exception of studies dealing with marijuana use, are fairly consistent. Marijuana use will first be discussed, and much attention will be devoted to this particular drug since it is the illegal drug used most frequently

Etiology and Consequences

by adolescents. Numerous investigators have reported consistent associations between marijuana use and a range of biological consequences.[59] Thus, for instance, marijuana appears to result in impairment of short-term memory, pulmonary function, and immune system functioning. In contrast to the findings of studies dealing with the consequences of marijuana for physical functioning, which are pretty consistent, results dealing with the impact of marijuana use on psychosocial functioning are somewhat inconsistent and are not as clearly understood. Over the last 20 yr, a number of investigators have noted that marijuana can result in the "amotivational syndrome." As noted by Koop,[60] this term refers to a "... pattern of loss of energy, diminished school performance, harmed parental relationships and other behavioral disruptions" (p. iv). In contrast to those who have found that marijuana use has an impact on aspects of the amotivational syndrome, other investigators have failed to find that marijuana results in decreased academic performance and academic achievement, as well as other aspects of the amotivational syndrome.[61] Although the literature is quite spotty, it does appear that marijuana may affect family relations; for instance, Hendin, et al.[62] reported that marijuana use served to heighten distance in the parent–adolescent relationship. As regards peer relations, there is some evidence that marijuana has an impact on friendship networks. According to Kandel,[28] similarity in drug use between friends exists prior to the relationship and may in part be considered a causative factor in the association. Nevertheless, as pointed out by Kandel, marijuana use does lead to associating with peers who are drug users. There is also a well-known association between marijuana use and delinquent behavior, resulting in fights, automobile theft and accidents, and truancy. Some users also become involved in criminal drug sales and distribution networks. These findings concur with those findings discussed below concerning the effects of marijuana use on personal responsibility.

The question of distinguishing occasional use from heavy use and abuse is now being investigated with more interest than previously. In addition, another current research issue is polydrug abuse, which can synergistically worsen the effects of marijuana use alone. Although some occasional users may suffer no adverse longitudinal effects, some go on to become heavy users or abusers, and some turn to polydrug abuse. Polydrug abuse can, depending on the particular drugs used, interfere significantly with adolescent growth and development, and hence with further maturation into adult life.

The authors of this chapter have examined the effects of marijuana use on both intrapersonal and interpersonal functioning in both Black and White adolescents. The sample for this particular study was first seen when they were in ninth and tenth grades and then again two years later. It was found that regular use of marijuana by young high school students had a detrimental impact on their personalities, attitudes, and behaviors, as well as on their relationships with their parents. In addition, marijuana users tended to associate more often with both deviant and drug-using peer groups. Taken as a whole, the results therefore implied that use of marijuana on a weekly basis or more may have interfered with the adolescents' sense of personal and social responsibility, may have impeded the relationship with their parents, and may have led to the adolescents becoming involved with nonachievement-oriented, deviant, and drug-using peers. It is especially noteworthy that it was in the area of personal responsibility that marijuana use by high school students had its greatest impact. Regular marijuana use, especially among Whites, was associated with greater tolerance of deviance and lower motivation to achieve. These results therefore lend some support to the notion of the amotivational syndrome, which includes such personality attributes as indolence, little interest in productivity, and lack of interest in academic issues or activities.[63-65] Although the psychopharmacological impact of marijuana is not entirely understood, one theory that has been espoused is that tetrahydrocannabinol, which is a major component of marijuana, has some sedative effect on the central nervous system, which results in a blunting of responsivity and an accompanying loss of motivation.[66]

As noted previously, the findings noted above are consistent with those of other investigators who have looked at high school students and have indicated that marijuana use does have an effect on motivation; however, they are inconsistent with those investigators who have looked at college populations[61] and reported no adverse effects for marijuana use. It may be that marijuana use causes problems for younger students, but not for older students, since younger students can be considered more vulnerable both psychologically and physiologically, and therefore are more likely to be susceptible to the harmful impact of marijuana. Regular use of marijuana is also related to a decrease in the sense of social responsibility, but does not appear to result in greater depressive mood. In general, it appears that marijuana use has an impact on those personality dimensions that also are associated with predicting later drug use. Thus, it may be that regular

Etiology and Consequences

marijuana use decreases personal and social responsibility, and this decreased personal and social responsibility results in an increased frequency of marijuana use, thus creating a feedback loop.

Regular use of marijuana also has an impact on interpersonal functioning. For example, regular use of marijuana appears to result in a decrease in the mutual attachment between parent and child. This may result in a serious condition, in that the more frequently involved marijuana users may miss crucial socialization experiences. Marijuana also appears to result in an increase in associating with youngsters who are both deviant and who themselves use drugs. Although in some adolescents light or experimental use of marijuana may not be problematic, it does appear that more serious involvement and heavier use affects both intrapsychic and interpersonal functioning. Of course, heavy drug use is the usual necessary precursor for drug abuse, with its associated morbidity.

As regards the use of other drugs, such as alcohol, amphetamines, and cocaine, the findings are more consistent. Drug use and abuse may have short-term consequences, such as automobile accidents, absenteeism, and deleterious health sequelae. Short- and long-term consequences of drug use and abuse include a wide range of intrapsychic, personal, and interpersonal difficulties.[25] In a recent study, Newcomb and Bentler[3] mapped out links between early drug use and precocious adolescent development reflected in early marriage, family-rearing, and participation in the work force to the neglect of the pursuit of further education. Adolescent polydrug use interfered with the achievement of a number of adolescent developmental tasks, which resulted in later difficulties in role acquisition, such as maintaining a marriage. However, according to Kandel, although drug use does not appear to have an effect on occupational attainment, drug use is associated with discontinuous work careers and delayed entry into conventional family roles.[67–69]

It is interesting to note that adverse consequences of some drugs appear to be gender-related. For instance, Robbins[70] reported that the consequences of higher levels of alcohol and drug abuse for psychosocial problems in general were greater for men than for women. Furthermore, the association between substance abuse and intrapsychic problems was greater for women than for men, whereas the relation between substance abuse and social functioning was greater among men.

Overall, drugs may be used by adolescents to cope with internal stresses or external demands, thereby depriving them of developing the resources to deal with the developmental tasks of adolescence. As noted above, some users of illegal drugs are also involved with criminal drug-connected enterprises. Although recognition and specification of the consequences of the use of a number of different drugs by adolescents has been made, future advances in this area require longitudinal studies that follow youngsters from adolescence into adulthood. A number of such longitudinal studies are in progress and important results are beginning to emerge.[3,67,69]

Conclusion

Adolescent substance use and abuse must be viewed in the light of the adolescent's interactions and relationships with family and peers who are not substance users, as well as with those who are; the causal factors mentioned in Fig. 1 all play a part in the psychosocial etiology of drug use. Moreover, mutual parent–adolescent attachment and identification protects against adolescent substance use, as does association with nonsubstance-using peers. Parental conventionality and adherence to tradition are related to a nonconflictual and affectionate parent–adolescent relationship, which leads to increased identification with the parents. This in turn is related to increased adolescent conventionality and association with nondrug-using peers, resulting in adolescent nonuse of drugs. This whole psychosocial process has its roots in the parent–child bonds formed in early childhood and in the quality of the child's psychosocial adjustment. It is likely that a strong parent–child bond leads to lasting internalization of parental values, behavior, and attitudes, and to the development of responsible, conventional, and nonrebellious attitudes towards societal norms. Adolescents with a history of such strong parent–child bonds grow to have enhanced feeling of self-control, and the ability, self-esteem, and maturity to solve problems reasonably and successfully.

In contradistinction, childhood drug-prone personality traits, such as aggression, and unfavorable childhood experiences, such as parental sociopathy, can influence the development of adolescent drug-prone personality traits and an inadequate and noxious parent–child bond. Such children and adolescents often show poor self-control, greater aggression, and poor academic achievement, with an increased risk for drug use.

As concerns the issue of drug use vs heavy use or abuse, although occasional drug use in an emotionally and physically healthy adolescent may not interfere with development or lead to harm every time, such use under

Etiology and Consequences

certain circumstances certainly increases the risk of harmful interactions, and is a necessary prerequisite for heavy use or abuse. No adolescent becomes a heavy user or drug abuser suddenly; rather, there is a gradual and insidious increase in use in vulnerable adolescents, which in some results in heavy drug use or abuse.

During development there are, however, a number of temporal points and several psychosocial areas in which interventions to increase protective influences against risks for drug use and to ameliorate drug use can be effective. It is important to keep in mind the risk and protective factors involved in family, peer, and environmental interactions during childhood and adolescence for a more comprehensive understanding of drug use. Another example is that sibling mutual attachment marked by nurturance, little conflict, and mutual identification protects adolescent males against drug use.

To summarize, family factors correlated with adolescent drug use, not necessarily in order of importance, include:

1. Relative lack of parental supervision, less involvement and control, and low familial goal-directed behavior;
2. A weak parent–child mutual attachment;
3. Conflictual parent–child relationship;
4. Intrafamilial tension and conflicts in adolescence;
5. Parental and sibling tolerance of deviant, illegal, or unconventional behavior;
6. Parental and sibling deviant, legal or illegal drug behavior;
7. Parental and sibling unconventionality, aggression, or social isolation;
8. Parental psychopathology or poverty; and
9. Parental divorce, death, or abandonment.

Future investigations should be expanded to include the study of children and families from a variety of ethnic backgrounds, such as Black, Hispanic, and Asian. It should be remembered that peer drug use and peer support for drug use and deviant behavior are among the most important predictors of adolescent drug use. Moreover, environmental factors play a role in the adolescent's drug use.

As noted above, this group has also examined the consequences of marijuana use on intrapersonal and interpersonal functioning.[71] In contrast to work on some of the biomedical consequences of marijuana use, findings cited in the literature on the psychosocial effects of marijuana have been inconsistent, and more research in this area is needed, especially as concerns the impact of marijuana use on casual, infrequent users. It is clear, however, that, from an insufficient appreciation of the risks of marijuana use 20 yr ago, with some professionals even proposing its use for a variety of reasons, the field has moved to a widespread recognition of marijuana's potential for adverse impact on psychosocial and intrapsychic functioning. In contrast to marijuana use, there is general agreement that the psychosocial and psychophysiological effects of heavy use of alcohol and other illicit drugs are deleterious.

The findings of Brook et al.[71] suggest that regular marijuana use has a detrimental effect on psychosocial domains of personality and behavior, perceived parent–adolescent relationships, and perceived peer factors. Although on some of the personality measures some ethnic differences were present, generally marijuana use was found to adversely effect the adolescent's personal and social responsibility, and to increase the adolescent's involvement with nonachievement-oriented deviant or rebellious peer groups. These findings did support an association between marijuana use and the "amotivational syndrome" described by a number of investigators. Marijuana use tends to be self-perpetuating, since the initial personality changes resulting from its use increase the likelihood of continued use. Although marijuana is not a physiologically addictive drug, it can be described as habituating, in this way.

In studying the causes and consequences of drug use, it would be of great assistance if some of the results that are emerging from the field of developmental psychopathology could be integrated. For instance, as noted by Rutter,[72] researchers should attempt to incorporate the developmental level of the child as a moderator variable in their models. Level of development can be assessed in a number of diverse ways including, but not limited to, different psychological stages or phases and different physiological stages. It would be of great value to explore the relationship between familial and extrafamilial factors and drug use in the context of alternate stages or processes. Another variable that has been incorporated in more recent studies is that of the child's sex. It would be important to develop models that determine whether the predictors of drug use are similar or different for males and females.

At the present time, it seems clear that the initiation and maintenance of drug use and abuse are each determined by a complex set of interactions of psychosocial, familial, environmental, genetic, pharmacological, and psychiatric factors. This set of interactions is not the same for both initiation and continued use or abuse. Different people are vulnerable or at risk for drug use or abuse in different ways and at different times of life, dependent also on the influence of many environmental or biological influences. Such characteristics may be shared in common by members of various groups, which may facilitate measurement and the statistical validation and treatment of such influences. Vulnerability may be genetic, psychosocial, or psychiatric in nature, or may depend for a particular person on a combination of such factors. People at risk for drug use or abuse also manifest a number of other personality or behavioral characteristics, often pathological, at least under some circumstances. For best results, prevention or treatment efforts must employ methods to achieve a drug-free state, although such efforts must take into account the particular vulnerabilities of certain individuals or groups of people. Early identification of children and/or families at risk can allow for the optimal early introduction of protective or treatment efforts, and for the individualization of such efforts, whether at a psychosocial, familial, medical-psychiatric, environmental, or societal level.

To conclude, additional theory and interdisciplinary research is needed on the nature, development, and consequences of drug use. It seems clear that one conceptual model is not sufficient to explain the development and consequences of drug use. Broader frameworks, such as one using an interactional perspective, might prove more suitable. What is also needed is the development of models, such as those presented in this chapter, that attempt to explain drug use and drug abuse. The advantages of the models approach is that models provide direct empirical tests of specific influences that promote adolescent drug use. Models examine several domains and integrate these into a chain of influences to indicate how drug use is initiated and continues. Models, of course, need to include many influences that are likely to impinge on the youngster's drug use, such as hereditary factors, personality, peer, parental, sibling, school, and broader cultural influences. The advantage of the models approach is that it can be tested directly. Longitudinal studies can assess the degree to which the directions of influence are plausible, so that the specific paths leading to drug use can be identified and replicated.

Acknowledgments

This research was partially supported by grant DA02390 and by Research Scientist Development Award DA00094, Level II, from the National

Institute on Drug Abuse. The assistance of both Ann Gordon and Dorothy Marion is gratefully acknowledged.

References

[1] J. S. Brook, D. W. Brook, M. Whiteman, A. S. Gordon, and P. Cohen (1990) *The Psychosocial Etiology of Adolescent Drug Use and Abuse. Genetic Psychology Monographs* **116**, 20.

[2] R. Jessor and S. L. Jessor (1977) *Problem Behavior and Psychosocial Development* (Academic, NY).

[3] M. D. Newcomb and P. M. Bentler (1988) *Consequences of Adolescent Drug Use: Impact on the Lives of Young Adults* (Sage Publications, Newbury Park, CA).

[4] D. B. Kandel, R. C. Kessler, and R. Z. Margulies (1978) Antecedents of adolescent initiation into stages of drug use: A developmental analysis, in *Longitudinal Research on Drug Use: Empirical Findings and Methodological Issues* (D. B. Kandel, ed.), Hemisphere, Washington, DC, pp. 73–99.

[5] H. B. Kaplan, S. S. Martin, R. J. Johnson, and C. A. Robbins (1986) Escalation of marijuana use: Application of a general theory of deviant behavior. *J. Health Soc. Behav.* **27**, 44–61.

[6] J. E. Donovan and R. Jessor (1985) Structure of problem behavior in adolescence and young adulthood. *J. Consult. Clin. Psychol.* **53**, 890–904.

[7] D. B. Kandel (1975) Stages in adolescent involvement in drug use. *Science* **190**, 912–914.

[8] J. S. Brook, M. Whiteman, and A. S. Gordon (1982) Qualitative and quantitative aspects of adolescent drug use: Interplay of personality, family, and peer correlates. *Psychol. Rep.* **51**, 1151–1163.

[9] J. S. Brook, I. F. Lukoff, and M. Whiteman (1977) Peer, family, and personality clomaines as related to adolescents' drug behavior. *Psychol. Rep.* **41**, 1095–1102.

[10] J. S. Brook, M. Whiteman and A. S. Gordon (1983) Stages of drug use in adolescence: Personality, peer, and family correlates. *Dev. Psychol.* **19**, 269–277.

[11] C. R. Cooper, H. D. Grotevant, and S. M. Condon (1983) Individuality and connectedness in the family as a context for adolescent identity formation and role-taking skills, in *Adolescent Development in the Family* (H. D. Grotevant and C. R. Cooper, eds.), Jossey-Bass, San Francisco CA pp. 43–59.

[12] E. W. Labouvie and C. R. McGee (1986) Relation of personality to alcohol and drug use in adolescence. *J. Consult. Clin. Psychol.* **54**, 289–293.

[13] D. Magnusson (1988) *Individual Development from an Interactional Perspective: A Longitudinal Study* (Lawrence Erlbaum Associates, Hillsdale, NJ).

[14] R. A. Zucker and E. S. L. Gomberg (1986) Etiology of alcoholism reconsidered: The case for a biopsychosocial approach. *Am. Psychol.* **41**, 783–793.

[15] P. M. Bentler and M. D. Newcomb (1986) Personality, sexual behavior, and

drug use revealed through latent variable methods. *Clin. Psychol. Review* **6**, 363–385.

[16]J. A. Stein, M. D. Newcomb, and P. M. Bentler (1987) An eight-year study of multiple influences on drug use and drug use consequences. *J. Pers., Soc. Psychol.* **53**, 1094–1105.

[17]J. S. Brook, M. Whiteman, A. S. Gordon, and P. Cohen (1986a) Dynamics of childhood and adolescent personality traits and adolescent drug use. *Devel. Psychol.* **22** 403–414.

[18]J. S. Brook, M. Whiteman, A. S. Gordon, and P. Cohen (1986b) Some models and mechanisms for explaining the impact of maternal and adolescent characteristics on adolescent stage of drug use. *Devel. Psychol.*. **22**, 460–467.

[19]R. Jessor, A. Chase, and J. E. Donovan, (1980) Psychosocial correlates of marijuana use and drinking in a national sample of adolescents. *Am. J. Public Health* **70**, 604–613.

[20]E. J. Kay, A. Lyons, W. Newman, D. Mankin, and R. C. Loeb (1978) A longitudinal study of the personality correlates of marijuana use. *J. Consult. Clin. Psychol.* **46**, 470–477.

[21]J. A. Wingard, G. J. Huba, and P. M. Bentler (1980) A longitudinal analysis of personality structure and adolescent substance use. *Personality and Individual Differences*, **1**, 259–272.

[22]A. I. Alterman, ed. (1985) *Substance Abuse and Psychopathology* (Plenum, NY).

[23]E. J. Khantzian (1985) The self-medication hypothesis of addictive disorders: Focus on heroin and cocaine dependence. *Am. J. Psychiatry* **142** (11), 1259–1264.

[24]E. R. Swaim, E. W. Oetting, R. W. Edwards, and F. Beauvais, (1989) Links from emotional distress to adolescent drug use: A path model. *J. Consult. Clin. Psychol.* **57** (2), 227–231.

[25]A. T. Jersild, J. S. Brook, and D. W. Brook (1978) *The Psychology of Adolescence*, 3rd Ed. (Macmillan, NY).

[26]D. Baumrind and K. A. Moselle (1985) A developmental perspective on adolescent drug use. *Advances in Alcohol and Substance Use* **5**, 41–67.

[27]D. B. Kandel (1980) Drug and drinking behavior among youth. *Ann. Rev. Sociol.* **6**, 235–285.

[28]D. B. Kandel (1985) On process of peer influences in adolescent drug use: A developmental perspective. *Advances in Alcohol and Substance Abuse* **4**, 139–163.

[29]E. R. Oetting and F. Beauvais (1987) Peer cluster theory, socialization characteristics, and adolescent drug use: A path analysis. *J. of Counseling Psychol.* **34** (2), 205–213.

[30]M. Penning and G. E. Barnes (1982) Adolescent marijuana use: A review. *Int. J. Addict.* **17**, 749–791.

[31]J. S. Brook, M. Whiteman, D. W. Brook, and A. S. Gordon (1984) Paternal determinants of female adolescent's marijuana use. *Devel. Psychol.* **20**, 1032–1043.

[32]J. S. Brook, M. Whiteman, A. S. Gordon, and D. W. Brook (1984) Identification with paternal attributes and its relationship to the son's personality and drug use. *Devel. Psychol.* **20**, 1111–1119.

[33]J. D. Hawkins, D. M. Lishner, and R. F. Catalano Jr. (1985) Childhood predictors and the prevention of adolescent substance abuse, in *Etiology of Drug Abuse: Implications for Prevention* (C. L. Jones and R. J. Battjes, eds.)(DHHS Publication No. ADM 85-1335), National Institute on Drug Abuse, pp. 75–126.

[34]E. Kaufman (1985) *Substance Abuse and Family Therapy* (Grune & Stratton, Orlando, FL).

[35]R. Needle, H. McCubbin, and J. Lorence, (1985) A test of nonrespondent bias in a family-based study: A research note. *Int. J. Addict.* **20**, 763–769.

[36]R. Needle, H. McCubbin, M. Wilson, R. Reineck, A. Lazar, and H. Mederer (1986) Interpersonal influences in adolescent drug use: The role of older siblings, parents and peers. *Int. J. Addict.* **21**, 739–766.

[37]R. H. Coombs and K. Coombs (1988) Developmental stages in drug use: Changing family involvements. *J. Chem. Dependency Treatment* **1**, 73–98.

[38]E. Kaufman and L. Borders (1988) Ethnic family differences in adolescent substance use. *J. Chem. Dependency Treatment* **1**, 99–121.

[39]J. S. Brook, M. Whiteman, A. S. Gordon, and D. W. Brook (1990) The role of older brothers in younger brothers' drug use viewed in the context of parent and peer influences, *J. Genet. Psychol.* **151**(1), 59–75.

[40]J. F. Dunn, R. Plomin, and D. Daniels (1986) Consistency and change in mother's behavior toward young siblings. *Child Dev.* **57**, 348–356.

[41]J. S. Brook, M. Whiteman, D. W. Brook, and A. S. Gordon (1989b) Sibling influences on adolescent drug use: Older brothers on younger brothers. Manuscript submitted for publication.

[42]E. F. Coccaro, L. J. Siever, H. M. Klar, G. Maurer, K. Cochrane, T. B. Cooper, R. C. Mohs, and K. M. Davis (1989) Serotonergic studies in patients with affective and personality disorders: Correlates with suicidal and impulsive aggressive behavior. *Arch. Gen. Psychiatry* **46** (7), 587–599.

[43]M. D. Newcomb (1988) *Drug Use in the Workplace: Risk Factors for Disruptive Substance Use among Young Adults* (Auburn House, Dover, MA).

[44]M. R. Yarrow, C. Z. Waxler, and P. M. Scott (1971) Child effects on adult behavior. *Devel. Psychol.* **5**, 300–311.

[45]E. Kaufman and P. Kaufmann (1977) Multiple family therapy: A new direction in the treatment of drug abusers. *Am. J. Drug and Alcohol Abuse* **4** (4), 467–478.

[46]S. S. Kellam, C. H. Brown, B. R. Rubin, and M. E. Ensminger (1983) Paths leading to teenage psychotic symptoms and substance use: Developmental epidemiological studies in Woodlawn, in *Childhood Psychopathology and Development* (S. B. Guze, F. J. Earls, and J. E. Barrett, eds.), Raven, NY, pp. 17–47.

[47] J. Block, J. H. Block, and S. Keyes (1988) Longitudinally foretelling drug usage in adolescence: Early childhood personality and environmental precursors. *Child Dev.* **59**, 336–355.

[48] R. J. Johnson and H. B. Kaplan (1988) Gender, aggression, and mental health intervention during early adolescence. *J. Health Soc. Behav.* **29** (1), 53–64.

[49] K. G. Jöreskog and D. Sörbom (1988) *LISREL VII: A Guide to the Programs and Applications* (SPSS, Chicago, IL).

[50] S. Scarr and R. McCartney (1983) How people make their own environments: A theory of genotype environment effects. *Child Dev.* **54**, 424–435.

[51] L. J. Siever, H. Klar, and E. F. Coccaro, (1985) Psychobiologic substrates of personality, in *Biologic Response Styles: Clinical Implications* (L. J. Siever and H. Klar, eds.), American Psychiatric Press, Washington, DC, pp. 38–66.

[52] D. W. Goodwin (1979) Alcoholism and heredity: A review and hypothesis. *Arch. Gen. Psychiatry* **36**, 57–61.

[53] M. Bohman, S. Sigvardsson, and C. Cloninger (1981) Maternal inheritance of alcohol abuse: Cross-fostering analysis of adopted women. *Arch. Gen. Psychiatry* **38**, 965–969.

[54] C. Cloninger, M. Bohman, and S. Sigvardsson (1981) Inheritance of alcohol abuse: Cross-fostering analysis of adult men. *Arch. Gen. Psychiatry* **38**, 861–868.

[55] G. M. Barnes, M. P. Farrell, and A. Cairns (1986) Parental socialization factors and adolescent drinking behaviors. *J. Marriage and Family* **48**, 27–36.

[56] D. Baumrind (1985) Familial antecedents of adolescent drug use: A developmental perspective, in *Etiology of Drug Abuse: Implications for Prevention* (C. L. Jones and R. J. Battjes, eds.) (Research Monograph No. 56), National Institute on Drug Abuse, Rockville, MD, pp. 13–44.

[57] A. Norem-Hebeisen, D. W. Johnson, D. Anderson, and R. Johnson (1984) Predictors and concomitants of changes in drug use patterns among teenagers. *J. Soc. Psychol.* **124**, 43–50.

[58] R. J. Pandina and J. A. Schuele (1983) Psychosocial correlates of alcohol and drug use of adolescent students and adolescents in treatment. *J. Stud. Alcohol* **44** (6), 950–973.

[59] R. C. Petersen (1980) Marijuana Research Findings: 1980 (HHS publication No. ADM80-1001, III-IV). National Institute on Drug Abuse, Washington, DC.

[60] C. E. Koop (1982) Introductory statement, in *Marijuana and Health: Ninth Report to the U. S . Congress from the Secretary of Health and Human Services* (HHS publication No. ADM82-1216). National Institute on Drug Abuse, Washington, DC.

[61] A. C. Miranne (1979) Marijuana use and achievement orientations of college students. *J. Health Soc. Behav.* **20**, 194–199.

[62] H. Hendin, A. Pollinger, and R. B. Ulman (1981–1982). The functions of marijuana abuse for adolescents. *Am. J. Drug Alcohol Abuse* **8** (4), 441–456.

[63]S. Burman (1971) Marijuana: A study of the toxicity drug reaction among adolescents. *Medical Annals of the District of Columbia* **40,** 142–144.

[64]H. Kolansky and W. Moore (1971) Effects of marijuana on adolescents and young adults. *JAMA* **216,** 486–492.

[65]W. McGlothlin and L. J. West (1968) The marijuana problem: An overview. *Am. J. Psychiatry* **125,** 126–134.

[66]D. Janowsky, D. L. Klopton, T. P. Leichner, A. A. Abrams, L. L. Judd, and R. Pechnick (1979) Interpersonal effects of marijuana: A model for the study of interpersonal psychopharmacology. *Arch. Gen. Psychiatry* **36** (7), 781–785.

[67]D. B. Kandel and K. Yamaguchi (1987) Job mobility andn drug use: An event history analysis. *Am. J. Sociol.* **92,** 836–878.

[68]K. Yamaguchi and D. B. Kandel (1985) On the resolution of role incompatibility: A life event history analysis of family roles and marijuana use. *Am. J. Sociol.* **90,** 1284–1325.

[69]D. Kandel, P. Mossel, and R. Kaestner (1987) Drug use, the transition from school to work and occupational achievement in the United States. *Euro. J. Phys. of Ed.* **II,** 337–363.

[70]C. Robbins (1989) Sex differences in psychosocial consequences of alcohol and drug abuse. *J. Health Soc. Behav.* **30,** 117–130.

[71]J. S. Brook, A. S. Gordon, A. Brook, and D. W. Brook (1989a) The consequences of marijuana use on intrapersonal and interpersonal functioning in black and white adolescents. *Genetic, Social, and General Psychology Monographs* **115,** 351–369.

Training Teachers for Substance Abuse Prevention

Susan J. Fordney and Randall M. Jones

Results of a 1986 national survey of experts in the field of alcohol and other drug abuse prevention summarized the basic information and skills thought to be necessary for teacher effectiveness in this area.[1] It was concluded that a marriage between knowledge and skills is imperative if teachers are going to make a difference with students in substance abuse prevention. Past efforts in prevention that relied solely on dissemination of factual drug information have not significantly impacted patterns of drug use.[2] Nor has teacher knowledge of drugs resulted in effective strategies for working with youth in prevention. Differences in student learning styles make the use of one type of drug prevention, such as the didactic presentation of material, unrealistic in meeting individual needs.[3] Children who may be at greater risk for substance abuse are often the same students who, because of learning deficiencies, are unable to benefit from drug prevention that is solely informative in design.

Teacher training in the early 1970s emphasized gaining knowledge of the effects or consequences (e.g., pharmacological, psychological, and behavioral) associated with various substances. Coincidentally, the primary focus of school-based prevention activities during this period was drug education (i.e., if students were more knowledgeable, they would change their behavior). Hence, the argument that teachers needed drug education in order to teach it was both logical and timely.[4] As evidence accumulated, prevention specialists documented the effectiveness of this approach in increasing drug-related knowledge, while simultaneously affecting attitudes in the desired direction. The underlying assumption linking knowledge and attitudes to behavior, however, has eluded empirical support—knowledge and attitude shifts failed to impact behavior.[5-8]

How, then, is having information about drugs and related material helpful to the teacher and ultimately to the students? Knowledge may provide the teacher with increased confidence to broach the subject of drugs in the classroom. It is unlikely that educators will want to bring up a topic for discussion about which they have little knowledge and understanding. It would seem then that teachers who are adequately informed about drugs and other pertinent material will have more credibility with students who frequently know more about drugs than teachers.

In general, it may be useful for the teacher to be familiar with commonly used drug types and their effects. Understanding and awareness of the historical and sociological perspectives of drug use patterns can help the teacher to be less narrow and judgmental in presenting drug information. Consequently, students may be better able to assess objectively current influences that impact their decisions to use or not use drugs. Knowledge of community resources that can assist classroom efforts in prevention is essential.[9] Hopefully, teachers who are able to integrate state-of-the-art prevention concepts and relevant learning experiences into existing curricula increase the likelihood that the message will be heard.

Training in those skills that help teachers to identify students who may be experiencing problems with drugs or who are at risk of abusing drugs is necessary given the realities of today's classrooms. This training, however, must be predicated on the assurance that teachers have the required knowledge of existing resources and procedures to address the topic adequately. Identifying students who are in trouble, but having no idea of how to be helpful, creates impossible dilemmas in the lives of teachers.

Lastly, understanding of how health-enhancing behavior patterns in combination with other prevention strategies contribute to drug abuse resistance is another important component of substance abuse prevention.[10] Teachers who possess this knowledge are more apt to share this information with students and create classroom experiences that reinforce healthy behavior.

Characteristics of Teachers Effective in Prevention

Having briefly reviewed some of the knowledge helpful to teachers in substance abuse prevention, a discussion of the characteristics and skills required of the teacher to take this information and make it relevant for students seems pertinent. Most of these skills are behaviors that should be seen in any quality educator.

From the student perspective:

> Good teachers are able to go beyond academics. They realize the powerful effect of the psychological climate in their classrooms. They understand the developmental level of their students. They appreciate the young adolescents' sensitivity to their interpersonal relationships with adults. They interact with their students with warmth, genuineness, empathy, acceptance, and understanding. The preferred teacher creates a psychologically supportive climate in his (or her) classroom. He conveys a sense of empathy, of caring about students' needs (sometimes beyond academics). He is perceived as being fair showing neither favoritism nor prejudice. He respects his students and knows them well, gives appropriate assignments, is accepting of their efforts, and grades fairly from the students' viewpoint. He communicates well, explains things well, listens well, and makes himself available to students. And, he is thought of as good-humored, nonthreatening, easy-to-talk-to, and nice.[11]

The preceding student profile of the "ideal" teacher is not discrepant from our notion of the "ideal" prevention educator. For both, the teacher is aware of and respects individual differences and needs. This stance is communicated consistently by an interpersonal style that exudes warmth, genuineness, empathy, acceptance, understanding, respect, fairness, courtesy, and concern for others. Teachers who meet these criteria will have a greater impact upon student decisions to use and abuse substances than teachers who believe their role is simply one of transmitting information, whether they're involved in prevention education or not. Skills that promote a positive student-teacher relationship also foster a classroom climate where it is permissible to be oneself and express one's views in a context that is nonjudgmental and respectful. Good teachers exude acceptance of self and others by demonstrating a willingness to listen without judgment, and by sharing appropriate feelings and thoughts that contribute to the learning experience. Teachers must be willing to examine their own values, attitudes, and behaviors in regard to substance abuse prior to entering the classroom.

Learning Appropriate Teacher-Student Communication

Effective communication skills are critical if educators are going to be able to engage students in meaningful discussions and activities that complement substance abuse prevention. Some of these skills are the same facilities needed by students to strengthen a position of self-control among peers and other influences. Teachers who are congruent and model the behaviors they are trying to develop in their students are more likely to influence the behaviors of students than those who say one thing but do another.[12]

What communication skills are we talking about and how do they relate to substance abuse prevention? Language factors are important. The actual words used by the teacher affect student response. For example, teachers who use personal pronouns make it clear that they are expressing their own beliefs and thoughts. Contrast, "Everyone knows that kids who use drugs are weak and have low self-esteem," with, "I believe that drug use may be a way of avoiding uncomfortable feelings." Which of these statements are students more apt to hear and respond to? The first sounds judgmental, and either insists on agreement or sets up defensiveness. The latter is clearly a personal opinion and seems to invite others to share their opinions and/or beliefs. Self-talk appears to be an important predictor of behavior.[13] Encouraging students to use language that reinforces the idea that the responsibility for their beliefs, attitudes, and behavior lies with them is important in substance abuse prevention. Oftentimes when drug users talk about their reasons for use, they speak as though these behaviors are outside of their control and not a consequence of personal choice. Careful selection of language reinforces personal responsibility for thoughts, feelings, and actions. The use of open-ended questions—questions that cannot be answered with a simple yes or no—are powerful in the discussion of life issues, such as drug use. When a student is asked a question such as, "What does that mean for you?" an opportunity is created to reflect and come closer to self-understanding in a particular area.

Connecting with children means that teachers are able to give feedback to students in a manner that is objective and steers away from personal assaults.[14] This is important in substance abuse prevention, since many adolescents stop listening when they feel judged. Students are more apt to explore their beliefs and feelings if they are acknowledged in the classroom.[15] Teachers can do this by showing that they have heard what a student has said by paraphrasing the student's remarks. It is important not to analyze a student's statements or create solutions for the individual. This may rob the student of the opportunity for self-exploration, and the development of critical thinking and problem-solving skills that are necessary for personal growth and development as well as drug prevention.

Fostering Student Growth and Development

It is not enough, however, to be a good communicator and to develop a classroom climate that is conducive to learning and positive interaction. Teachers must also create for students specific learning opportunities, and activities for cognitive, social, and emotional development. We know from research in substance abuse prevention that feeling good about oneself and having knowledge of drug effects is not enough to promote abstinence.[16] It is through the development of life skills that the young person is empowered to move effectively in the world. Skills, such as values clarification, problem solving, decision making, and communication, in the context of accurate information and a supportive environment help students to make choices that are healthy.

Modeling Healthy Attitudes and Choices

The teacher as a role model is an important contribution to prevention.[17] By demonstrating respect, genuineness, honesty, and personal self-care, teachers may influence their students to follow suit. If the act of teaching is one of love and self-expression, it may convey the most powerful message teachers can send to their students. This type of behavior relays an attitude that, "I count—my work and life have meaning. I find joy in being in the classroom. I like to work with young people." Students who are most at risk of abusing drugs, or who are already doing so, frequently lack meaning in their own lives and question their self-worth. Teachers who, through their own behavior, demonstrate an appreciation for life and for each individual are critical for effective school-based prevention efforts.

Preparing Teachers for Larger Roles in Student Lives

What does this mean for teacher-education programs? If the problem of drugs is relevant for schools and if the teacher is a potentially powerful factor in substance abuse prevention, what then should be done in the training of teachers to best prepare them for this role? Historically, when there was a new area of emphasis thought to be important for teacher preparation, often a single course was developed. This may not be feasible or desirable in many colleges of education. Basic prevention content and skills are more effectively transmitted to students when integrated into appropriate coursework throughout the entire teacher-preparation program.[18] Substance abuse education is complex and requires an interdisciplinary approach that incorporates elements of psychology, pharmacology, sociology and counseling techniques among others.[19] Public school classrooms are in desperate need of teachers who are broadly trained and who have developed effective interpersonal skills to work with youth. All of this training need not take place in specific courses. Student teachers can benefit from increased exposure to youth and real-life experiences in the classroom. They must become involved with children early in their training in order to assess how well they enjoy the challenge of teaching. Field experiences, seminars, volunteer programs, and computer-based instruction are possible avenues for bridging the gap between teacher training and classroom reality.

Providing a Knowledge Base

Student teachers must become aware of the extent of the drug problem and other related risk behaviors, relevant research, and state-of-the-art prevention strategies. Much of this can be handled through traditional teaching methods, such as lecture, outside readings, and guest speakers. Relevant content can be integrated into introductory course work, but should not be delivered without taking into consideration the previously mentioned attitudes and behaviors of an effective teacher. Just as the public-school teacher is not likely to make a difference in substance abuse prevention without using well-developed interpersonal skills, a college-level teacher educator will be much less effective without a foundation in communication.

Given the numbers of children who are using drugs or who are impacted by families where substance abuse is a problem, it is imperative that student teachers receive training in identification and referral skills. Be-

Substance Abuse Prevention

cause of such problems as drug abuse, teenage pregnancy, dropouts, and poverty, schools and teachers are faced with the critical challenge of interfacing with a range of community resources. The training for how to refer students to appropriate services and utilize these resources should begin in teacher-education programs.[20]

Obviously, if faculty members are going to deliver this type of training, they need to develop these skills as well. Teacher-education programs that combine classroom content with actual observation, real classroom dilemmas about drug-related problems, and case studies of at-risk youth in classroom settings prepare potential teachers for some of the "real" situations that occur in today's schools.

Supporting Innovative Teaching Methods and Interactions

A variety of instructional approaches in prevention are needed in classrooms today. Many of our youth at risk for substance abuse and other problem behaviors do not respond well to traditional teaching methodology.[21] These children often do better in cooperative learning environments where peer leadership is utilized. Interpersonal relationships form the basis of learning in the classroom. Student teachers need to be trained in those skills that empower them to interact effectively with a wide variety of personalities among children, peers, administrators, and parents. Some of the most promising prevention programs are peer-led,[22] and student teachers need study and practice in how to implement these learning situations in the classroom. The skills developed by students in these types of learning experiences are extremely important in substance abuse prevention, even if the content is not specific to drugs.

Wise choices about drug use require critical-thinking abilities. Prospective teachers need instruction and practice throughout their training in activities and interactional strategies that increase the opportunities for young students to think critically.

Encourage Self-Examination by Students and Faculty

Individuals aspiring to become teachers must also be willing to explore their own values. Teacher-education programs need to assist students in self-exploration of personal choices regarding drug use. If this is true for students in teacher-preparation programs, it goes without saying that college instructors must be willing to develop these skills and self-understandings if they are to be effective role models for prospective teachers. Just as we ask young people to examine attitudes and values regarding drug use, it is important for teachers in training to explore their own. Typically, little time is spent in teacher-education programs to raise awareness of values—most critically those values that may get in the way of being able to work effectively with children who are of different cultural backgrounds, beliefs, and values. Teacher educators must create experiences in which prospective teachers are required to demonstrate empathy and tolerance for individual differences.

If teachers are to make a difference in substance abuse prevention—and we believe they can—they must receive the most relevant training from mentors who model the skills they are teaching. Teacher educators must demonstrate in their attitudes, beliefs, and most importantly their behavior what they expect to see in their students. They must create experiences for student teachers to be exposed to children and actual classrooms early in their training. They must involve these future teachers in practice activities that simulate classroom methods and contribute to student development in skills and knowledge supportive of prevention and healthy lifestyles.

No doubt, the issue of teacher training cannot be resolved until:

1. The educational system recognizes that substance abuse is a serious problem for our society at large, and more specifically, a barrier to quality education (i.e., student substance use and abuse reduces the effectiveness of the schools in accomplishing their primary objectives);
2. Schools, and more importantly, teachers unite in a concerted and committed effort focused upon eradicating substance use; and
3. Successful school programs are recognized, rewarded, and publicized. In lieu of achieving these goals, teacher training for substance abuse prevention will probably run a gamut that parallels the plethora of packaged curricula, often yielding little or no impact on student substance use and abuse.[24-26]

Fortunately, we are moving in the right direction. There is clearly heightened public awareness concerning substance use and associated problems as evidenced by the 1987, 1988, and 1989 Gallup polls, which revealed that "use of drugs" was the most important issue facing public schools. Federal monies for "drug-free schools" have clued the educational system as to its role in prevention. In addition, the federally funded regional centers are promoting "school team" trainings to address the nature and extent of the problem, to foster team cohesiveness through team-building activities, and to teach the basic elements of action planning such that school teams can identify school-specific problems, produce a sequenced plan of action, and monitor the effectiveness of their efforts. As these initiatives progress, it is imperative that school programs share their successes and failures so all schools can benefit. In the meantime, efforts to train teachers in prevention education would probably do well to parallel efforts to train teachers who are effective in general.

References

[1] R. M. Jones and J. E. Organist (1987) *Smith Substance Abuse Education Project Teacher Characteristics and Skills Identification: Implications for Curriculum Modification Within the College of Education* (University of Arizona, AZ), unpublished manuscript.

[2] G.F. Jaker (1985) *Lessons Learned: A Review of the Research in Drug Education* (Minnesota Prevention Resource Center, MN).

[3] R. H. Blum, E. Blum, and E. Garfield (1976) *Drug Education: Results and Recommendations* (D. C. Heath and Company).

[4] R. F. Aubrey (1971) Drug education: Can teachers really do the job? *Teachers College Record* **72,** 417–422.

[5] S. Eisman, J. Robinson, and V. Zapata (1984) A multi-disciplinary approach for teacher effectiveness training in drug education. *Journal of Drug Education* **14,** 4, 357–367.

[6] M.S. Goodstat (1986) School-based drug education in North America: What is wrong? What can be done? *J. Sch. Health* **56,** 7, 278–281.

[7] R. Jessor (1986) Predicting time of onset of marijuana use: A developmental study of high school youth. *J. Consult. Clin. Psychol.* **44,** 125–134.

[8] K. Pickens (1985) Drug education: The effects of giving information. *Journal of Alcohol and Drug Education* **30,** 3, 32–44.

[9] R. H. Blum, E. Blum, and E. Garfield (1976) *Drug Education: Results and Recommendations* (D. C. Heath and Company).

[10] C. L. Perry and R. Jessor (1985) The concept of health promotion and the prevention of adolescent drug use. *Health Ed. Q.* **12,** 2, 169–184.

[11] L. Veaco and C. Brandon (1986) The preferred teacher: A content analysis of young adolescents' writings. *Journal of Early Adolescence* **6,** 3, 221–229.

[12] R. E. Calmes (1984) Teachers as models in the middle and secondary schools. *Journal of Early Adolescence* **4(3),** 199–202.

[13] D. Meichenbaum (1979) *Cognitive Behavior Modification: An Integrative Approach,* Plenum, NY.

[14]S. Miller, D. Woekman, E. Numally, and C. Saline (1982) *Straight Talk: A New Way to Get Closer to Others by Saying What You Really Mean* (Publishers, Inc), The New American Library, NY.

[15]R. R. Carkhuff and B. G. Berenson (1976) *Teaching as Treatment: An Introduction to Counseling to Psychotherapy*, Human Resource Development Press, Inc., Amherst, Mass.

[16]G. F. Jaker (1985) *Lessons Learned: A Review of the Research in Drug Education* (Minnesota Prevention Resource Center, MN).

[17]A. Bandura (1977) *Social Learning Theory* (Prentice-Hall, Englewood Cliffs, NJ).

[18]H. J. Cornacchia, D. E. Smith, and D. J. Bentel (1978) *Drugs in the Classroom: A Conceptual Model* (C. V. Mosby, St. Louis, MO).

[19]D. R. Crippen (1983) Substance use-abuse and cognitive learning: Suggested approaches to viable drug education programs. *Journal of Instructional Psychology* **10(2)**, 74–82.

[20]J. V. Hamby and L. J. Shirley (1988) The role of teacher educators in at-risk youth issues. (Paper presented Teacher Education Conference, Myrtle Beach, SC).

[21]M. S. Goodstat (1986) School-based drug education in North America: What is wrong? What can be done? *J. Sch. Health* **56**, 7, 278–281.

[22]C. Perry, C. Klepp, A. Halper, K. Hawkins, and D. Murray (1986) A process evaluation study of peer leaders in health education. *J. Health Ed.* **56**, 62–67.

[23]G. J. Botvin (1983) Prevention of adolescent substance abuse through development of personal and social competence, in *Preventing Adolescent Drug Abuse: Intervention Strategies* (T. J. Glynn, C. G. Leukefeld, and J. P. Ludford, eds.), Monograph 47, National Institute on Drug Abuse Research, Rockville, MD.

[24]J. M. Moskowitz (1983) Preventing adolescent substance abuse through development of personal and social competence, in *Preventing Adolescent Drug Abuse: Intervention Strategies* (T. J. Glynn, C. G. Leukefeld, and J. P. Ludford, eds.), Monograph 47, National Institute on Drug Abuse Research, Rockville, MD.

[25]E. Schaps, R. DiBartolo, J. M. Moskowitz, C. S. Palley, and S. Churgin (1981) A review of 127 drug abuse prevention program evaluations. *J. Drug Issues* **11**, 17–43.

Adolescent Alcohol and Drug Treatment Outcome

Sandra A. Brown, Mariam A. Mott, and Mark G. Myers

Adolescent Alcohol and Drug Treatment Outcome

In recent years there has been a dramatic rise in the national concern over youth alcohol and drug use. Along with this enhanced awareness of adolescent alcohol and drug use has come a substantial increase in the number of treatment programs available for adolescent substance abusers. Teens in treatment all report a history of heavy alcohol use, but the vast majority use drugs in addition to alcohol. Often, it is this overlay of hard drug use and abuse that brings the teen's problems to the attention of others who initiate the treatment process. Thus, in contrast to other chapters in this alcohol-focused text, our examination of teen treatment outcome focuses on the composite of alcohol and drug abuse.

Despite the recent proliferation of adolescent alcohol and drug treatment programs, limited empirical data exists on clinical samples of teens in treatment, and even less is known about the long-term course for adolescents following treatment for substance abuse. A great deal is known about adult alcohol and drug abuse treatment outcome; however, this knowledge is only generally related to treatment or prognosis for adolescents, because teens are differentially impacted by substance abuse and dependence.

Further, adolescents are in the process of mastering different developmental tasks compared to adults.

Our knowledge of alcohol and drug use in the general adolescent population is also expanding, providing a better understanding of risk factors associated with initiation of alcohol and drug use and abuse among youth. However, findings from adolescent school samples cannot be easily generalized to substance-abusing adolescents in treatment. The majority of adolescents who enter alcohol and drug treatment programs often fail to attend school and experience frequent suspension or expulsion. Consequently, teens with the most disruptive alcohol and drug use patterns may be underrepresented in national studies examining junior high and high school populations. Additionally, alcohol and drug problems with an early onset severe enough to warrant treatment suggests there may be differences in the course of use and abuse for these teens relative to adolescents able to maintain their participation in school. Further, the consequences of multiple drug use may emerge relatively quickly, whereas the effects of heavy alcohol use may take longer to manifest themselves.

What is perhaps one of the most difficult methodological problems in this area is the lack of consensus regarding what constitutes problem drinking or drug use for teens. New assessment procedures specific to adolescents are being developed, but definitions of problem use have been derived most often from measures designed for adults and have varied across studies, thereby restricting comparisons. Although many researchers (e.g.,[1]) recommend simultaneous consideration of drug use when studying adolescent alcohol use and abuse, often research continues to measure alcohol use in isolation.

With these caveats in mind, the present chapter will address several theoretical and methodological issues related to the study of treatment outcome for teen problem drinking and drug use. The review of the literature in the area also draws on data from nonclinical adolescent reports and adult treatment outcome studies because of the limited data available on adolescent treatment outcome. The first section of the chapter will provide an overview of theoretical and methodological issues pertinent to the assessment of adolescent treatment outcome. The second section presents a discussion of our research on adolescent alcohol and drug abuse treatment outcome, with a particular focus on several domains considered important in the study of such outcome for teens. Along with alcohol and drug use following treatment, we will consider social functioning, psychosocial stress, coping skills, overall emotional health, family interaction, and functioning in school and work.

Teen Treatment Outcome Studies

Most of the data available for teen treatment outcome was collected at a time when few drug and alcohol treatment programs were designed specifically for adolescent clients. A survey by the National Institute of Drug Abuse[2] estimated that approx 20% of those in treatment for alcohol or drug abuse in the US were 19 yr old or younger and found that only 5% of the programs surveyed had teens comprising more than 50% of their clientele. Beschner and Friedman[3] note that since few residential alcohol and drug treatment programs are specifically designed for adolescents, teens are likely to receive the same treatment as adults. With the increase of drug-involved teenagers from the middle and upper socioeconomic levels, newly established programs have been created to more specifically address the age-related needs of adolescents. Despite advertising a broad range of therapeutic services, the policies of these programs appear to reflect a lack of scientific evidence regarding optimal therapeutic combinations for treating chemically dependent adolescents.[4]

Among the few systematic attempts to evaluate which methods are most effective in treating adolescent drug abusers, the three largest studies[5-7] are descriptive in nature. Sells and Simpson[5] analyzed information collected by the Drug Abuse Reporting Program (DARP) on 5,406 adolescents four to six yr following admission to treatment using an "intake only" group for comparison. The DARP programs were targeted to adult opioid abusers; therefore, the extent to which efforts were made to specifically reduce alcohol or other drug use is not clear. Significant reductions in the use of opiates and criminal activities were reported across the treatment environments surveyed. However, findings from this sample indicated that adolescents still used alcohol and marijuana extensively one year following treatment. In particular, Black teens were reported to increase their level of marijuana use, and the level of such use remained constant among Anglo teens. Additionally, alcohol use appeared to increase slightly among Black 18- and 19-yr-olds.

Another large scale descriptive study of adolescent treatment programs was conducted by Rush.[6] Using data from the Pennsylvania Data Collection System on 4,738 teens, Rush examined variables potentially predictive of treatment outcome at discharge, comparing residential therapeutic communities with Drug-Free Outpatient Programs (DFOPs). A composite score based on education, training, and employment was used as an outcome measure labeled "productivity." For teens in residential therapeutic communities, a greater length of time in treatment was the greatest predictor of improvement in productivity, whereas time in treatment was negatively related to productivity gains for adolescents in the DFOPs. Rush concluded that those who remain longer in outpatient treatment are more likely to have more severe problems and are less capable of achieving gains in productivity. The residential therapeutic community adolescents had been more heavily involved in drug use and criminal activities prior to entering treatment than those in the DFOPs, thus limiting conclusions that can be drawn regarding the efficacy of the different treatment modalities.

Hubbard and colleagues[7] conducted the third major study of adolescent treatment outcome. Two-hundred forty adolescents in six cities were interviewed one year posttreatment for the Treatment Outcome Prospective Study (TOPS). Comparisons were made between residential and outpatient programs for adolescents who remained in treatment at least three mo. Teens who participated in residential programs reported better one-yr outcomes in that daily marijuana use dropped sharply (79% prior to treatment vs 12% at the one-yr followup), and heavy alcohol use decreased, as did involvement in illegal activities. Comparisons of pretreatment with one-year followup information from teens who were treated in DFOPs revealed less involvement in criminal activity following treatment and fewer heavy alcohol users, but showed a greater percentage of daily marijuana users (58% posttreatment compared to 48% pretreatment).

A more recent survey was aimed at examining client characteristics associated with successful treatment.[8] Friedman and his colleagues analyzed data for over 5000 adolescents treated in outpatient clinics and reported that length of time in treatment, being White, fewer previous admissions, and having a primary drug problem other than marijuana significantly predicted posttreatment reduction in drug use.

The relatively positive outcomes reported in the aforementioned studies must be viewed with caution. These studies are by and large descriptive, with no control or comparison groups, and provide limited information on reliability. Further, the data selected for examination are generally designed to evaluate adult treatment programs, and thus may fail to include variables important to the understanding of adolescent outcome. In addition, some of the data come from older teens who participated in adult treatment programs, thus limiting relevance to current adolescent programs that attempt to provide services better tailored to the needs and developmental level of younger abusing teens. Given the important cognitive, social, and emotional differences across adolescent age groups (e.g., 14- and 15-yr-olds vs

18- and 19-yr-olds), the applicability of these findings to all adolescents in treatment for alcohol and drug use is questionable at best. Overall however, the treatment programs studied appear to reduce hard drug use among teens but have a more limited impact on levels of alcohol and marijuana use.

Little attention has been directed to client-treatment matching among adolescent alcohol and drug abusers (an area just underway in adult populations), but two Scandinavian studies have investigated client characteristics of teens which are related to outcome following substance abuse treatment. Holston[9] found that an absence of legal problems in the year preceding first treatment, no alcohol problems at the time of first treatment, being female, coming from a broken home, and lack of an alcoholic father during the teen's childhood accounted for 25% of the outcome variance at one to six year following treatment. Taking a different approach, Benson[10] examined teens who continued alcohol and drug use following treatment. In this study, relapsing adolescent males tended to display more truancy, whereas female relapsers more commonly had one or more alcoholic parents, and all relapsers deviated more from school careers than abstainers.

In sum, adolescent alcohol and drug treatment outcome research is currently in its infancy. As is typical of studies in a new area, investigations to date have generally been descriptive rather than controlled investigations, and may have reported findings based on measures derived from adults rather than assessment instruments developed specifically for an adolescent population. There is a great need for controlled studies with well-defined treatment protocols examining teen-specific pretreatment and posttreatment outcome variables. These studies would allow clearer understanding of the clinical course for adolescent treatment samples and the investigation of client-treatment matching utility among teens.

Lessons from Adult Alcoholism Treatment Outcome

Given the dearth of studies on adolescent treatment outcome, most of the current alcoholism treatment outcome information available comes from studies of adult treatment. The limitations regarding generalizability noted above prohibit direct application of adult findings to adolescents, but the results from adult studies provide a unique opportunity for comparison, and have fostered theoretical development in the field of treatment outcome research in general. Further, adult studies have examined in more detail the efficacy of alcoholism treatment and the relationship of pre- and posttreatment variables to outcome.

Adult alcoholism treatment success, when measured as abstinence from drinking, has typically been modest. One-year abstinence rates range from 25% or less for chronic alcoholics seen at public treatment facilities, to 50% or better for subchronic alcoholics treated in private treatment facilities.[11] Longitudinal studies of alcoholic adults have typically focused on the effects of pretreatment patient characteristics and treatment variables on posttreatment drinking outcomes. Patient characteristics indicative of higher functioning are generally most predictive of positive treatment outcomes, with research suggesting that younger, married, employed professionals achieve greater levels of abstinence following treatment (e.g.,[12,13]). Other predictors noted across studies of adult alcoholism treatment outcome include more limited initial symptomatology and psychopathology (particularly, level of dependence and antisocial personality disorder; e.g.,[14]), better social support systems (e.g.,[15]), fewer neuropsychological deficits, and affective problems such as depression (e.g.,[16]), and more recently, coping skills (e.g.,[17,18]) and alcohol reinforcement expectancies (e.g.,[19,20]). Among adults in treatment for alcohol dependence, abuse, or dependence on other drugs tends to be associated with poorer prognosis.[21,22] The above associations are particularly noteworthy with respect to adolescents in that most teens in treatment are polydrug abusers,[23] and there appears to be a higher incidence of concomitant psychopathology and family dysfunction among teen abusers than among adults (e.g.,[24–26]).

In concert, the above noted predictors of treatment outcome account for only a modest portion of outcome variance. Estimates range from 10–30% of outcome variance predicted by pretreatment factors (e.g.,[18]). Consequently, posttreatment environmental factors have also been examined in an attempt to improve the prediction of adult alcoholism treatment outcome. Billings and Moos[18] reported that alcoholics abstinent following treatment experience fewer psychosocial stressors and use more cognitive and behavioral coping strategies than relapsed alcoholics. More recently, Brown and colleagues[27] reported that highly threatening and chronic stressors significantly increase risk for relapse. Recovering alcoholics have also been found to make more effective use of coping strategies and social supports to successfully manage the posttreatment stressful life events that they face.[15,28]

In sum, treatment outcome studies focusing on adult alcoholic populations suggest that outcome varies depending on the population studied and the definition of successful outcome. Studies to date show no advantage of inpatient treatment over outpatient treatment despite great differences in cost,[29] yet it is not clear that such studies are examining the same populations (i.e., type of treatment may relate to severity of alcohol dependence). Although patient characteristics are found to relate to treatment outcome, there is little agreement among investigators on the best approach to measure some of these variables (e.g., level of motivation). Overall, despite a greater volume of research on adult alcoholics, a variety of methodological problems limit the confidence with which conclusions can be drawn.

Clinical Features of Adolescent Abusers

Outcome results for adults give direction to adolescent abuse research, but there are several reasons why generalization to adolescents may be misleading. First, in adult alcoholism outcome studies, use of illegal drugs is typically associated with poorer prognosis (e.g.,[30]); however, virtually all teens in treatment use multiple drugs. For example, 55% of the adolescents in one investigation reported primary marijuana use, whereas alcohol was the secondary substance of abuse for 33% of adolescents entering drug treatment programs.[3] Other investigators find that teen alcohol and marijuana abusers also used more than three other substances regularly,[31] and that teens in treatment are typically using three different drugs immediately prior to treatment entry.[23] Second, alcohol and drug dependence among adolescents may have different developmentally salient features and maintenance characteristics than adults. For example, motivation for use may differ[32] and pretreatment dependence symptomatology may have a more restricted range in the adolescent population since the medical effects of chronic alcohol/drug abuse are seldom observed. Third, adolescents may have less control over posttreatment experiences or resources compared to adults (e.g., being sent to residential treatment programs, financial dependence on parents/guardians). Fourth, influential factors such as exposure to life stressors and vulnerability to social and physical consequences may vary with age and biological as well as social developmental stages. Thus, although teens are less likely to experience severe medical consequences compared to adults, they may be more likely to have disrupted the educational process, thereby limiting long-term career options.[33]

Another significant difference between adolescent and adult abusers emerges in studies of relapse. Although relapse rates may appear comparable for teens and adults, the process of relapse may be quite different.[23,34] Adult relapse to a variety of addictive behaviors is typically preceded by negative affect, interpersonal conflict, or social pressure (e.g.,[35,36]). In contrast, a recent study of substance abusing teens in treatment[23] finds a majority of teen relapses occurring in the face of social pressure, with limited reference to negative emotional states. This finding highlights a difference in relapse precipitants between teens and adults, and suggests that relapse prevention efforts for teens must consider the unique aspects of their experience.

Similarly, the study of teen alcohol and drug abuser coping skills has just begun, and further highlights the importance of the independent study of treatment outcome for adults and adolescents. For example, in an investigation of perceived efficacy of various coping options, Brown and Stetson[37] identified differences between adolescent and parent views of how teens should cope with pressure to drink alcohol. Additionally, the use of cognitive coping strategies has been associated with abstinence in adults (e.g.,[17,35]), but not in teenagers. Cognitive coping efforts have not emerged as more prevalent among adolescent abstainers following treatment.[38] Instead, a study of self-generated coping responses to a high risk relapse situation[34] found that behavioral strategies that appear to be useful in social pressure situations best discriminate abstaining from relapsing teens. Thus, teens, perhaps by virtue of differences in development or exposure to different relapse risk situations, appear to utilize fewer cognitive coping strategies and more behavioral coping efforts as protection from relapse.

Other factors suggesting generational or age differences in abuse come from research indicating that adolescents may perceive alcohol reinforcement differently than do adults.[32] Anticipated reinforcement from alcohol or other drugs may play an important role in mediating decisions to drink or use following treatment (see[39] for review;[40]). Studies of expectations of the effects of consuming alcohol suggest that adolescent motivation for drinking diverges from adult motivation, and that distinct etiological factors play a role in influencing continued drinking among teens relative to adults.[40,41]

Alcohol expectancies also have demonstrated utility in predicting outcome following treatment among alcohol abusers. Brown[19] found that alcohol expectancies were related to outcome at one year following alcoholism treatment in a sample of adult male alcoholics. A consistent negative linear relationship was found between individual alcohol expectancies and measures of success following treatment, such that higher positive expectancies resulted in poorer treatment outcome. In particular, the expectancy of Tension Reduction evidenced the largest correlation with abstinence.

Similar findings have been found among adolescents following treatment for alcohol and drug abuse. Brown[40] measured alcohol expectancies among adolescents during treatment and at six months following treatment, and found that expectancies changed over time. Teens expected more enhancement of social behavior and less cognitive and motor improvement from alcohol at six months posttreatment than they reported during the treatment program. Additionally, there was a differential change across time on one expectancy, Altered Social Behavior, depending on treatment outcome. Both relapsers and abstainers reported higher social change expectancies at six months following treatment, but relapsers increased their scores to a significantly higher level over time than did abstainers. Thus, relapsing teens may be relying on alcohol to change their social functioning, whereas abstainers did not return to their former social patterns.

Each of the previously mentioned factors has been associated with outcome for adults and has only begun to be systematically investigated among clinical samples of adolescent abusers. Despite the paucity of information on the posttreatment course of addiction in adolescents, differences between adolescent and adult abuse following treatment are becoming apparent. Given such differences, it is clear that more detailed study of treatment outcome and the process of change among adolescents is merited.

Longitudinal Studies of Adolescent Drinking

Much of what is currently known about adolescent alcohol abuse comes from longitudinal studies of teens in national school samples. The degree to which the longitudinal patterns observed in the general adolescent population parallel the course of use and abuse among adolescents who receive treatment has not yet been determined. However, findings from longitudinal studies of this nature may act to highlight domains of functioning sensitive to variations in alcohol or drug use by teens.

Adolescent research implicates peer, family, sociocultural and personality factors in the onset of drinking, heavy consumption, and later problems with alcohol (e.g.,[23,25,42]). Further, as Donovan and Jessor note, other types of problem behaviors and attitudes place the adolescent "at risk" for alcohol problems during adolescence or young adulthood.[42] Longitudinal studies of adolescent alcohol use have focused predominantly on general junior and senior high school samples of adolescents. In a recent review,[43] 80 such investigations were identified, with the vast majority compromised because of methodological problems. Of the methodologically sound studies, certain patterns have emerged which indicate that age of initial use has decreased, use of cocaine and other stimulants has risen, and negative consequences of drinking have remained constant.

The recent longitudinal efforts of Newcomb and Bentler[33] highlight the multidimensional nature of the teen "drug use lifestyle" and the wide ranging patterns of use and consequences of alcohol and drug involvement for young adult functioning. In a sample of 654 teens followed for eight yr, heavy drug use during adolescence was found to be associated with a variety of negative consequences during early adulthood, including impaired social relationships and physical and psychological disturbances. Additionally, such drug use interfered with normal maturational processes prominent during this developmental period. According to Newcomb and Bentler, the consequences of adolescent alcohol use on functioning during young adulthood were less severe. Alcohol use during adolescence was reported to decrease relationship problems and property crime involvement, and increase positive affect among young adults. Further, patterns of both alcohol and other drug use were found to vary across the time intervals examined.

These results are consistent with the longitudinal findings of Kandel and colleagues.[25] These authors explored the impact of continued illicit drug use on several domains of functioning as a large cohort of high school adolescents entered into young adulthood. They found that use of a particular drug in the past was the best predictor of its future use. Additionally, illicit drugs had an impact on conventional behaviors, such as participation in major social roles. These drugs had an adverse effect on continuity of employment and marriage, and an enhancing effect on delinquency, especially participation in theft. Users of illicit drugs were also characterized by unstable work histories and higher rates of divorce. Thus, in nonclinical samples of teens, alcohol and drug use appears to fluctuate significantly over time and differ markedly in consequences during early adulthood.

The applicability of such findings to teens in treatment for alcohol- and drug-related problems is uncertain. Most teens in treatment in our studies report nonattendance at school (98%), suspension or expulsion (51%), or dropping out of school (40%), and therefore may be underrepresented in school samples. Additionally, an early onset of drug and alcohol problems of sufficient severity to merit treatment suggests there may be differences in the course of abuse or consequences in late adolescence and young adulthood in treatment samples compared to teens not receiving treatment. Whereas the consequences of adolescent drug use may be evident in a few years (in young adulthood), effects of heavy alcohol use may be slower to emerge and thus not appear in surveys of school age adolescents or young adults. In fact, the peak risk period for onset of recurrent major life problems resulting from alcohol does not appear until the third decade of life. Finally, fluctuations in drinking patterns are not uncommon among adults, even adult alcoholics.[44] Thus, longitudinal studies in the general adolescent population provide possible direction for the examination of the clinical course for substance abusing teens, but these results may not be directly applicable to adolescent treatment populations.

Methodological Issues

In addition to the aforementioned problems with outcome literature on adolescent alcohol and drug abuse treatment, several methodological issues hamper studies in this field. One difficult issue faced by researchers in the area of the addictions is that of outcome classification. Traditional models of addiction have viewed any use of alcohol or drugs following treatment as failure.

More recent multidimensional approaches to relapse (e.g.,[45]) view this process as dynamic and prefer to distinguish between lapses (i.e., isolated occurrences of substance use) and relapse (i.e., return to pattern of abusive use). Whereas quantitative measures of alcohol and drug use such as quantity and frequency of use may partially address this issue, functioning in other life domains may be equally important in understanding treatment outcome as well as the process by which adolescents are able to maintain behavioral and lifestyle changes. A variety of aspects of day-to-day functioning, including interpersonal, psychological, physical, financial, and occupational status, are expected to change as a consequence of treatment (and are targeted as areas of change in adolescent treatment programs). Unfortunately, there is currently no generally agreed upon system for defining outcome for these qualitative features, nor is there agreement as to when such qualitative aspects of functioning are best assessed. This heterogeneity in the field is reflected in disparate definitions and measures of treatment outcome, as well as considerable variability in when (at which time points) outcome is measured. The net effect of such variability is difficulty in comparing findings across treatment outcome studies.

A second related area of difficulty for outcome researchers concerns reliability and validity of treatment outcome information. Alcohol and drug abusers tend not to be good historians, which may reflect not only distortion caused by the low social desirability of some of these behaviors, but also drug-produced changes in cognitive functioning (e.g., memory impairment). Physiological measures aid in determining recent alcohol and drug intake, but retrospective recall of quantity and frequency of consumption appears to be less reliable even among adults. The use of significant others (e.g., additional resource people) to corroborate outcome and consumption information improves the validity of such data, but is still subject to retrospective recall bias. Some measures of outcome can be considered "objective" (e.g., legal problems, job difficulties, expulsion from school, and so on); however, other domains of functioning (e.g., affective state) may be more susceptible to distortion because of compromised neuropsychological functioning of alcohol and drug abusers.

A third, and often overlooked, methodological issue with regard to the study of adolescent treatment outcome is the heterogeneity of substance abusing samples. Alcohol and drug abusers often display significant symptoms of other psychiatric disorders. For example, an elevated incidence of affective disorders, anxiety disorders, and a variety of personality disorders has been reported among adult alcoholics and drug abusers in treatment.[21] Similarly, certain types of psychiatric disorders appear to be associated with alcohol and drug abuse during adolescence.[24] Although symptom patterns may change rapidly during the first few weeks of treatment,[46,47] diagnoses are most often made within a few days of entry into treatment programs. Thus, the accuracy of diagnoses may vary from study to study and the incidence of concomitant psychopathology is often difficult to compare across studies. A recent study[48] examined the frequency and severity of Conduct Disorder in a sample of teens in treatment. The authors found that conduct disorder type behaviors are highly prevalent among adolescents in treatment for substance abuse; 95% of the sample met DSM III-R criteria for Conduct Disorder. Of note, however, for a significant portion (48%) of the sample, delinquent behavior was secondary to involvement with alcohol and other drugs. There were two distinct groups of adolescents: Those with Conduct Disorder that was secondary to their drug and alcohol involvement (e.g., stealing to get money for drugs, burglarizing while under the influence), and those teens who met criteria for Conduct Disorder that was independent of substance involvement. Teens with an independent diagnosis of Conduct Disorder engaged in more deviant behaviors that have a low frequency of occurrence in the general adolescent population (e.g., cruelty to others, stealing with confrontation, and initiating fights).

It is vital to consider this heterogeneity when assessing alcohol and drug treatment outcome, since concomitant psychopathology will impact on individual functioning both in terms of creating additional risks for relapse and limiting one's ability to cope in potential relapse situations. Adolescent alcohol and drug abuse treatment outcome studies to date have often failed to consider this issue when examining clinical outcomes. Thus, selecting samples free of accompanying psychopathology or assessing and considering such heterogeneity are necessary strategies for improving teen outcome research.

The second section of this chapter summarizes findings from our longitudinal study of adolescent alcohol and drug abusers in treatment. Teens selected for inclusion in this project were consecutive admissions at three inpatient adolescent substance abuse treatment programs in southern California. Teens were screened to include those meeting DSM-III-R criteria for substance abuse or dependence. Teens were excluded from study if they met criteria for another major psychiatric disorder (e.g., major depression) prior to the onset of alcohol or drug abuse, did not have a resource person (typically parent or guardian) to provide independent corroboration of functioning, or lived more than 50 miles from the research site. After obtaining independent consent from teens and parents (or legal guardians), each family member participated in separate confidential structured interview and assessment sessions during the third week of adolescent treatment, and at six and twelve months following discharge from the inpatient program. Ninety-eight percent meeting criteria for inclusion in the study agreed to participate. Followup rates for the six- and twelve-mo assessments were 97 and 95%, respectively.

Adolescent Treatment Outcome

One question that remains largely unanswered is the extent to which treatment programs are effective for substance-abusing adolescents. In one of the few treatment outcome studies available utilizing adolescents, Brown and colleagues[23] found that nearly two-thirds of the sample (64%) relapsed during the first three months following treatment. An additional 7% had their initial relapse during the fourth through sixth month after treatment. Thus, in this study, relapse rates among adolescents were similar to those found among adults with much more extended histories of substance abuse and dependence (e.g.,[49]).

These findings have been replicated in an independent sample of adolescents in treatment for substance abuse.[50] At six month following treatment, teens were classified into one of three outcome groups. Abstainers were defined as teens who consumed no alcohol and no drugs during the six-month followup period. Minor relapsers were defined as teens who reported only transient lapses, with no more than a total of 30 d of alcohol or drug use during the six mo following treatment. Major relapsers were defined as teens who returned to heavy use or once again reported recurrent problems secondary to their alcohol or drug use. Of the original adolescents in treatment, 33% reported no alcohol or drug use in the first six months following treatment. One quarter (24%) of teens fell into the minor relapse categorgy, and 43% were considered major relapsers. Thus, the abstinence rate in this study is relatively consistent with rates observed in other adolescent treatment samples (e.g.,[23]).

As noted previously, only limited information is available regarding the characteristics of relapse situations among adolescents. In one of the few studies available utilizing adolescents, Brown and colleagues[23] examined relapse precipitants among 75 adolescents between the ages of 12 and 18. The majority of initial adolescent relapses following treatment occurred in the company of other people (90%), and 73% of the relapses contained either no abstention models or no abstention models who were considered "close" friends of the adolescent. Initial relapses typically occurred in the afternoon or evening (87%), either at a friend's house (29%), out of doors (14%), or in the teen's home (11%). The most frequently reported activity during the relapse episode was socializing (49%) but 20% of the relapses occurred when the main purpose of the gathering was alcohol or drug use. Relapse was most common while socializing with pretreatment friends (44%).

In keeping with the relapse categorization of Marlatt and Gordon,[51] relapse episodes were also scored for social pressure (i.e., direct offer of alcohol or drug), negative affective state (e.g., anger, frustration, depression), and interpersonal conflict. In contrast to the Marlatt and Gordon scoring system, which attempts to define the primary precursor to relapse, if any of these situations was evident it was scored as a precursor. Using this classification system, 60% of the adolescents reported social pressure prior to use, 33% reported a negative affective state as an immediate precursor to relapse, and interpersonal conflict was identified in 27% of relapse episodes. Thus, the social and environmental context features appear particularly salient in initial adolescent alcohol and drug relapse. Social factors appear to predominate posttreatment relapse among adolescents, both in terms of pressure to drink or use, and in provision of models of alcohol and drug use.

Posttreatment Psychosocial Functioning

Clearly, social, environmental, and psychological factors play a role in precipitating relapse among adolescent substance abusers.[23] Identifying the relative importance of these factors in treatment outcome is a first step toward targeting modifiable psychosocial domains and therefore enhancing the rate of favorable outcome. Cross-sectional and longitudinal studies of adolescents suggest a number of psychosocial domains which may be particularly relevant to the study of adolescent alcohol and drug treatment outcome. In particular, functioning with peers, psychosocial stress, coping skills, overall emotional health, family factors, and functioning in school and/or work have been associated with protracted abuse or remission of abuse. Each of these domains will be briefly reviewed below.

Social Functioning

The presence or absence of social support is a potentially important correlate of adolescent substance abuse as well as treatment outcome. Social support can be conceptualized as coping assistance,[52] or as the active participation of significant others in an individual's stress management efforts.[53] Social support might act as coping by helping the teen to change the situation, to change the meaning of the situation, to change his/her emotional reaction to the situation, or to change all three. In essence, this approach suggests that support works like coping by changing or eliminating the primary sources of threat to the individual. An individual's efforts at stress management can be supplemented and strengthened by the guiding participation of others in those efforts.[53]

There is evidence that, in the absence of adequate social supports, individuals turn to alcohol or other drugs in an attempt to cope with stress.[54,55] For example, teens with limited social support networks may find relating to others a difficult task which is alleviated or avoided through alcohol or drug use. Holden, Brown, and Mott[56] found that the number and type of social supports available to adolescents was related to both parental and teen alcohol and drug abuse status. Teens with alcoholic parents were less likely to identify their parents as a source of support than teens with nonabusing parents. This was true regardless of whether the adolescent him/herself was abusing alcohol or drugs. Teens who were themselves abusing relied on friends more, and parents less, than demographically comparable nonabusing teens. Additionally, abusing teens in this study tended to report fewer supports than nonabusing teens.

With regard to social support and treatment outcome, studies conducted among adults verify the role of social support in abstinence efforts. For example, Billings and Moos[18] reported that more supportive posttreatment environments were associated with better outcome after treatment. Brown[19] found that greater social support was related to increased length of abstinence among alcoholic veterans during the first year following treatment for alcohol problems. Likewise, Westermeyer and Peake[44] reported that poor treatment outcome was partly the result of the absence of a stable spouse or family environment.

Outcome studies utilizing adolescents also support a relationship between social resources and substance use following treatment. Vik, Grizzle, and Brown[57] found that the teen's perception of his/her social network when entering treatment was related to substance use status three mo following treatment. Teens who remained abstinent throughout the followup period typically described their social network as more supportive and less similar to themselves than teens who relapsed. This finding is important, since social factors are particularly salient in adolescent relapse, both in terms of pressure to drink or use, and in providing models of alcohol and drug use.[23]

In a more comprehensive study examining outcome six months following treatment for adolescent substance abuse, Brown and colleagues[50] found that teens who remained abstinent following treatment reported significantly more supports, as well as significantly higher satisfaction with those supports, compared to teens who returned to abusive levels of consumption. Additionally, abstainers reported new friends (friends made following treatment) as being significantly more helpful in efforts to remain abstinent following treatment than did major relapsers. Preliminary analyses examining one-yr outcome in the same sample yielded a similar pattern of a greater number of social supports, greater satisfaction with those supports, and greater perceived helpfulness of new friends for abstainers compared to teens who returned to substance abuse.

The available research on adolescent treatment outcome and social resources thus suggests that abusing adolescents are likely to have fewer social supports than nonabusing peers, and that the availability of satisfactory social supports, particularly nonabusing peers, appears to be an important correlate of success following treatment.

Psychosocial Stress

The presence of stress is another psychosocial factor that may influence the clinical course of adolescent substance abuse following treatment. While the relationship between stressful life events and alcohol treatment outcome has been well documented in the literature, the majority of studies have been conducted with adult populations.[58] These studies have shown an elevated incidence of negative life events among adult alcohol and substance abusers in treatment.[59] Further, undesirable life events have been related to relapse following treatment for alcohol and substance abuse, and to levels of depression among adult alcoholics.[18,60,61] Of note, severely threatening or chronic stress that is unrelated to alcohol use may pose particular risk for relapse among adult abusers.[27]

Far fewer studies have examined the relationship between stressful life events and substance abuse among adolescents. Pandina and Schuele[1] found a relationship between negative life events and Substance Use Inventory scores in a large sample of adolescent students and chemical dependence treatment participants. In another study, McCubbin and colleagues[62] found a significant correlation between the number of life events experienced by the family and adolescent substance abuse, even after events related to substance abuse were deleted from the analysis. A third study conducted by Duncan[63] suggested that higher levels of stress may actually precipitate alcohol and drug abuse by adolescents. Brown[58,64] has explored the relationship between stressful life events and substance use among adolescents. In one study by Brown,[58] three groups of adolescents were compared: adolescents in treat-ment for substance abuse, adolescents who had a parent in treatment for alcohol abuse, and nonabusing adolescents from the community with no family history of substance abuse. Results indicated that although all groups were comparable in the number of positive life events reported, adolescents in treatment and those with a parent in treatment had more negative life events than nonabusing teens without a family history of alcoholism. This pattern of findings was replicated in a more recent study,[64] which examined life events in relation to teen alcohol/drug use status and parent alcohol/drug use status. In this sample of 130 teens, all groups were relatively comparable in the number and subjective rating for positive life events. However, abusing teens reported more negative life events, and rated those stressful experiences a more undesirable, than nonabusing teens.

The evidence thus suggests a relationship between negative life events and substance abuse among adolescents, even when controlling for sociodemographic differences across groups. Since the data are correlational, however, it is impossible to determine the extent to which stressors precede substance abuse or are concomitants of abuse, or whether substance abuse precipitates certain life stressors. One way to clarify the relation of psychosocial stress and teen abuse is to examine life events that occur independently of alcohol or drug use following treatment. If relapsing adolescents report more negative life events that are independent of their substance use than do abstaining teens, this would support the hypothesis that stressful events may act to precipitate a return to substance use. Conversely, if relapsing and abstaining teens report a comparable number of negative life events that are independent of substance use, the hypothesis that abuse promotes stressful life events would be supported.

As part of an ongoing longitudinal study, we examined the relationship between life events and outcome at six months following treatment for adolescent substance abuse. It has been noted[27] that research exploring the relationship between life events and outcome has typically been confounded by the failure to separate out stressful events that are related to alcohol or drug use. Consequently, we eliminated from analyses events that were definitely or probably related to adolescents' posttreatment substance use, and compared the number and subjective ratings of life events in three outcome groups: abstainers, teens who experienced only transient alcohol or drug use episodes (minor relapsers), and teens who returned to heavy or abusive levels of substance use following treatment (major relapsers).

Abstainers reported more positive life changes than teens returning to heavy drug use (major relapsers). There were also significant group differences for the number of negative life events experienced following treatment, but, contrary to expectation, major relapsers reported fewer negative life events than abstainers. Thus, at six mo following treatment, abstaining teens report a greater number of stressful life events in general than do major relapsers. Although the reason for this finding is unclear, it may be that abstainers are going through several psychosocial changes, both positive and negative (e.g., more changes in peer relations; more changes in daily or social activities), as a function of remaining abstinent. In contrast, the posttreatment functioning of major relapsers may be less disrupted, since they have generally returned to their pretreatment patterns of social functioning and patterns of abuse.

Coping

As noted previously, coping factors have been hypothesized to play a central role in the addiction relapse process.[65,66] The cognitive-behavioral model of relapse[51] posits that certain situations increase the probability of relapse. High-risk relapse situations are those appraised as stressful (primary appraisal), and for which the person's coping resources may be inadequate (secondary appraisal). This model and others[45,55] further suggest that drug or alcohol use may be a strategy used to cope with stressful situations. Thus, a poverty of coping responses may lead to secondary appraisal of increased threat or demand in a high risk situation, and therefore, a greater likelihood of alcohol or other drug use. Specifically, relapse is conceptualized as a response to emotional discomfort (emotion focused coping) caused by the high-risk situation.[66] This approach suggests that a larger coping repertoire, including both problem-focused and emotion-focused strategies, would reduce the overall appraisal of stress by providing methods of managing the situation and enabling utilization of a response other than drug or alcohol use.[51]

Recently, Myers and Brown[34,38] examined coping efforts of substance abusing adolescents in relapse situations following treatment. Six months after treatment for substance abuse, adolescents described the most stressful situation in which they successfully abstained from drinking and drug use. The teens also rated a hypothetical situation which was previously identified as a common relapse precipitant for adolescent alcohol and drug abusers.[23] As expected, the teen outcome groups did not differ in appraisal of difficulty or type of coping employed (problem- and emotion-focused coping) in the self-generated high-risk situation in which all teens successfully abstained. However, significant appraisal and problem-focused coping response differences were reported for the hypothetical high-risk situation. Teens with better outcomes (i.e., abstainers and minor relapsers) viewed the hypothetical situation as more stressful, and reported more problem-focused efforts, than did major relapsers. Thus, teens did not differ in their coping efforts when they appraised a personal relapse risk situation as stressful, but displayed both primary appraisal and coping differences in standardized risk situations. The authors noted that these findings support the cognitive-behavioral model of relapse.[38] Specifically, teens with better outcomes following treatment have a heightened vigilance for relapse risk as well as more flexibility in their coping repertoire.

Emotional Health

Overall emotional functioning is an additional factor that may be related to adolescent substance use, as well as to successful outcome following treatment. However, to date, little research is available examining emotional and psychological functioning and outcome among clinical samples of substance abusing teens. As part of an ongoing longitudinal study, we examined these areas of functioning in our sample of substance-abusing adolescents at six months[50] and one year following treatment. Emotional difficulties following treatment (e.g., emotional or psychological problems requiring hospitalization; significant psychiatric major depressive episode or incapacitating anxiety) and self-esteem were examined in relation to alcohol and drug use outcome.

There were no significant differences across the three outcome groups (abstainers, minor relapsers, and major relapsers) for a composite measure of emotional difficulties six months and one year following treatment. The absence of a significant finding may be due to the overall low frequency in our sample of the more serious psychological symptoms, given the exclusion of concomitant psychopathology within the sample of teens selected for study. There were, however, significant differences in self-esteem following treatment. Teens who returned to heavy or abusive drinking and/or drug use reported significantly lower self-esteem than either abstainers or minor relapsers.

Our finding of posttreatment differences in self-esteem is especially noteworthy, since the three outcome groups reported comparable levels of self-esteem during treatment. It appears that self-esteem for abstainers and minor relapsers increased in the first six mo following treatment, whereas the self-esteem measures for major relapsers did not significantly change. Self-esteem also continued to increase for abstainers up to the one-year time point, but not for major relapsers. Thus, self-esteem changes following treatment are related to treatment outcome, with improvements in self-esteem associated with continued abstinence.

Genetic Risk and Family Modeling Influence

Substantial literature, including family, twin, and adoption studies, documents the importance of genetic factors in lifetime risk for alcoholism.[67] Cloninger and colleagues[68] also argue that the clinical course of the addiction is different for alcoholics with a family history of alcoholism compared to alcoholics without such a family history. Thus, it is possible that family history of addiction may relate to the clinical picture of adolescent alcohol and drug use following treatment. This relationship may manifest itself in several ways: Genetic predisposition, exposure to familial models of abuse, general family disruption, or interactions of these factors.

Based on the available evidence for genetic predisposition to alcoholism, it may be hypothesized that individuals with a strong genetic loading would not only be more susceptible to developing addictive disorders initially, but would also be more likely to return to substance abuse following treatment. This prediction is tempered by the apparent lack of relationship between genetic predisposition and initial rates of consumption in offspring of alcoholics (e.g.,[69-71]). Preliminary analyses in our sample of substance-abusing adolescents do not support a relationship between family history and early treatment outcome.[72] There was no significant relationship between outcome at six months following treatment (abstinence, minor relapse, or major relapse) and family history of either alcoholism or substance abuse.

Genetics alone cannot fully account for the transmission of alcoholism and drug abuse.[73,74] Exposure to parental drinking, which is often confounded in descriptive studies of family history of alcoholism, appears to be an additional risk factor in the development of alcoholism.[74-76] It has been suggested[77] that environmental factors may operate independently as well as in interaction with genetic factors in placing an individual at risk for the development of alcoholism. Similarly, family modeling may play an important role in relapse following treatment for adolescent substance abuse. It is essential, therefore, that both environmental and genetic contributions are considered when evaluating familial risk for adolescent substance use and abuse, as well as risk for relapse following treatment.

With regard to the role of familial modeling of substance use in adolescent relapse following treatment, Brown and colleagues[50] compared pretreatment lifetime exposure to abusing models in the family across teen outcome groups at six months following treatment. Since our study is ongoing and longitudinal, preliminary analyses were also conducted on lifetime exposure variables for outcome one year following treatment. The outcome groups differed in total pretreatment lifetime exposure to both alcohol and drug use in their families. In all analyses, abstainers reported the least lifetime exposure to drinking and drug-using family models, whereas major relapsers reported the greatest exposure to abusive family models. Thus, although genetic risk for alcoholism was not associated with early relapse following adolescent alcohol and drug treatment, level of pretreatment exposure to alcohol-abusing models in the family was linked to poorer outcome.

The finding that exposure to abusing models is associated with poorer outcome was corroborated using peer models as well. Abstaining teens reported that a greater proportion of their friends were either nondrinkers or currently abstaining from alcohol (92% at six months, 85% at one year); minor re-lapsers reported an intermediate percentage of their friends were not drinking (54% at six months, 52% at one year); and major relapsers reported the lowest percentage of nondrinking peers (21% at six months, 20% at one year). The same pattern held true for peer drug use following treatment. Abstainers reported the greatest percentage of their friends were not using drugs (95% at six months, 92% at one year), minor relapsers reported an intermediate percentage (71% at six months, 78% at one year), and major relapsers reported the smallest proportion of their friends were not using drugs (33% at six months, 29% at one year). These findings are particularly notable, since there were no differences across the teen outcome groups in reported friends' drinking and drug use patterns prior to treatment.

Interestingly, although there were differences between the three teen outcome groups with regard to posttreatment peer substance use and lifetime exposure to alcohol and drug-using models in the family, there was no consistent relationship between parental use of alcohol or drugs during the followup period and adolescent outcome six months and one year following treatment. Thus, among adolescents, familial exposure to abusing models seems to be related to initiation of alcohol and drug use, but not necessarily to short-term outcome following treatment. Peer modeling, however, seems to be related both to earlier alcohol and drug use and to successful outcome following treatment.

Family Interaction

The nature of the familial environment, particularly characteristic interaction, is a third family factor that may be related to general adolescent functioning, as well as to adolescent substance abuse and outcome following treatment. Within the general adolescent population, research suggests that family environment is related to overall adjustment. Kurdek and Sinclair[78] found that successful adjustment (as measured by high goal directedness, low severity of psychopathology, and few school problems) was related to low family conflict, high relationship, and high personal-growth dimensions of family environment. These relations between family functioning and adolescent adjustment appear to hold true across diverse family structures (e.g., intact families, single mother families, and stepfather families).

Even among alcoholic families, environmental factors appear to influence the risk that the children will develop alcoholism themselves. For example, Wolin and colleagues[79] found that children from alcoholic families are less likely to become alcoholic themselves if family members are able to maintain family rituals such as Christmas activities or regular mealtimes, and to keep these times relatively stress-free.

Family environment also appears to be related to adolescent substance use. For example, adolescent children who report a lack of closeness, support, and affection from their parents are more likely to begin to use drugs, and to maintain the abuse of drugs.[80] Other family factors that have been associated with adolescent alcohol or drug abuse include parent-adolescent conflict (see[81] for review) and lack of family cohesiveness (see[82] for review). Conversely, it has been generally found that a positive, loving bond between parent and child is linked to a reduced likelihood of the child's drug use.[82]

Although limited research is available exploring the relationship between family environment and adolescent treatment outcome, data from our laboratory suggest that parent and adolescent perception of family environment is significantly related to outcome. For example, using the Family Relationship Index (FRI) of the Family Environment Scale,[83] the perception of Expressiveness within the family (of both positive and negative content) was associated with adolescent outcome. As expected, parents of abstaining teens reported the highest levels of expressiveness in their families, parents of minor relapsers reported intermediate levels, and parents of major relapsers reported the least expressiveness in their families.

As another measure of family environment, we have compared adolescents' perceptions of family helpfulness in efforts to remain abstinent following treatment. Again, teen perception of familial support was significantly different for the teen outcome groups across followup time points. Teens who abstained or experienced minor relapses rated their families as significantly more helpful than did teens who returned to alcohol and drug use on a regular basis. This result parallels the finding that family members of abstainers also participated in more treatment program-sponsored aftercare meetings in the six months immediately following discharge than did family members of relapsers.

In summary, family functioning appears to be an important variable in initiation of adolescent substance use and in the progression from use to abuse. Additionally, our longitudinal data suggest that relations within the family, particularly as reflected in expressiveness by family members and willingness to support abstinence efforts, are related to early success following adolescent substance abuse treatment.

School, Work, and Activities

Another area of functioning expected to be related to changes in alcohol and drug use following treatment is participation in traditional adolescent roles, including school, work, and social/recreational activities. Other researchers (e.g.,[25,84]) have indicated that, within the general adolescent population, continued illicit drug use has an impact on participation in major social roles (e.g., employment, romantic involvement or marriage, and work) by young adulthood. Similarly, it may be hypothesized that return to abusive or problematic levels of substance use following treatment will be associated with impaired functioning in these areas.

We have tested this hypothesis in our sample of adolescents at six months following substance abuse treatment.[50] Based on structured interview questions gathered separately from teens and parents during followup interviews, composite scores were created for school/academic functioning (e.g., current grades in school, attitude toward school, and academic problems in school) and recreational/occupational functioning (e.g., frequency of dating, participation in sports or other recreational activities, and steady employment). In order to rule out the possibility that posttreatment differences were merely an artifact of level of pretreatment functioning, we compared pretreatment functioning in these areas for the abstaining, minor relapser, and major relapser outcome groups of adolescents. While there were no differences across the three groups on any of the pretreatment variables, groups did differ in school functioning as early as six mo following treatment. Major relapsers demonstrated significantly poorer functioning in school whereas abstainers were functioning at the highest level in that environment. Interestingly, the outcome groups did not differ on pretreatment recreational or occupational measures and also were not different on these dimensions at six-month followup.

In summary, our longitudinal data for adolescent alcohol and drug abuse treatment outcome support the notion that continued drug use following treatment is related to impairment in school functioning. The failure to find significant outcome differences in successful involvement in work, recreation, and social activities is not particularly surprising since adolescent substance use generally takes place in social situations (e.g.,[23]) and may involve opposite-sex peers (in terms of dating or participation in group activities). Thus, a return to alcohol and drug use in the early period following treatment would not necessarily impair or disrupt functioning on this domain, especially if the other peers also use alcohol or other drugs. It is unclear whether this time period is sufficient for changes on these dimensions to become evident in adolescents. However, the extent to which functioning in major interpersonal and occupational roles becomes impaired over more extended periods of time has not been assessed for well-defined clinical samples of substance abusing teens.

Summary and Conclusions

The clinical course of adolescent alcohol abuse can be understood only when concomitant use of other drugs is considered. Since teens typically enter treatment after problems with other drugs compound alcohol use and its related problems, we have focused on posttreatment patterns of change for the modal polysubstance abusing teen. Findings from adult treatment programs and nonclinical samples of adolescents provide direction to the study of adolescent alcohol and drug treatment outcome, but there are important differences across these populations that highlight the unique needs and problems of substance abusing teens in treatment.

Heretofore, detailed examination of outcome for teen-specific treatment has been conducted over relatively short periods of time. Thus, these results may not reflect the long term impact of intervention efforts with adolescent alcohol and drug abusers, nor the long term consequences of substance abuse that begins during adolescence. In particular, although polydrug use effects on life course may be prominent by young adulthood, the long term risk for continued alcohol abuse may not be fully evident until years later. Clearly, research on the long term course for adolescents who have participated in treatment for alcohol and drug abuse is necessary to understand the impact of addictive behaviors on the accomplishment of developmental tasks and to clarify the significance of the heterogeneity of psychopathology within clinical samples.

With these concepts in mind, there are several general findings that have already emerged from studies of substance abusing teens. Relapse rates for teens appear to be comparable to those reported for adults with much longer addiction histories. Additionally, in the first year after treatment, teens are more likely to continue alcohol or marijuana use than other hard drug use, suggesting that teens may not view these substances or their effects as deleterious compared to those of other drugs. The process of relapse for adolescents has features clearly distinct from that of adult addiction relapse.

For example, social pressure is the predominating precursor to teen relapse, and a sense of vigilance in one's appraisal of potential relapse risk is an important correlate of early success after treatment. Additionally, although cognitive coping strategies seem to be particularly useful for adults, among adolescents the application of behavioral coping efforts seems to be more critical to early abstinence.

Clearly, the initial year following adolescent alcohol and drug abuse treatment is a stressful time for teens who are able to maintain abstinence. This group experiences more life changes (both positive and negative) and has more disruption in its social networks than teens reverting to alcohol and drug use. Fortunately, abstaining teens also experience enhanced self-esteem and improvement in both family- and school-related functioning during this time period. Such findings highlight the stressfulness of the process of change and maintenance of new lifestyles for teens following treatment.

In addition to the emerging evidence regarding the clinical course for teen substance abusers following treatment, research efforts have drawn attention to important methodological issues in the study of addiction during adolescence. In particular, the quantitative and qualitative measurements used in the study of adult treatment outcome may not be appropriate for adolescents. Efforts to assess the cyclic nature of adolescent relapse have not yet begun. Further, the reliability and validity of self-report measures for teens has not been well assessed, and we do not know the significance of various forms of concomitant psychopathology for long-term outcome. These questions and others help to encourage continued research in the area of teen alcohol and drug abuse treatment outcome.

References

[1] R. Pandina and J. Schuele (1983) Psychosocial correlates of alcohol and drug use of adolescent students and adolescents in treatment. *J. Stud. Alcohol* 44(6), 950-973.

[2] National Institute of Drug Abuse (1983) *Main Findings for Drug Abuse Treatment Units: Data from the National Drug and Alcoholism Treatment Utilization Survey (NDATUS)*. Department of Health and Human Services, Rockville, MD.

[3] G. Beschner and A. Friedman (1985) Treatment of adolescent drug abusers. *Int. J. Addict.* 20, 971–993.

[4] E. Rahdert (1988) Treatment services for adolescent drug abusers: Introduction and overview. In *National Institute of Drug Abuse Research Report*. Department of Health and Human Services Publication no. (ADM)88-1523. Supt. of Docs., US Govt. Printing Office, Washington, DC, pp 1–3.

[5] S. Sells and D. Simpson (1979) Evaluation of treatment outcome for youths in

the Drug Abuse Reporting Program (DARP): A followup study, in *Youth Drug Abuse: Problems, Issues and Treatment* (G. Beschner and A. Friedman, eds.), Lexington Books, Lexington, MA.

[6]T. Rush (1979) Predicting treatment outcomes for juvenile and young adult clients in the Pennsylvania substance-abuse system, in *Youth Drug Abuse: Problems, Issues and Treatment* (G. Beschner and A. Friedman, eds.), Lexington Books, Lexington, MA.

[7]R. Hubbard, E. Cavanaugh, S. Graddock, and J. Rachel (1983) *Characteristics, Behaviors and Outcomes for Youth in TOPS Study.* Report submitted to National Institute on Drug Abuse, Contract No. 271-79-3611. Research Triangle Institute, Research Triangle Park, NC.

[8]A. Friedman, N. Glickman, and M. Morrisey (1986) Prediction of successful treatment outcome by client characteristics and retention in treatment in adolescent drug treatment programs: A large scale cross-validation. *J. Drug Ed.* **16**, 149–165.

[9]F. Holsten (1980) Repeat followup studies of 100 young Norwegian drug abusers. *J. Drug Issues* **10**, 491–504.

[10]G. Benson (1985) Course and outcome of drug abuse and medical and social condition in selected young drug abusers. *Acta Psychiatr. Scand.* **71**, 48–66.

[11]P. Nathan (1986) Outcomes of treatment for alcoholism: Current data. *Ann. of Behav. Med.* **8**, 40–46.

[12]P. Orenstein and J. Cherepon (1985) Demographic variables as predictors of alcoholism treatment outcome. *J. Stud. Alcohol* **46**, 425–432.

[13]A. Wiens and C. Menustik (1983) Treatment outcome and patient characteristics in an aversion therapy program for alcoholism. *Am. Psychol.* **38**, 1089–1096.

[14] J. Hesselbrock, V. Hesselbrock, T. Babor, J. Stabenau, R. Meyer, and M. Weidenman (1984) Antisocial behavior, psychopathology and problem drinking in the natural history of alcoholism, in *Longitudinal Research in Alcoholism* (D. Goodwin, K. Van Dusen, and S. Mednick, eds.), Kluwer-Nijhoff, Boston, MA, pp. 197–214.

[15]R. Moos, J. Finney, and W. Gamble (1982) The process of recovery from alcoholism: II. Comparing spouses of alcoholic patients and matched community controls. *J. Stud. Alcohol* **43**, 888–909.

[16]M. Schuckit (1983) Alcoholism and other psychiatric disorders. *Hosp Community Psychiatry* **34**, 1022–1027.

[17]G. Litman, J. Eiser, N. Rawson, and A. Oppenheim (1979) Differences in relapse precipitants coping behavior between alcohol relapsers and survivors. *Behav. Res. Ther.* **17**, 89–94.

[18]A. Billings and R. Moos (1983) Psychosocial processes of recovery among alcoholics and their families: Implications for clinicians and program evaluators. *Addict. Behav.* **8**, 205–218.

[19]S. Brown (1985) Reinforcement expectancies and alcoholism treatment outcome after a one year follow-up. *J. Stud. Alcohol* **46(4)**, 304–308.

[20] S. Brown, A. Millar, and L. Passman (1987) Utilizing expectancies in alcoholism treatment. *Psychol. Addict. Behav.* **2(2)**, 59–65.

[21] R. Meyer (1986) *Psychopathology of Addictive Behavior* (Guilford, New York).

[22] M. Schuckit (1984) Prospective markers for alcoholism, in *Alcoholism: Longitudinal Research and Analysis* (D. Goodwin, K. Van Dusen and S. Mednick, eds.), Kourver-Nykoff Publishing, New York.

[23] S. Brown, P. Vik, and V. Creamer (1989) Characteristics of relapse following adolescent substance abuse treatment. *Addict. Behav.* **14**, 291–300.

[24] L. Robins (1986) The consequences of conduct disorder in girls, in *Development of Antisocial and Prosocial Behavior* (Olweus, J. Block and M. Radke-Yarrow, eds.), Academic Press, Orlando, FL.

[25] D. Kandel, M. Davies, D. Karus, and K. Yamaguchi (1986) The consequences in young adulthood of adolescent drug involvement. *Arch. Gen. Psychiatry* **43**, 746–754.

[26] R. Jessor (1985) Adolescent problem drinking: Psychosocial aspects and developmental outcomes. *Proceedings: NIAAA-WHO Collaborating Center Designation Meeting and Alcohol Research Seminar* (L. Towle, ed.), Public Health Service, Washington, DC, pp. 104–143.

[27] S. Brown, P. Vik, J. McQuaid, T. Patterson, and I. Grant (in press) Severity of psychosocial stress and outcome of alcoholism treatment. *J. Abnorm. Psychol.*

[28] R. Moos, J. Finney and D. Chan (1981) The process of recovery from alcoholism: I. Comparing alcoholic patients and matched community controls. *J. Stud. Alcohol* **42**, 383–402.

[29] P. Nathan and A. Skinstad (1987) Outcomes of treatment for alcohol problems: Current methods, problems and results. *J. Consult. Clin. Psychol.* **55**, 332–340.

[30] M. Schuckit (1985) The clinical implications of primary diagnostic groups among alcoholics. *Arch. Gen. Psychiatry* **42**, 1043–1049.

[31] E. Farley, Y. Santo, and D. Speck (1979) Multiple drug-abuse patterns of youths in treatment, in *Youth Drug Abuse: Problems, Issues and Treatment* (G. Beschner and A. Friedman, eds.), Lexington Books, Lexington, MA.

[32] B. Christiansen, M. Goldman and S. Brown (1985) The differential development of adolescent alcohol expectations may predict adult alcoholism. *Addict. Behav.* **10**, 299–306.

[33] M. Newcomb and P. Bentler (1988) *Consequences of Adolescent Drug Use.* (Sage Publications, Newberry Park, CA).

[34] M. Myers and S. Brown (1990) Coping responses and relapse among adolescent substance abusers. *J. Substance Abuse* **2**, 159–171.

[35] G. Marlatt and J. Gordon (1985) *Relapse Prevention* (Guilford, New York).

[36] S. Shiffman (1986) A cluster-analytic classification of smoking relapse episodes. *Addict. Behav.* **11**, 299–308.

[37] S. Brown and B. Stetson (1988) Coping with drinking pressures: Adolescent versus parent perspectives. *Adolescence* **23**, 297–301.

[38]M. Myers and S. Brown (in press) Coping and appraisal in potential relapse situations among adolescent substance abusers following treatment. *J. Adol. Chem. Depend.*

[39]M. Goldman, S. Brown, and B. Christiansen (1987) Expectancy theory: Thinking about drinking, in *Psychological Theories of Drinking and Alcoholism* (M. Blane and K. Leonard, eds.), Guilford, New York, pp. 181–226.

[40]S. Brown (1988) *Do expectancies mediate post-treatment drinking decisions?* Paper presented at the American Psychological Association annual meeting, Atlanta, GA.

[41]B. Christiansen, G. Smith, P. Roehling, and M. Goldman (1989) Using alcohol expectancies to predict adolescent drinking behavior after one year. *J. Consult. Clin. Psychol.* **57**, 93–99.

[42]J. Donovan and R. Jessor (1985) Structure of problem behavior in adolescence and young adulthood. *J. Consult. Clin. Psychol.* **53**, 890–904.

[43]C. Johnson (in press) Prevention and control of drug abuse, in *Public Health and Prevention Medicine* (Maxey-Rosenau, eds.)

[44]J. Westermeyer and E. Peake (1983) A ten year follow-up of Native Americans in Minnesota. *Am. J. Psychiatry* **140**(2), 189–194.

[45]K. Brownell, G. Marlatt, E. Lichtenstein, and G. Wilson (1986) Understanding and preventing relapse. *Am. Psychol.* **41**(7), 765–782.

[46]S. Brown and M. Schuckit (1988) Changes in depression among abstinent alcoholics. *J. Stud. Alcohol.* **49**(5), 412–417.

[47]S. Brown, M. Irwin, and M. Schuckit (in press) Changes in anxiety among abstinent male alcoholics. *J. Stud. Alcohol.*

[48]S. Brown, A. Gleghorn, and M. Schuckit (1989) Conduct disorder among adolescent substance abusers. Unpublished manuscript.

[49]W. Hunt, L. Barnett, and L. Branch (1971) Relapse rates in addiction programs. *J. Clin. Psychol.* **27**, 455–456.

[50]S. Brown, M. Mott, and M. Myers (1989) Adolescent drug treatment outcome: Correlates of success. Submitted for publication.

[51]G. Marlatt and J. Gordon (1980) Determinants of relapse: Implications for the maintenance of behavior change, in *Behavioral Medicine: Changing Health Lifestyles* (P. Davidson and S. Davidson, eds.), Brunner/Mazel, New York, pp. 410–452.

[52]R. Lazarus and S. Folkman (1984) *Stress, Appraisal, and Coping.* (Springer, New York).

[53]P. Thoits (1986) Social support as coping assistance. *J. Consult. Clin. Psychol.* **54**(4), 416–423.

[54]M. Tucker (1982) Social support and coping: Applications for the study of female drug abuse. *J. Soc. Issues* **38**(2), 117–137.

[55]T. Crutchfield and W. Grove (1984) Determinants of drug use: A test of the coping hypothesis. *Soc. Sci. Med.* **18**(6), 503–509.

[56]M. Holden, S. Brown, and M. Mott (1988) Social support network of adolescents: Relation to family alcohol abuse. *Am. J. Drug Alcohol Abuse* **14(4)**, 487–498.

[57]P. Vik, K. Grizzle, and S. Brown (1989) Social resource characteristics and adolescent substance abuse relapse. Submitted for publication.

[58]S. Brown (1987) Alcohol use and type of life events experienced during adolescence. *Psychol. Addict. Behav.* **1(2)**, 104–107.

[59]J. Mules, W. Hague, and D. Dudley (1977) Life change, its perception, and alcohol addiction. *J. Stud. Alcohol* **38(3)**, 487–493.

[60]H. Rosenberg (1983) Relapsed versus non-relapsed alcohol abusers: Coping skills, life events, and social support. *Addict. Behav.* **8(2)**, 183–186.

[61]I. Grant, J. Yager, H. Sweetwood, and R. Olshen (1982) Life events and symptoms. *Arch. Gen. Psychiatry* **39**, 598–605.

[62]H. McCubbin, R. Needle, and M. Wilson (1985) Adolescent health risk behaviors: Family stress and adolescent coping as critical factors. *Family Relations* **34**, 51–62.

[63]D. Duncan (1977) Life stress as a precursor to adolescent drug dependence. *Int. J. Addict.* **12(8)**, 1047–1056.

[64]S. Brown (1989) Life events of adolescents in relation to personal and parental substance abuse. *Am. J. Psychiatry* **146(4)**, 484–489.

[65]G. Marlatt (1978) Craving for alcohol, loss of control, and relapse: A cognitive-behavioral analysis, in *Alcoholism: New Directions in Behaviorial Research and Treatment* (P. Nathan, G. Marlatt and T. Loberg, eds.), Plenum, New York.

[66]G. Marlatt (1985) Relapse prevention: General overview, in *Relapse Prevention* (G. Marlatt and J. Gordon, eds.), Guilford, New York, pp. 3–344.

[67]M. Schuckit (1988) Reactions to alcohol in sons of alcoholics and controls. *Alcoholism: Clin. Exp. Res.* **12(4)**, 465–470.

[68]C. Cloninger, M. Bohman, and S. Sigvardsson (1981) Inheritance of alcohol abuse: Cross-fostering analysis of adopted men. *Arch. Gen. Psychiatry* **38**, 861–868.

[69]M. Schuckit and S. Sweeney (1987) Substance use and mental health problems among sons of alcoholics and controls. *J. Stud. Alcohol* **48**, 528–534.

[70]A. Alterman, R. Bridges and R. Tarter (1986) Drinking behavior of high risk college men: Contradictory preliminary findings. *Alcoholism* **10**, 305–310.

[71]J. Knop, T. Teasdale, F. Schulsinger, and D. Goodwin (1985) A prospective study of young men at high risk for alcoholism: School behavior and achievement. *J. Stud. Alcohol* **46(4)**, 273–278.

[72]S. Brown (1989) *Family history of alcoholism and adolescent relapse factors*. Paper presented at the Annual Meeting of the Research Society on Alcoholism.

[73]R. Cadoret, E. Troughton, T. O'Gorman, and E. Heywood (1986) An adoption study of genetic and environmental factors in drug abuse. *Arch. Gen. Psychiatry* **43**, 1131–1136.

[74]W. Reich (in press) Children of alcoholics: Environmental correlates. *Br. J. Addict.*

[75]G. Barnes (1977) The development of adolescent drinking behavior: An

evaluative review of the impact of the socialization process within the family. *Adolescence* **12,** 572–589.

[76]R. Tarter and K. Edwards (1988) Psychological factors associated with the risk for alcoholism. *Alcoholism: Clin. Exp. Res.* **12(4),** 471–480.

[77]K. Sher (1987) *What we know and do not know about COAs: A research update.* Paper presented at the MacArthur Foundation Meeting on Children of Alcoholics, Princeton, NJ.

[78]L. Kurdek and R. Sinclair (1988) Adjustment of young adolescents in two-parent nuclear, stepfather, and mother-custody families. *J. Consult. Clin. Psychol.* **56(1),** 91–96.

[79]S. Wolin, L. Bennett, D. Noonan, and M. Teitelbaum (1980) Disrupted family rituals: A factor in the intergenerational transmission of alcoholism. *J. Stud. Alcohol* **41(3),** 199–214.

[80]D. Kandel (1978) Convergences in prospective longitudinal surveys of drug use in normal populations, in *Longitudinal Research in Drug Use: Empirical Findings and Methodological Issues* (D. Kandel, ed.), Hemisphere-John Wiley, Washington, DC.

[81]R. Needle, T. Glynn, and M. Needle (1983) Drug abuse: Adolescent addictions and the family, in *Stress and the Family* (R. Figley and H. McCubbin, eds.), Brunner/Mazel, New York, pp. 37–52.

[82]J. Hundleby and G. Mercer (1987) Family and friends as social environments and their relationship to young adolescents' use of alcohol, tobacco, and marijuana. *J. Marriage and Fam.* **49,** 151–164.

[83]Moos (1986) *Family Environment Scale Manual* (2nd Ed.). (Consulting Psychologists Press, Palo Alto, CA).

[84]M. Newcomb and P. Bentler (1988) Impact of adolescent drug use and social support on problems of young adults: A longitudinal study. *J. Abnorm. Psychol.* **97(1),** 64–75.

Index

A
Abortion, 185
Abstainers, 203, 390
Abstinence, 133, 303
Abstinence teaching, 135
Acculturation, 154
Adolescent
　drinking, 381
　drug use, 339
　mortality, 21
　population, 374
　treatment outcome, 385
Adult alcohol treatment outcome, 377
Adult Children of Alcoholics, 250
Age, 236
Al-Anon, 250
Alcohol, 167, 182
　dependence, 177
　prevention, 1
Alcoholic beverage consumption and prices, 228
Allocentrism, 152
Amphetamines, 180
Analytic design, 52
Anticipatory guidance, 24
Arousal, 80

B
Baptist, 235
Beer, 228
Behavior attention, 86
Behavioral
　change research, 2
　models, 254
　psychologists, 316
Beverage prices and consumption, 224
Billboards, 231
Black, 192
　women, 193
　youth, 263
Brigham Young University, 139

C
Care, 197
Cessation of drug use, 301
Challenge of program evaluation, 99
Childhood factors related to adolescent drug use, 345
Church of Jesus Christ of Latter-Day Saints, 133
Circumstantial drug use, 30
Cocaine, 174, 190
Common-law partner, 171
Communication skills, 366
Community
　context, 109
　involvement, 158
　level intervention, 155
Comparative ability of DIS to detect clinical diagnosis, 58
Compliance, 199
Compulsive drug use, 30
Conduct disorder, 384
Coping, 391

Counter anxiety, 134
Cultural background, 45
Culturally appropriate drug
   abuse treatment, 155

D
Data
   collection forms, 116
   collection procedures, 268
Depression and antisocial
   personality disorders, 173
Diagnosis and management of
   substance abuse, 19
Diagnostic interview schedule, 46
Discrepant information, 75
Disease models, 250
Driver education programs, 6
Drug
   abuse intervention ideas, 155
   Abuse Reporting Program, 375
   prevention, 110
   treatment and family life, 294

E
Economic
   and regulatory variables, 224
   disincentives, 9
Education, 28
Educational campaigns, 211
Emotional health, 392
Environmental protections, 10
Evolution of substance abuse, 31

F
Familialism, 152
Family
   formation, 289
   interaction, 394
   interactions, 245
   interaction research, 246
   involvement, 158
   oriented treatment, 249

   systems models, 252
   treatment of alcoholism, 245
Fetoxic, 189
For kids only: What You Should
   Know About Marijuana, 79

G
Gender
   differences, 199
   differences in alcohol use, 168
   differences in polysubstance use, 170
   roles, 154
Genetic
   factors, 344
   risk, 392
Girls Club Inc., 100
Girls Clubs of America's Friendly
   PEERsuasion Program, 95

H
Hallucinogens, 180
Health and economic consequences
   of substance abuse, 21
Health warning labels, 8
Heroin, 171, 270, 276, 281
Heroin users, 291
Hispanic drug abuse, 151
Husband, 171
Hyperprolactinemia, 186

I
Immediate intervention:
   early stages of abuse, 37
Implementation, 129
Implications for drug abuse
   prevention campaigns, 89
Improving current treatment
   approaches, 160
Incentives, 159, 319
Incentives, lotteries, and
   competitions, 313

Index

Income, 236
Individual differences, 88
Innovative teaching methods, 369

L
Laboratory tests to identify substances of abuse, 38
LDS, 133

M
Major relapsers, 390
Marijuana, 176, 189, 351
Material reinforcers, 317
Media interventions, 7
Medical history, 35
Medium, 88
Message style, 88
Methadone maintenance, 172
Minority women, 191
Monitoring system, 111
Mormons, 133
Multiple media, 159

N
National Institute on Alcohol Abuse and Alcoholism, 1
Native Americans, 139
Natural experiments in alcohol prevention, 3
Nontreated users, 288
Normative hypothesis, 137

O
Opiates, 172, 180
Organizational factors, 316

P
Paradoxical alcohol use, 136
Patterns of drug use, 264, 269
PCP, 274, 278
Person known to be abusing substances, 36

Physical examination and laboratory findings, 35
Physician guidance, 8
Posttreatment psychosocial functioning, 387
Predisposing factors for substance abuse, 27
Primary care practitioner, 19, 23
Printed materials, 159
Protestants, 136
Psychiatric hospitals, 192
Psychoactive drugs, 193
Psychosocial consequences of marijuana use, 350
Psychosocial stress, 389
Punishments and penalties, 10

Q
Questionnaire items relevant to substance abuse, 33
Questions concerning drugs for the school aged child, 29

R
Recognition of the substance abuser, 29
Regression diagnostics, 223
Regulation on alcoholic beverage consumption, 223
Regulations, 224
Reinforcement programs, 318
Relapse, 315
Religiosity, 142
Reproductive compromise, 187
Respeto, 153
Restricted availability, 9
Retail transaction prices, 224
Role models, 159

S
S.A.V.E., 145
School context, 107

School, work, 396
School-based interventions, 6
Selection approaches, 1
Self-examination, 369
Sensation seeking marijuana use, 73
Sexual activity, 186
Simpatica, 153
Single parent, 190
Skin conductance, 84
Smoking, 288
Social
    attainment, 291, 297
    -control approaches, 8
    functioning, 387
    -support approaches, 11
Socialization, 343
Socialization approaches, 6
Spanish, 48, 194
Stress, 181
Sunday sales, 230
Surgeon General's Workshop on Drunk Driving, 3
Symptoms and signs, 36

T
Teach, 97
Teacher, 364
Teen treatment outcome studies, 375
Television, 7
Temptations, 316
Tourism, 236
Training teachers, 363
Treatment
    outcome, 195, 200
    behavior, 263, 279
    effects, 195
    entry, 298
    experiences, 284
    histories, 281

U
University of Washington, 139
Utah, 135

W
Wine, 228
Women, 167, 184
Worksite smoking, 313